William Henry Welch

AND THE

Heroic Age of American Medicine

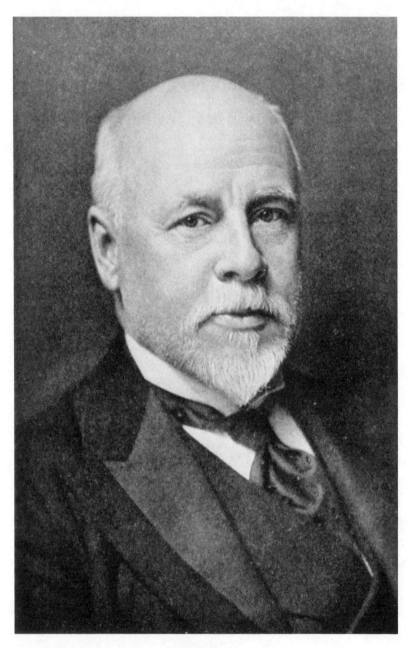

William Henry Welch

William Henry Welch

AND THE

Heroic Age of American Medicine

BY

Simon Flexner *and* James Thomas Flexner

The Johns Hopkins University Press

Baltimore and London

Copyright 1941 by Simon Flexner and James Thomas Flexner
Copyright renewed 1968 by James Thomas Flexner and
William W. Flexner
Foreword © 1993 The Johns Hopkins University Press
All rights reserved
Printed in the United States of America on acid-free paper

Originally published in 1941 by The Viking Press, Publishers,
New York
Johns Hopkins edition, 1993

The Johns Hopkins University Press
2715 North Charles Street
Baltimore, Maryland 21218-4319
The Johns Hopkins Press Ltd., London

In honor of their grandfather, James Carey Thomas, founding
trustee of The Johns Hopkins University and School of Medicine,
and their father, Simon Flexner, who always felt a great loyalty to
the Hopkins, William Welch Flexner and James Thomas Flexner
have generously waived royalties on copies of this book distributed to
members of The Johns Hopkins Medical and Surgical Association.

Library of Congress Cataloging-in-Publication Data

Flexner, Simon, 1863–1946.
    William Henry Welch and the heroic age of American medicine/
by Simon Flexner and James Thomas Flexner.—Johns Hopkins ed.
        p.   cm.
    Originally published: New York: Viking Press, 1941.
    Includes bibliographical references and index.
    ISBN 0-8018-4501-7 (hc)
    1. Welch, William Henry, 1850–1934.   2. Physicians—United
States—Biography.   3. Medical teaching personnel—United
States—Biography.   I. Flexner, James Thomas, 1908–   .
II. Title.   [DNLM: 1. Welch, William Henry, 1850–1934.
2. Physicians—biography.   WZ 100 W4417F 1941a]
R154.W32F6   1993
610'.92—dc20
[B]
DNLM/DLC
for Library of Congress
                                                            92-13529

To the Memory of

EMELINE WELCH WALCOTT

1847 - 1910

Contents

Contents

Illustrations

Foreword to the
1993 Johns Hopkins Edition

William Henry Welch and the Heroic Age of American Medicine, by Simon Flexner and James Thomas Flexner, was first published in 1941. Welch, who had died in 1934, was already a legend. Although the "Heroic Age" itself may have dimmed, Welch's contribution to medical education has grown in luster. Indeed, the model of medical education initiated at Johns Hopkins in the last decade of the nineteenth century, with Welch at its center, gradually became the national norm.

How all this came about is a fascinating story, as is the illuminating picture of this remarkable man. It is a happy circumstance that this book is being brought back into print. One hundred years after the opening of the Johns Hopkins University School of Medicine, there is need for a critical re-examination of medical education as some of the principles Welch fought for are slowly fading.

In the later half of the nineteenth century, German institutions were at the cutting edge of medical research. Welch, a young medical graduate, went to Strasbourg, Leipzig, and Breslau, and worked with such emerging giants of the new era as von Recklinghausen, von Leyden, Ludwig, and Cohnheim.

Daniel Coit Gilman, president of the new Johns Hopkins University and his close collaborator in planning, John Shaw Billings, were on the prowl for talent to staff the future medical school. Not altogether by chance, Billings met Welch in Leipzig; an evening in Auerbach's Keller, where Goethe's Faust was reputed to have been beguiled by the devil, sealed the intellectual bond. No words whispered by Satan, the Flexners suggest, could have been sweeter than those of Billings extolling the vision of the new Johns Hopkins; Welch eventually became the first full-time faculty member of the School of Medicine.

Welch's life unfolds in this book. His ideas and the scope of his vision have made a lasting impact on many institutions and people. In 1884 Welch wrote to Gilman from Germany, "I have been particularly impressed with the hygienic institute which is the pride of the Medical School in Munich. I hope we may have a similar institute in Baltimore." Largely through Welch's efforts, the Johns Hopkins School of Hygiene and Public Health was established thirty-three years later; as its first director, Welch made an indelible imprint.

A distinguished foreign scholar, when offered the professorship of pharmacology at Johns Hopkins in 1885, stipulated that he be allowed also to engage in private practice. The trustees made the fateful decision to decline his condition, thereby affirming the full-time system which was extended to include the core clinical faculty in 1914, under Welch's leadership.

In a speech in 1894, Welch said that "physiological chemistry means much more than what is usually taught in our medical schools," then described his view of this vital forerunner of clinical medicine. What is generally not known is that the strongest entrance requirements to the new Johns Hopkins Medical School, as imposed by Mary Garrett as a condition of her munificent financial gift, were in fact originally outlined by Welch: a bachelor's degree, adequate preparation in biology, chemistry, and foreign languages (German and French), and a four-year medical course. (Welch, however, was not involved in Mary Garrett's major bombshell, that women be admitted on the same terms as men.) These stipulations, together with the manner of instruction shaped by Gilman, Billings, Welch, Osler, and Mall, immediately set this new medical school apart from all others.

In 1925 Welch wrote, "My dream has been a central library for the Medical School, Hospital and School of Hygiene and in connection with this an endowed chair of the history of medicine." He assumed reluctantly, because of his age, the first chair of the History of Medicine at Hopkins in 1929. This volume is replete with other institutions touched by his genius, including the Rockefeller Institute (now the Rockefeller University), the

Association of American Physicians, the Maryland State Board of Health, and the Peking Union Medical College.

The Flexners pay tribute to Welch's personality as well. "Moving in a highly controversial field toward revolutionary ends," they write, "he was always gentle, never raising his voice above the tone of ordinary talk. He was to win affection and admiration until he became, first to his associates and then to younger scientists everywhere, in common parlance the beloved 'Popsy.'" President Herbert Hoover was the principal speaker at a widely broadcast ceremony honoring Welch on his eightieth birthday in 1930—a fitting cap to a remarkable career.

The Flexners, father and son, belong to a family that itself has made, and continues to make, many contributions to medicine. Simon Flexner, who died in 1946, studied medicine at the University of Louisville. As in many schools of the time, medical education was largely limited to lectures; and Flexner, having secured access to a microscope, was self-taught in pathology when he became a student of Welch's in 1890, several years before the Johns Hopkins University School of Medicine opened. He became a fellow in 1891 and an associate professor in Welch's department in 1895.

After Flexner was offered the chair in pathology by the Medical College of Cornell University in 1898, Hopkins promoted him to professor of pathological anatomy. The following year he accepted the professorship of pathology at the University of Pennsylvania. Appointed the first head of the Rockefeller Institute in 1901, Flexner held the position until his retirement in 1935. For five years he also served as a trustee of the Johns Hopkins University. Many contributions to medicine distinguished his career, including Flexner's antimeningococcus serum and discovery of the Flexner dysentery bacillus. Simon Flexner was a leader of American scientific medicine.

James Thomas Flexner is the author of more than twenty books on American history, and his work has been translated into more than twenty languages. He is a former president of the American Center of PEN, the international writers organization, and of the Society of American Historians. Winner of a

National Book Award and a Special Pulitzer Prize Citation—one of five given in the Pulitzer's seventy-five years—James Thomas Flexner is also the recipient of the Gold Medal of the American Academy and Institute for "eminence in biography."

Thomas B. Turner, M.D.

William Henry Welch

AND THE

Heroic Age of American Medicine

CHAPTER I

The Dean of American Medicine

"DR. WELCH is our greatest statesman in the field of public health," said the President of the United States, and all over the world scientists heard his words in pleasure and agreement. The celebration of the eightieth birthday of William Henry Welch was being broadcast by America's major networks, and across the ocean by two short-wave sending stations. A London station was standing by to retransmit it over the British Isles and on into the Continent.[1]

The portly, genial bachelor who sat at President Hoover's side in Washington on that afternoon in 1930 had long been called "the dean of American medicine," but, as this celebration revealed, his influence was much greater than national. Not only had large meetings of scientists gathered in more than a score of American medical centres, but over the seas research workers in many lands were crowded about radio transmitters. Simultaneous ceremonies were being staged in London by the School of Hygiene and Tropical Medicine, in Paris by the Pasteur Institute, in Geneva by the Health Section of the League of Nations, and in Tokyo by the Kitasato Institute. Later that day Chinese physicians gathered to honour Welch at the Peiping Union Medical College. Formal meetings, however, were only part of the activities inspired by Welch's birthday. As wireless messages and telegrams that hurried to Washington demonstrated, innumerable scientists and laymen in their homes, even some as far away as Sydney, Australia, made it a point to tune in.

Listeners everywhere knew that this celebration, unique in the annals of American medicine, was a historical landmark, for it indicated a major change in American life. Throughout the North American continent the radio spoke in majestic institutions given over to medical science, in hospitals that dominated the skylines of cities, in research laboratories equipped with the costly paraphernalia of a new art. Fifty years before such buildings did not exist; only the wildest visionary could have imagined the chambers in which now reverberated the name of William Henry Welch. A revolution, more important perhaps than the revolutions created by politics or war, had taken place, and, as speaker after speaker emphasized, Welch, more than any other American, had inaugurated the new era of healing in the land.

Among the Litchfield hills in rural Connecticut a group of old people sat on front benches in the crowded Norfolk town library listening to the ceremony that honoured the man they remembered as a child—a boy who was given to baseball, sledding, and practical jokes. If these contemporaries of the physician had tried to tell their grandchildren what was the state of medicine when Welch was a child, the youngsters could hardly have believed their ears, so complete was the change that had taken place.

At Yale, where Welch had been taught theological reasoning and had dreamed of becoming a professor of Greek, teachers and students listened, but few were aware that when Welch had walked those halls as an undergraduate, science had hardly existed in the college curriculum. They would have been amazed had they been told that as a commencement orator Welch had defended revealed religion against the encroachments of the inductive method, for the environment that had urged Welch into this speech was dead now as the Age of Bronze.

A hundred miles down the Atlantic seacoast, in the city of New York, the President's words moved smoothly through the air into the great hall of the College of Physicians and Surgeons. When, fifty-five years before, Welch had been a medical student in the single small building on Twenty-Third Street that then housed that college, half the subjects his listeners now taught or studied—the very bases of modern medical education—were unknown. Practical instruction was limited to dissection and an occasional clinic; all the rest was talk. By the hour Welch had listened to didactic orators who explained how to deal with diseases in a traditional manner. Although a few of the more advanced professors owned microscopes, they would never have dreamed of allowing students to use such complicated instruments.

Struggling with the atmosphere, radio waves pushed faintly into German air. Here it was, in a very different Germany, that Welch had experienced a revelation. Under a succession of great discoverers, including Ludwig, Cohnheim, and later Koch, he learned the sciences that were to give a new foundation to the healing arts. And when his empty pocket brought his student years to a close, he returned across the Atlantic with his eyes fixed on a vision: America too must become the home of medical science. It seemed a mad vision to his friends, and even to himself in moments of depression, for not a single medical school on the entire continent possessed a laboratory devoted to the basic science of pathology, and, so far as he could learn, no American physician had ever made a living in the way he was determined to do, by teaching and scientific work alone.

During 1878 Welch founded America's first pathological laboratory at the Bellevue Hospital Medical College, whose professors were now listening to the radio, a laboratory so successful that in a few months another was founded at the College of Physicians and Surgeons. A gap had appeared in the dike, and through it the flood-waters of modern medical science began to roll over the North American continent. Soon Welch was given his great opportunity: called to Baltimore as the first appointee to the faculty of the yet embryonic Johns Hopkins Medical School, he led in the organization of a new type of institution which set a standard that the older schools were gradually induced to follow. Advances now taken for granted were regarded as wildly radical when initiated by the Hopkins in those not distant days: high entrance requirements, including a knowledge of foreign languages; a four-year graded course, instruction in the laboratory, an emphasis on basic sciences, the fostering of research.

Through the amazingly full collections of original documents that have come down to us, we may follow a great change in American life and thinking which took place in less than fifty years. From the single laboratory Welch founded as a young man we shall see other laboratories grow; we shall see young men trained under his direction become fruitful investigators, influential in raising American medical science until it played a major part in the science of the world. We shall see the reforms Welch sponsored, in co-operation with such men as Sir William Osler, alter the practice of medicine, go into all the homes of the land. We shall see the progress of medical science produce a reaction among ill-informed people that changed Welch into a general, fighting in the national legislature to preserve the new knowledge and the new techniques from destruction. The battle won, we shall see the state itself altering its processes to further the health of the people.

Philanthropic foundations, long unconcerned with the physical well-being of the nation, entered the lists at last, and soon the support of scientific medicine became their greatest single interest.[2] Advances once almost inconceivable were now actual possibilities, but always there was the need of wisdom to guide and determine. Welch was called in for counsel, and when new ventures were finally undertaken, he was often persuaded to lead them. At the advanced age of sixty-six, and again ten years later, he broke new trails as the first director of pioneering institutions. Thus, step by step, American medical science was strengthened and raised, until, by the time he was eighty, the vision Welch had seen as a young man was realized as a concrete whole.

In the hundreds of years since the settling of America, the tide of medical knowledge had always moved across the Atlantic from east to west; the most fertile American doctors had received their training abroad, even as Welch had done. But before this man was very old, new tides appeared in the current of knowledge. American discoveries, American institutions and aims flowed back across the Atlantic, as well as across the Pacific to China and Japan. Then, little by little, foreign students began turning up in American medical schools, foreign research workers in the laboratories of the New World. It was not by chance that scientists everywhere listened to the ceremonies on the eightieth birthday of Welch. Their participation in the honouring of the dean of American medicine was as inevitable then as it would have been impossible fifty years before.

There was more than an official note in the ceremonies held on Welch's eightieth birthday; the speeches delivered and the editorials written all over the globe radiated affection for the great man being honoured. Everywhere he was referred to by the familiar name of "Popsy."

The attitude of his pupils is revealed in a letter written to him by Lewellys F. Barker on a previous occasion: "We Anglo-Saxons find it difficult to express adequately our feelings to those to whom we are most sincerely attached, but I do desire to say to you, today, dear Dr. Welch, what I think you already well know, that I regard you as my intellectual father and that no son could, I believe, have stronger feelings of gratitude and of filial affection. . . . The term of endearment, so commonly used by your assistants and pupils, was happily chosen. ' 'Tis a happy thing to be the father unto many sons,' especially when they are bound to you by so many and such strong bonds as those that hold your sons.' You have known how to show a tender fatherly regard for us, and I wish you could fully know how it has been, and is, appreciated."

Welch had many eccentricities and foibles on which affection might fix a tender smile. It was typical of him that on the morning of the international celebration he placed a cornflower, given him by the wife of an old friend, in his buttonhole, obscuring the ribbon of the Distinguished Service Medal, and that when an army officer in full regalia rushed up to object to this heinous breach of decorum Welch removed the flower with a docile apology belied by the twinkle in his eye.

It was typical of him that when he stood before the microphone that was to broadcast his words to scientists everywhere, he found that he could not see to read, since he had misplaced his glasses. While the world waited and seventeen hundred people in the hall watched uneasily, he began going systematically through his clothes. Finally, after a prolonged search over his capacious person, he reached into his right trouser pocket and, to the relief of everybody, pulled out the spectacles. Unhurriedly he placed them on his nose.

And it was typical of him that the speech on which he finally launched was perfect for the occasion: "Did I accept merely as a personal tribute these words of praise and this manifestation of appreciation and good will marked by this large and distinguished gathering and by meetings elsewhere, I should be overpowered with a sense of unreality depriving me of utterance, but I shall assume, as I feel that I am justified in doing, that by virtue of certain pioneering work and through over a half-century of service I stand here to represent an army of teachers, investigators, pupils, associates, and colleagues, whose work and contributions during this period have advanced the science and art of medicine and public health to the eminent position which they now hold in this country. . . .

"If I have handed on any intellectual heritage to pupils, assistants, and associates, whose work and achievements have been the greatest satisfaction and joy of my life, it is derived from that which I received from my own masters. America is now paying the debt which she has owed so long to the Old World by her own active and fruitful participation in scientific discovery and the advancement of the science and art of medicine and sanitation. . . . It is perhaps not too much to claim that America has taken a position of leadership in the application of the new knowledge to the prevention of disease and to personal and public hygiene.

"But, my friends and hearers . . . so much more remains to be done than has been accomplished, the problems awaiting solution are so numerous and pressing, above all, the better utilization of existing knowledge and the need of more knowledge are so obvious and so urgent that our mental attitude should be far removed from satisfaction with existing conditions."

CHAPTER II

Shadows Cast Before

I

THE story of William Henry Welch's ancestors is an integral part of the story of our national life, and at the end of the eighteenth century it became a history in miniature of American medicine. Rarely has a man sprung from a line in which were so deeply implanted the seeds of his own future accomplishment. It is, of course, impossible to determine how much a man's heredity influences his career, but certainly there is more than coincidence in the similarity between Welch and many of his forebears.

Philip, who began the Welch line in this country, was in 1654 kidnapped from Ireland by Cromwell's soldiers; at the age of eleven he was sold in Boston harbour for a nine-year term as an indentured servant. He showed a spirit of independence much greater than his fellows when, four years later, he refused to work any longer in his master's fields unless he were paid, staging what some writers call the first strike in New England's history. The upshot is not entirely clear, but in any case Philip became free as a young man, fought the Indians in King Philip's war, and left a numerous progeny.

Philip's great-grandson, Hopestill Welch, established the family in Norfolk, Connecticut, when he moved there in 1772 from the town of Windham. He was a blacksmith, a small man of prodigious strength. It is said that when he joined Israel Putnam's company during the French and Indian war his commander, observing his size, asked scornfully what he could do. Hopestill bared the blacksmith's muscle of his right arm and replied that he could lick any man in the company. During the Revolution he had an opportunity to display his physical prowess, for he accompanied Benedict Arnold on the march to Quebec that was one of the most arduous marches in American

9

history, and he was among the few who came back alive. He lived to be eighty-seven, dying the same year as his wife, who was eighty-two. Longevity was early a characteristic of the Welches.

All Hopestill's thirteen children—ten daughters and three sons—grew to maturity, some living to a great age. Seven became pioneers, emigrating to the Western Reserve and beyond. Of the three boys, the eldest followed his father's trade and the other two began a family tradition by becoming doctors. One, Hopestill, junior, died young, but the other, Benjamin, lived to a respected old age as "the beloved physician" of Norfolk, and became the grandfather of William Henry Welch.

The year of Dr. Benjamin Welch's birth, 1768, was an important one for American medicine, since it saw the founding in Philadelphia of the first medical school on the continent; this innovation, which was much disapproved of by the body of the profession, had no influence on his education. Following the custom of many generations, Benjamin was apprenticed, while hardly more than a lad, to a local doctor. His preceptor, Dr. Ephraim Guiteau, was the first physician to reside in Norfolk and is believed to have enjoyed a large reputation that attracted students from other states. Benjamin lived in his master's house, made up his drugs, accompanied him on his rounds, and held the bowl into which the patients were bled. If Dr. Guiteau's library contained more than one or two antiquated medical texts he was a very unusual physician for his period, and it is quite possible that young Benjamin had no source of information except his preceptor's recipes, which Dr. Guiteau in turn had learned from his preceptor.

When Benjamin received his licence to practise from the Litchfield County Medical Society, he was as well prepared as most of his colleagues, for at that time all the medical schools in America had graduated about a hundred men. Benjamin married Dr. Guiteau's daughter, succeeded to his practice, and remained the leading, and often the only, physician in Norfolk until his death at the age of eighty-two. In addition to carrying out the arduous duties of country practice, he was active both in the church and in politics, holding at different times nearly every office in the gift of the town. A student of books, he was of a disposition eminently kind, yet capable of great firmness on occasion. But there was one art in which he was lacking— the art of collecting money, a deficiency which he transmitted to one at least of the five sons who followed in his professional footsteps.

His first wife, Louisa Guiteau, bore him eight children, and all of the three sons who survived became doctors. The eldest, Asa Guiteau Welch, studied with his father, but by the time the second, Benjamin Welch, junior, was old enough to begin his labours, medical schools had been accepted as a part of American life; he went to the Yale Medical Institution in New Haven and spent an additional year at Jefferson Medical College in Philadelphia to perfect himself in anatomy and surgery. Medical degrees soon became so important that even the most experienced apprentice-trained doctors had to get them somehow. In 1838, after many years of successful practice, Benjamin Welch, senior, was on the advice of the local medical society given an honorary medical degree by Yale, and about the same time his eldest son, Asa, received one from the Berkshire Medical Institute at Pittsfield, Massachusetts, from which the third son, James Welch (1807–1886), had just been graduated.[1]

After the death of his first wife Dr. Benjamin, senior, married Elizabeth Loveland of Glastonbury who, at thirty, was younger than one of her stepchildren. She bore two sons, both of whom grew up to be physicians. The elder of these was to be the father of William Henry Welch.

Born December 10, 1818, William Wickham Welch grew up in the house where his father and two of his brothers practised medicine. At an early age he was sent to the Yale Medical Institution. Since in those days medical schools were designed merely to supplement apprentice training—every student had to have a preceptor—he spent the periods between his terms of lectures studying with his elder brother Benjamin. When he was graduated in 1839, he was still under twenty-one and had to wait for his diploma until he reached his majority. He was later playfully to speak of having begun practice "when I was a boy." Even while he was at Yale he had won such a reputation as a physician that the citizens of the neighbouring town of South New Marlboro offered to discourage any other physician from settling with them if he would promise to come to their community after his graduation. William Wickham, however, settled down in Norfolk as assistant to his father, his elder brothers having sought larger opportunities elsewhere. Since Benjamin, senior, was now old, the burden of the family practice soon fell on his son's shoulders. William Wickham was already a very successful physician when, in the fall of 1843, he visited Hillsdale, New York. It was a fateful visit, for there he met Emeline Collin, who was to be the mother of William Henry Welch. Their marriage mingled two different strains, both of which were to reappear in their famous son: the easy-going matter-of-factness of the physician Welches and a more sensitive quality, delicate, poetic, not so closely allied with the everyday world.

II

Emeline Collin had the American honour of being born in a log cabin, although she left it while yet a baby. She traced her ancestry back to Paul Collin, a Huguenot exile who fled to Rhode Island about 1695. Early in the eighteenth century the family moved to Hillsdale, where they were among the earliest settlers. Emeline's father, Henry Collin, and her mother, Nancy McAlpin, were married in that town in 1814; they immediately set out in a two-horse wagon loaded with household equipment for the frontier region of Ontario, New York, where they lived in a succession of log huts in the vicinity of Benton. In the last of these Emeline was born on September 25, 1822.

The girl spent her childhood in a community that was rapidly changing from arduous frontier to comfortable back country; while her father rapidly amassed more acres, she lived the happy life of a child on a prosperous farm. But when she was ten, her mother died; three years later her father followed. An orphan now, she was handed back and forth between her relatives at Hillsdale and Fayetteville, New York. A little sheaf of her child-

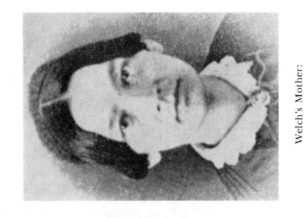

Welch's Mother:
Emeline Collin Welch

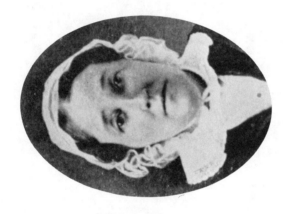

Welch's Grandmother:
Elizabeth Loveland Welch

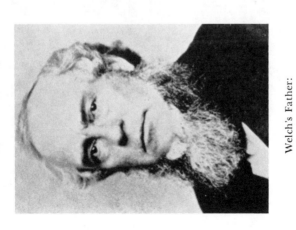

Welch's Father:
William Wickham Welch

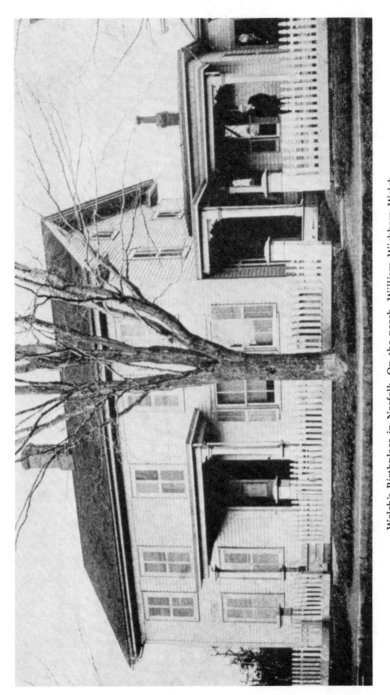

Welch's Birthplace in Norfolk. On the porch, William Wickham Welch hood scribblings has come down to us; they show that at an early age she sought relief from her loneliness by recording her hopes and fears in writing. We find four different versions, dated between 1837 and 1839, of a bad dream that seems to have haunted her continually:

On yon dark blue sea swiftly glides a noble vessel freighted with the wealth of another shore and with happy hearts who go to meet endeared friends from whom absence has long severed them. Now no angry wave impedes their peaceful course. The sun beams brightly upon the sea-worn voyagers and even as a speck in the distance they perceive their destined port. Every heart beats high with hope, every eye sparkles with pleasure, every countenance is lighted with smiles. All partake of the general pleasure.

But now what means that frowning cloud? Will it destroy their bright expectations? Will it forever blast their future happiness? The gloom increases. The fearful, deafening sound of thunder and the vivid flashes of lightning add terror and grandeur to the awful scene. Despair bids pleasure fly and sheds its sombre influence over every heart. Gloom commands every smile to depart and enthrones itself on every brow. Yet a faint, glimmering hope remains. They are near the shore—may they not by their exertions reach it 'ere the dreaded storm arrives? Their exertions, their prayers prove futile. The storm has already reached them. The last hope is extinct. Cruel fate has destined for them a watery grave. They are lost!

Bright indeed had been their anticipations, but how sad the reality. Such are our lives. We look through the mazy scenes of futurity and see a fair, sunny spot, and there we expect to obtain pure, unsullied happiness. We hasten onward, and when finally we have reached that spot, our fond dreams of happiness vanish, and leave us overshadowed by the dark clouds of a cold reality.

In a notebook of school themes we find one on *Home*. Having described Fayetteville, she adds: "But dear as it is, yet is it not my *native home*. . . . The friends I there loved are now *no more*, and the fair, sunny days of childhood have left but a sad remembrance."

Emeline loved to write. As several of her essays show, she romanticized herself as the beautiful female scholar of some story, whose bright hair was hidden under a hermit's hood and whose ardent heart was absorbed in worshipping the muses. But always behind this vision is the possibility that a change of fate will enable her to throw back the hermit's cowl and allow her hair to fly free. "Yes, I will go and behold the boasted beauties of Greece and Italy . . . I will mingle in the gay circles of France; in fine nothing worthy of the least attention shall escape my observation."

In the meantime Emeline tried to be as learned as she could. She wrote a long argument in which one of the characters—a young lady who has secluded herself "from all society and the fascinating joys of life"—offers to prove "the materiality of sleep." Under the heckling of fellow-female intellectuals she announces: "I will conduct my argument, by a philosophical investigation, and call it under the following heads, viz.: Impenetrability, Extension, Figure, Divisibility, Inertia, and Attraction." These, the fair philosopher insists, are the attributes of matter, and she labours to show that they are the attributes of sleep as well.

The girl made excellent use of such educational opportunities as she had. When she was sent for her last term to the impressive Murdoch Place Academy in New Haven, she immediately led her class. Graduation, however, made little change in the external aspects of her life; she still moved back and forth between her grandparents in Fayetteville and her relatives in Hillsdale and Benton. Yet the passing of years seems to have calmed the conflict in her bosom. Her writings changed from extreme self-centred emotion to keen and dispassionate comedy of manners. A little playlet which is the most mature of her girlish efforts shows that she could write sparkling dialogue and reveal character with an amusing maliciousness.

Emeline was playing the part of an amused bystander at life's pageant when in the fall of 1843 she met William Wickham Welch, who was on a brief visit to Hillsdale. She made so deep an impression on the twenty-four-year-old doctor that, after his return to Norfolk, he sent her a stiff note full of embarrassed platitudes asking her if she would go for a ride with him, "spending part of the day"; he doubted if he could find time to spend a whole day. During this ride William Wickham proposed that they "continue our acquaintance with reference to forming at some future time a relation, at once the most intimate and enduring we can assume." The correspondence that followed gives us an insight into the diverse characteristics that William Henry Welch inherited from his parents.

The gentleness of his father is indicated in the letter he wrote to Emeline after his return to Norfolk: "I inferred from a remark of yours that you considered our acquaintance too limited to authorize a final decision. . . . Far be the wish from me, my dear Emeline, as far even as the power to induce you to violate any moral principle or conscientious scruples on my account. Be deliberate, be prayerful, asking the guidance of Him in whose hands are the destinies of us all, and whose all-wise and over-ruling providence we should recognize in all the events of our lives. And if you desire to assume new responsibilities and, I trust, enduring relations, and to share with me the joys and sorrows incident to life, giving me the *first love* of your heart, as I give you mine, please inform me of your decision as soon as convenient."

After a month of hesitation, Emeline, "implicity trusting to your sincerity, and confidently believing that you are *all* you seem," accepted the proposal of the young man she had seen only twice. "This decision is not made without long, deep, and even painful thought. I have faithfully sought guidance from Him in whose hands, truly, are all our destinies. . . . With generosity equal to your own, I leave you the privilege of changing your opinion in respect to myself, which I fear you may have occasion to do. You can, of course, imperfectly know my character. Indeed *I know not myself.* Left as I have been, even from childhood, with the dangerous privilege of having my own way, I tremble when I think what I may be, surrounded by the cares and responsibilities of life. I should surely despair were it not for the precious promise: 'My grace is sufficient for thee.' "

Dr. Welch was too busy with his practice to reply before two weeks had passed; then his letter was embarrassed and formal. "I need not assure you," he wrote, "of my persuasion that my affection has not been misplaced. . . . Think not that I contemplate the marriage state in the aspect of a sort of *fairy region* of *enchanted ground,* in which nothing reigns but undisturbed peace and unmingled happiness." After discussing the possible trials and disappointments of marriage, he expressed the faith that they could be overcome by love and "the blessing of Heaven." He added that he was so busy that he might not be able to see her again before their marriage, and begged her to set a date not too far distant.

Now that the formalities of proposal and acceptance were over, Emeline allowed her natural high spirits to bubble from her pen. She wrote from Fayetteville: "Allow me to introduce you this evening to our little family circle. A bright, blazing fire is burning upon the hearth, *so* bright, that were my pen a less stupid one it might be tempted to scribble 'sweet poetry.' Seated in one corner is my Grandfather, apparently musing upon a subject of vast moment, perhaps regretting that times have so sadly changed since he was a boy, or, maybe wondering what the weather will be on the morrow. In the other corner is my good Grandmother, very quietly keeping Saturday night. If you look upon her face as I do, you will discern traces of former beauty. And if you could look still deeper and read her character you would discover, not the traces of goodness, but goodness itself, and feelings, warm and fresh, as in the greenness of youth. Methinks I could well bear to grow old, were I sure of retaining the unclouded brow, and vigor and elasticity of mind that she has done. Seated near the stand upon which I am writing is *cousin David,* reading a learned treatise upon something (I can't say what). He is really looking very grave, as of course he should when thus engaged. 'Cousin Em' (alias myself), is certainly very strangely employed, writing with perhaps inexcusable, at least unprovoked, familiarity, to one whose name, even, has been but recently known. Strange, how strange, are the fitful changes of life. It seems but yesterday that I was a *knowing* school-girl, supposing I should soon reach the pinnacle of the famed 'Hill'; and the day before that I was a careless, light-hearted child. Today I *ought* to be what I am not, a thoughtful, dignified woman. And now, who, with Sibyl hand, will unfold the page of to-morrow, that I may read what is there written? Thanks to a kind Providence, no impious hand dare, or can lift the veil that conceals the morrow's sunshine or shade. So, depart from me, thou evil genius that wouldst tempt me to pry with idle curiosity into the hidden things of the future, for it is enough that He, who is faithful, has said, 'As thy day is, so shall thy strength be.' "

The end of the letter was less gay. Engaged to a comparative stranger, Emeline was terrified at the thought of marrying before she knew her fiancé better. She postponed indefinitely setting the day, but assured William Wickham that she would pray for guidance. Eventually Emeline's high-spirited chronicles of life in Fayetteville combined with her continued postponement of the wedding began to worry the good doctor, who was eager to get married and whose style of writing was naturally more constrained. Yet, he manifested his anxiety only between the lines; he rebuked her gaiety by stating his own dislike for society when she was absent. Emeline, however, was conscious of the slightest shading in his letters.

Concerning her reluctance to make the leap into marriage, she was frankly distressed; she was earnestly begging the Lord, she again told her fiancé, to solve her quandary. Indeed, Emeline had cause for her hesitation. How little she knew of the life she was expected to lead was shown when she wrote: "I was pleased with your allusion to your mother, for I have often wondered if she were still living, and a thousand times fancied how she looked." And yet after her marriage, her mother-in-law was to live in her house!

It seems clear that Emeline would have liked another interview before she took the irrevocable step, but it was not to be. Although the doctor expressed hope many times that he would be able to visit her, sickness in Norfolk always kept him busy with his patients. When William Wickham Welch finally made the trip to Hillsdale in November 1844, it was to get married.

Thus Emeline became the wife of a busy doctor who had little time to spend at home. One of William Wickham's letters described his routine. "Yesterday morning I commenced my day's work at 8 o'clock, first visiting Mrs. Beebe in Canaan, returning home, next rode to Mr. Saxton's and Norton and others. Next visited Mr. H. Roys, Bronson in Winchester, Humphry and M. Cowles, reached home at 11½ o'clock. I found myself in bed about 12 o'clock and in ½ hour *up,* feeling my way to the front door in search of the unceremonious disturber of my dreams, who all this time was insistently screaming 'Doctor, doctor!' (I have no doubt much to the annoyance of the neighbors as well as myself), and on raising the latch received a distressingly urgent call to ride 6 miles into Canaan. After a well nigh sleepless night, returned home, finding calls which have used up the day in attending to, and brought me home again this eve at 10 o'clock."

Soon Emeline herself needed her husband's attention, for she came down with a serious illness that exiled her to Saratoga Springs for the cure. "My dear husband," she wrote in July 1846, "I flatter myself that you would like to hear from me, even though I should tell you of *aches* and *pains.* To begin with, I must tell you how I felt after you left. I choked and swallowed for an hour to keep back the tears and yet they would come in spite of myself and Oh! how sad and discouraged I felt when I found that all my *old bad feelings* had returned. . . . I concluded that my disease had only been held in check by a pleasing excitement. . . . For your sake I am *intensely* anxious to recover. To be denied the privilege of contributing to your comfort causes a keener anguish than all the bodily pain I ever endure, and this feeling, I assure you, is not diminished by your uniform and generous kindness. My earnest prayer to God is that my life may be spared and my health restored, but I trust I not less earnestly pray that I may bow submissively and cheerfully to His will, whatever it may be. And Oh! my dear husband, may we commit all our ways unto Him, and enjoy the sweet consolation that we are in the care of *our Father* who afflicts not willingly His children, but for their good."

William Wickham replied: "I find myself this evening after a hard day's ride, solitary and alone, in our old kitchen with nothing of particular interest to divert my mind from you. . . . Do not borrow any trouble in regard to us at home, for we shall all get along after a fashion which I confess you would in many respects improve. When I would call for your aid and advice, and find no answer, I am comforted with the assurance that you are regaining your health, or at least are in the use of means for regaining it."

After three months of exile, Emeline returned home so much better that there was hope of her complete recovery, but complete recovery never came; she remained an invalid, suffering periods of great physical and mental anguish during which religion became so important to her that she could hardly bear the fact that her husband had never formally joined the church. Yet she was strong enough to become the mother of two children. On May 13, 1847, she gave birth to a daughter, Emeline Alice, known as Emma; and some three years later, on April 8, 1850, to William Henry Welch.

From then on her decline was rapid. Despite the best efforts of all the five Welch doctors, who often gathered for consultations at her bedside, she died on October 29, 1850, when her son was little more than six months old.

CHAPTER III

A Quiet Youth and a Crisis

I

THE disintegrating shock of his mother's death left the house in which William Henry Welch passed his childhood silent and lonely. His sister had been sent to live with an aunt at Winchester Center, six miles away, and his father no longer spent much time in the melancholy rooms where once Emeline had been his companion. The actual care of the child was entrusted to his grandmother, Elizabeth Loveland Welch, but she also was out of the house much of the time. While Dr. Welch attended to the physical needs of his neighbours, she attended to the spiritual; both were so busy helping the entire community that they had little time for their particular charge. A leading spirit in the Sunday School of which she was "Lady Superintendent," Mrs. Welch was known not only to William but to every child in the town as "Grandma Welch." When church members fell sick, she appeared at their bedside bearing calf's-foot jelly and a tract. And it was a rare ne'er-do-well who did not taste both of her charity and of her ability to deliver a sermon.

Her relation to her grandson, we gather, was a pious combination of benevolence and austerity. She loved to indulge the young; each Sabbath she presented every Sunday School pupil with a moralistic infant's journal entitled *The Dayspring,* and one of her youngest grandchildren remembers that the old lady never called without bringing her a present. On the other hand, the children seem to have found Grandma Welch's righteousness awe-inspiring. Crissey, the local historian of Norfolk, tells that when little William brought friends into the house for games, a sudden silence would fall "upon the group of playful and noisy children because Grandma had gone away to pray in her room."

Crissey comments that "daily and continued prayer was her habit."

When William was forced to stay at home he would escape from the emptiness of the house into the woodshed, where he imagined that certain sticks to which he had given human names were his friends; his favourite was a "Mrs. Gieke," with whom he played as if she were a doll. But he was usually able to avoid loneliness by going next door, just across a lawn divided by a white picket fence, to the home of his father's only full brother, John Hopestill Welch, a physician and William Wickham's partner. No death clouded this household; a large family of children played gaily all day long, and several were close to William in age.[1] The boy spent so much time there that the tradition has come down in John Welch's family that William actually lived in John's house. This was not so, although the boy probably envied the happy family life across the lawn; we are told that he moved a huge pile of stones for his cousins on condition that they would call him "brother." Certain it is that in three letters to him his cousin John Welch, junior, signed himself "your affectionate brother."

William early became inured to loneliness, laying perhaps the foundations for that self-contained reticence that was to characterize him during the rest of his life. His childhood, however, does not seem to have been unhappy; he was the epitome of the normal boy. Some of his admirers have tried to make out that he was a studious goody-goody—"Willie could not even whistle, but then he was not a whistly boy"; nothing seems to have been further from the truth. From the first a leader among his companions, he resorted to direct action when he believed it necessary. One of the earliest memories of his much younger cousin Alice is of William "holding his fist towards me and saying, 'Let me see you open it,' and when I tried to bite it he hit me and knocked out my first tooth."

The boy's mind, as his letters show, was concerned with ponies, parties, waiting for the maple-sugar season, and local gossip, particularly of fires and deaths. He wrote his sister with a delightful shiver of horror: "There was a woman died in Burville (a Mrs. Burr) very suddenly the other day she was eating and she died with the food in her mouth." Engaged in reading such stories as *The Secret Chamber,* he added to a letter concerned with nothing in particular the exciting sentence: "I hope you will be sure to burn this as soon as you have read it." Although the children had a Zouave troop which drilled occasionally on the village green, the Civil War was merely a minor excitement among the excitements of a small-town boyhood. The letters William exchanged with his companions are amazingly lacking in mention of it; even the victory was only commented on in passing. One of his friends wrote him: "I'll bet I would have given three cents to have seen Jeff Davis running off in his wife's petticoats."

Everything in the boy's environment made for a sense of peace and self-confidence. The Welches were a leading family, and in Norfolk family position was regarded as so important that its Congregational Church was the last in Connecticut to give up seating parishioners according to their social station. As the boy walked the streets, everyone he met knew that his small figure represented temporal power; the farmers touched their hats and asked without too much familiarity after his good father.

Looking back as an old man, Welch saw his childhood tinged with a rosy glow:

In the middle of the last century the New England towns, and none more so than this beautiful town of Norfolk, afforded the best which this country could offer in the way of heredity and environment for the upbuilding of that strength of character, that soundness of mind and of body, those moral and intellectual ideals which have been in the past (whatever the future may have in store for us) the determining forces in the development and prosperity of our country. . . .

The Norfolk of those and later days bore no resemblance to the "Main Street" depicted so realistically in that most depressing book by Sinclair Lewis. There was love of beauty so lavishly spread before our eyes in these Litchfield County hills and cultivated in our surroundings in flower-bed and lawn. There were singing schools and even then much of that love of music for which Norfolk has become so celebrated. We had or thought we had the best church choir of this region. The educational advantages were good for that time and intellectual interests were not lacking. There was a small circulating library and as we grew in years there was much reading of books. . . .

The outlook upon life may have been narrow, but upon the small altars the fire burned brightly. Our patriotism was stimulated by the fourth-of-July celebrations and orations and especially by the events of the Civil War. The days of the old Lyceum lecturers were not yet passed.

As in so many New England towns characters of strong individuality, sometimes even of marked personal idiosyncrasy, were developed. The religious faith which had come down from the fathers of the New England commonwealths was still strong, and the life of the church and of the town meeting was vigorous. The social atmosphere was that of genuine democracy, of mutual interests, of mutual helpfulness and kindliness, strikingly exemplified, I may be permitted to say, in the life of my father, the best type of country doctor. . . .

Our lives as children centered around the family, the church, the Sunday School, walks to the cemetery on Sunday afternoons—the only relaxation permitted on that day—the school, the village green, our games, our picnics in the old spring lot, our birthday parties. I was led to believe by my father, and I do not dispute it, that I owed everything in my start in life to my attendance at the Misses Nettleton's school, and I am sure that it was an excellent school of its kind.

This day school to which William was sent at an early age was kept by two sisters who were the entire faculty. Morals and manners played an important part in the curriculum: each pupil had to recite a verse of the Bible every morning and even the smallest tots were expected to know the names of the books of the Old Testament by heart. The boys as well as the girls were taught to sew on the pieced counterpanes popular in those days. "The favorite mode of punishment," Crissey tells us, "was to shut the misbehaved in the narrow back hallway, and leave them there in the dark until repentance came. The great honor was to be allowed to fill the water-pail at the spring, the other side of the brook, on the old parsonage grounds, and after trudging back with it, sometimes losing much in the return journey, to ladle the water out to the other scholars, in the large tin dipper provided for the purpose."

While he was at the Misses Nettleton's School, William, as was proper for a small-town boy, became fond of a little girl. She was Alice Eldridge, the daughter of the local minister, who had married one of the wealthiest women in Norfolk. Alice's several sisters were considered beautiful; but she was the harum-scarum one of the lot. When the others appeared primly in newly starched dresses, they were almost ashamed to be seen with Alice, who, even if her dress was newly starched, managed to button it up wrong and get it mussed in ten minutes. However, none of her sisters could compete with her in climbing trees.

When they were both old, Alice, then Mrs. Henry H. Bridgman, wrote Welch: "I went to you for help many times, being rather a rough little girl, in fights with boys, shouting and playing. I suppose because I was so healthy I could not resist being a tom-boy. But I flew to you in trouble and you were always there to help me. One little story: The boys told me I was not pretty, or gentle. I rushed to you and asked, 'Willy, am I not pretty?' (I was not, I squinted, my hair always cut very short.) You replied, 'You are the prettiest girl in Norfolk,' and I trusted you and really believed I was—deluded infant—and was sure I was, and said so, notwithstanding derisive shouts."

A story is still told in Norfolk which, if true, shows that William was not too greatly under the thumb of his charmer. Although Alice lived right next to the Misses Nettleton's School and he a quarter of a mile away, he once persuaded her to walk home via his house. Looking forward to an agreeable afternoon's stroll, the little girl agreed, but when they got to William's doorstep, he said a perfunctory good-bye and disappeared indoors.

Leaving the Misses Nettleton's School, William spent a year or so at Norfolk Academy, a more ambitious institution which attracted a few boarders from out of town. "The younger pupils," a former principal tells us, "were taught after a pretty well defined course, in reading, spelling, arithmetic, geography, grammar, and history, especially of the United States. . . . The object aimed at steadily and persistently was to lead the boys and girls to think for themselves; to look at the subject under consideration in a common-sense way." Mental discipline was considered more important than the amassing of facts.

At the age of thirteen the boy was sent to Winchester Institute, "a collegiate, military and commercial boarding seminary," at Winchester Center. "The discipline of the School," the announcement states, "will be mild and parental. . . . We shall endeavor to secure such obedience by appeals to the nobler faculties of the mind, and if possible induce the pupils to do right from choice. It is the aim of the Principal and his family to become familiarly acquainted with each pupil, and to surround all with the genial influences of a well-regulated Christian household. The School . . . is sufficiently retired to be free from all immoral local influences."

The principal, the Rev. Ira Pettibone, was the uncle with whom William's sister Emma had lived ever since their mother's death. During the boy's first term, she was in Winchester; by the time she moved away to Mount Holyoke Seminary, he was well used to the institution where his best friend, Frederic S. Dennis, was also a pupil. The atmosphere seems indeed to have been "mild and parental." The boys had ponies which they rode almost at will through the country lanes; they went on picnics and sleigh rides, and called on the children of the town much as if they were in their own homes.

Most of the instruction was in the hands of William's cousins, Ira Welch Pettibone and Benjamin Welch Pettibone. The former, who had been a colonel during the Civil War, conducted "military drill," a study which seems to have interested William less than his course in sewing. Describing to his sister the Christmas of his fifteenth year, William wrote: "I got a needle book, something I had long been wishing for." This present vied for delightfulness with a sugar dog from Allie Eldridge.

That his childish romance had not died is revealed by the many references in letters he received from his friends. Sam Dennis, for instance, kindly composed a document which he advised William to send to his "sweet hart." It read: "Dear Allie, My swetest of sweetest I love myself will you mary me at the oak on Saterday morning at 5 o'clock. Sweet sugar plum. From your atended [intended?] husband Will." A few months later Alfred M. Millard asked: "Have you seen Allie yet and is she as pretty as ever and besides I suppose you are in love with her, but keep on and you will some day have her for your wife." He signs this epistle: "Fish sh-sh, alias Alfred."

William's own letters of this period show that his major interest was not in his studies, but in the normal recreations of a healthy boy. He was encouraged in this attitude by his father, who believed that brainwork could easily be over-emphasized. "I was very much pleased," the doctor wrote his son, "to receive your letter and to learn that you want 'to go in with other boys in catching rabbits.' I hope you will be successful in catching the rabbits, for it is more pleasant to succeed than to fail in whatever we undertake to do, but whether you succeed or not in getting the rabbits, it will pay in the exercise in the open air it will give you. We must exercise in order to be strong and well, and if you do not establish a strong constitution, all the learning you can acquire will be worth but little. While you learn from the books all you can, I hope you will never lose sight of the necessity of growing up strong and healthy. If you at any time want 15 cts. as much as you did this now called for, and for as good an object, you may always expect to get it."

William reported in a letter to a friend: "We have got a ball club here, pay ten cents and you can be a life member. We play every night after school. . . . Fred and Sam, his brother, Pitcher and me room up in the third story. We have gay times up there." After the teachers were in bed, however, they occasionally sneaked out and slept in more romantic places. Fred Dennis, who kept a diary, noted: 'Slept in the cub-bar[d] in the school room with Welch for fun last night."

As a result of their study of Greek, the boys organized a comic secret society. A letter to William, signed "W. K. Harrison, Scribe," read as follows: "Most Honorable of the Greeks and worthy of all praise Your humble servant W. Harrison has taken the liberty to address your most exalted Majesty He received your most excelent epistle on Tuesday the fourth day of April 1865 and was much pleased as well as honored by it. The simplicity and grandeur of the style the loftiness of the tone and the exalted theme at once astonished, delighted and gladdened his heart. Why just to think of being so noticed and flattered by the most honorable of the Greeks is astounding to the mind."

Almost all the letters of William's classmates contain references to evangelical religion. Every boy is interested in which of his contemporaries have joined the church, and those who have not yet experienced the revelation of grace beg their friends to pray that it may be vouchsafed to them. A roommate is described as a gay fellow, "a Christian and a member of the church." A typical reference to Sunday in Fred Dennis's diary reads: "Pleasant day. Went to church 3 times. Mr. Pettibone preached two good sermons." The following notation is made without a hint of rebellion: "Snowed very hard indeed today my Father made me a life member of the American Bible Society for a birthday present."

That William was slow in professing his faith was a subject of concern at Winchester Institute and elsewhere. Early in 1864, his sister wrote him several exhortations, persisting even though he ignored the subject in his replies. Her pleadings must have borne great weight, since she seems to have taken the place in his affections of the mother he had never known; her letters were one of his greatest comforts. "I had waited all day Friday," he wrote her, "wishing the mail would come it seemed as if it never staid so long. But the longest day must have an end at last the mail came and with it your letter."

Nor were Emma's importunings the only ones he received; his classmates were receiving the sacrament in ever-increasing numbers, and his grandmother must have been deeply interested in his salvation. On the other side there was only the example of his father, who, although fundamentally religious, had even resisted the urging of his dying wife that he "build an altar in the home."

During March 1864, William announced at a revival meeting in his school that he had experienced grace, but, strangely enough, he failed to tell his sister. Having heard the news from another member of the family, she wrote him for verification. William replied: "There is indeed a great revival going on here I think about one hundred have expressed their determination of serving the Lord. Among them myself the reason I did not tell you was I was afraid I could not hold out but Emma I do mean to try and I hope I shall have an interest in your prayers that I may not falter and turn back. . . . You wanted to know my opinion of your going to Turkey [as a missionary]. I think I should rather have you labor nearer home."

Emma's next letter was an effusive pæan of joy: "How I wish I could see you to-night and tell you how *perfectly* glad I am that now another than an earthly love has filled the longing soul, stilled that vague yearning we always feel when conscious that after all the pleasures of earth there is but a blank. I wish I could tell you that always the yoke is easy and the burden light that it is but an easy thing to fight the good fight. But Alas! till the jasper gates stand ajar and we on the other side singing will the battle of life the stern strife of the present be over." She urged him to write their father "of your hope in the Savior. I am sure he will be very much rejoiced."

William was not so sure; he replied succinctly: "I have not yet written father of my hope." Then he added: "I feel now much happier than I ever have before. When I have been the happiest the thought would present itself 'this night thy soul shall be required of thee' and I thought am I prepared? I could not answer in the affirmative but now I hope I can."

William's difficulties, however, were not over. He had merely experienced a preliminary revelation; he had not taken the sacrament. Although his sister continually urged him to go further, he waited many months and listened to many exhortations before, on May 23, 1865, he was able to write her: "Alfred Millard and I joined the church here Sunday before last. I am determined to live a better life than I have ever done before. I feel that I have done many things that I ought not to have done and Emma you must always pray for me as I think you always do for I do [for] you." Then his letter turned to other matters. He never imitated the lyrical bursts of religious phraseology typical of his sister and his friends. However, his letters were almost always more reticent and self-contained. When only fifteen, he wrote truthfully: "I don't like to talk of myself as you well know."

II

William returned to Norfolk for his vacations. "We always had large family parties," his cousin Alice tells us, "especially at Thanksgiving and Christmas, and had the jolliest times imaginable. After great dinners all the older people—and as I remember them they were all tall, large, with white hair—would play games with the children. . . . It was a frequent occurrence for at least five or six Dr. Welches to be at the same dinner table. And we all inherited and imbibed a knowledge of medicine, I think."

William Wickham, himself fascinated with medicine, the son of a doctor, the nephew of another, and the brother of four doctors, always insisted that his own son should enter the family profession. William, however, expressed a repugnance to medicine. The continual stream of sick people cluttering up the house, the anguished knockings on the door at midnight, the moans that rose sometimes from his father's office, all these disturbed the sensitive child. Years later he told Dr. Harvey Cushing that he had been unable to bear the sight of blood or pain, that he had run away if a tooth were to be pulled in the family. He added that his father had failed to make him understand medical things.

William's relation with his father involves a seeming contradiction. We know that when he grew to maturity, he displayed many of the traits and idiosyncrasies of his elder; indeed, the passing of years seems increasingly to have brought out in William Henry Welch characteristics that were William Wickham's. Yet during his boyhood William was clearly not close to his father.

George T. Johnson, a local druggist who boarded in the Welch home during William's childhood, tells us that although he believed William Wickham was fond of his son, the physician rarely demonstrated affection. Dr. Welch was too busy attending to the community at large to pay attention to his child. "His love of humanity," a colleague remembers, "made all as dear to him as were his own household." When neighbours came to call, Dr. Welch, aware of the importance of a private interview in influencing people, would not allow the conversation to become general. "It made no difference if only his wife was present, the gentlemanly doctor with charming grace would rise and speak with 'By the way, sir, I wish to see you a moment,' and then usher you into an adjoining room and close the door."

William Wickham's day left him little time for his children, for he was an adept at the genial procrastination that was to characterize his son. He would sleep late and then hurry downstairs to his office, where he gossiped so long with his patients that it took him hours to examine a few simple ills. Finally, he returned to the main house for lunch, assuring the sufferers in his waiting room that he would be back in a moment. While the meal was being put on the table, he made his daily gesture of efficiency; he rang a bell and ordered the man of all work to harness his horse to the buggy at once; was he not almost ready to begin his rounds? All afternoon the buggy would remain in front of the house, the horse's head sinking lower and lower. The doctor was always detained by patients who came late and stayed long, while he advised them not only on health but on crops, politics, family affairs, manufactures, and the probable state of the weather. At about six o'clock he would stride out of his office and ring the big bell in the kitchen a second time. Again the hired man came running, but this time he was told to take the horse back to the barn, unharness him, feed him, reharness him, and tie him to the post again.

It was usually almost dark before the doctor started out with a well-filled lantern slung underneath the buggy and a Dalmatian dog running at the horse's heels; William Wickham was a night-owl, as his son was to be. Late passers would see a lantern swinging low, making crazy shadows, and then catch a glimpse of a flowing beard as the doctor rushed by behind one of his powerful horses. Often the doctor would be asleep as he travelled at a breakneck speed, but he knew the roads so well that he would awaken automatically at places where there were ditches or stones that had to be avoided. If he were not asleep, he could hardly resist stopping to speak to every passer-by he met, for all in the community were his patients and his friends. These conversations, usually long and intimate, were sometimes interrupted by his friend's asking him how much he owed for past medical services. Such a question never failed to fluster William Wickham Welch. "Oh, never mind now; we are in a hurry," he would reply as he whipped up his horse.

The doctor was an inveterate horse-trader, and the spirited steeds he drove were so famous in the countryside that on one occasion a race was arranged between one of his pairs and an equally famous pair belonging to Senator William H. Barnum of Salisbury; history does not record who won. Dr. Welch loved a good horse-race, and it is reported that the few times he ever demanded payment of a bill were when he needed money to attend the races at Hartford. He was sure to find some delinquent fellow-enthusiast at the station from whom he could collect, since almost everyone in town was in his debt.

He was always getting colts that ran away with him. On one occasion his horse returned alone late at night, dragging a broken harness. A searching party, we are told, "found his buggy, overturned, with the doctor pinned underneath. He raised two fingers, a characteristic gesture, and said, 'By the way, will some of you gentlemen be kind enough to turn this buggy over and let me out?'"

This large, bearded man who was so eccentric and gentle was greatly loved in the countryside, the more so because of the many funny stories that could be told about him. Patients gladly put up with the inconveniences caused by his peculiarities because they had complete faith in his skill; even as educators and scientists were later to put up with similar difficulties with his son. The citizens of Norfolk went to sleep after a long day of unattended illness confident that before morning the doctor would appear. But when the spirited horses galloped into the courtyard, the vigil might not yet be over. If the doctor were hungry, he would go into the pantry and eat whatever he could find. Then, if the well members of the family were still awake, the doctor would swap tales with them in the back parlour, or if a newspaper caught his eye, he would pick it up and read it, oblivious of all around him, for a half-hour or more before he remembered his patient and walked upstairs, his heavy tread resounding through the stillness.

But the instant he entered the sick-room the patient felt better. The art of healing seemed to surround his physical body like an aura; it was often not his treatment but his presence that cured. "One of his particular traits and characteristics," we are told, "was to do and say pleasant things in the sick-room." A colleague wrote: "His gentleness was almost feminine, and a delicacy of manner and sweet consideration for the inclinations and even whims of his patients never failed to make them good-natured. . . . He was to the invalid a cordial that aroused hopeful, happy feelings. . . . It was a trait of Dr. Welch's to make all feel that he was their true friend. . . . Dr. Welch was a deep thinker. How often have I seen him sit down at the bedside or in his office and ponder over his case. . . . His eyes were half closed, his head bowed, his fingers folded, and making a slow constant revolving motion with his thumb."

William Wickham Welch had the advantages of long tradition behind him. His father, whom he so greatly resembled, had begun practice in Norfolk in the 1780's; his much older brothers, too, had practised there and been successful. The community had implicit faith in "the Welch doctors."

Undoubtedly he had the control over the psychology of his patients that is imputed to the ideal country doctor; but what of the purely medical side of his practice? In 1857 he delivered the graduation address at the Yale Medical Institution, as his elder brother and preceptor, Benjamin Welch, had done in 1853. Although only four years separated the two orations, there was almost a half-century of difference in the points of view. Skilful physician as he was, Benjamin mingled his medical ideas with religious belief, building up a philosophical rather than a scientific argument.[2] William Wickham, on the contrary, denounced theorizing in medicine, as his son might have done. "All positive knowledge obtained . . ." he insisted, "has resulted from the accurate observation of facts." And in listing recent observations, he revealed a knowledge of new scientific developments amazing in a country doctor of his period, when American medical thought was largely isolated from Europe. Not only did he refer to auscultation, the technique of listening for sounds within the body, which was not to be mentioned in the Harvard Medical School catalogue for another eleven years; he also spoke of "the discovery of the cell theory with its results in physiology and pathology." These words were uttered a year before Virchow's book, *Cellularpathologie,* was issued in German, and three years before the first English translation. True, in 1855 Virchow had published his work in his German journal, but a diligent search of the ordinary channels by which American practitioners kept abreast of their period has failed to reveal the source of William Wickham's knowledge.

However, like most country practitioners of the time, Dr. Welch mingled traditional medicine with the scientific. He kept a ledger in which he recorded under the name of the disease remedies which other local physicians believed efficacious; he would note in the margin that it was the favourite prescription of Dr. So-and-so. Sometimes his "cures" seem bizarre to modern eyes. He was, for instance, particularly proud of his remedy for snake-bite: copper filings cut from a penny, dissolved in vinegar, and immediately applied to the wound. Of course the chemical thus produced, copper acetate, had no ef-

fect whatsoever, but the rattlesnakes of Connecticut are fortunately so small that they rarely give a fatal bite; William
Wickham was able to boast that he had "never lost a case."

As was again typical of his period, Dr. Welch believed in
drugging; George T. Johnson, the local pharmacist, says of his
prescriptions: "I remember some that he wrote which had in
them everything that he knew the name of." Elder citizens of
Norfolk tell that after examining a patient William Wickham
would call for a bowl and mix medicine in it, seeking to get
the right proportions by tasting the concoction as he went
along.

William Wickham, however, believed in the virtues of fresh
air, which many of his colleagues regarded as a deadly poison
for fever sufferers. The story is told that on passing the house
of a patient late one night he saw that the windows were, contrary to his instructions, all shut. He reined in his horse and
tore the window of the sick-room from the house, frame and all.
Placing it in his buggy beside him, he drove on, confident that
his patient would no longer disobey his orders.

William Wickham was a personal doctor, and he allowed his
personal tastes to carry him so far that he put off surgical operations for as long as his conscience would allow. Dr. Barber tells
us: "I believe he had a constitutional repugnance to operative
surgery, especially anything pertaining to gynecology, and of
this feeling, which I have often thought was due to his extreme modesty, he could never fully rid himself."

Not only did William Wickham carry on his arduous medical
practice; he played an important part in politics as well. A
staunch Republican, he was in 1852 a State Senator, and he
served many terms in the Assembly—1848, 1850, 1860, 1881—
where he finally became a senior member and thus ex-officio a
fellow of Yale College. During two of William's important
formative years, 1855–57, he was in Washington as a member
of the House of Representatives.

When Norfolk attempted to take part in the commercial
boom that swept New England after 1850, William Wickham
delightedly cast himself in the role of a captain of finance. He

became incorporator of a leather company and president of a woollen company; he manufactured Springfield rifles during the Civil War. These enterprises failed, but a hand-knitting manufactory set up in John Welch's house was successful, as was a power-knitting company based on a new type of machine whose inventor the Welch brothers had had the vision to back. In 1868 William Wickham, now vice-president of a savings bank, became an incorporator of the Connecticut Western Railway, which passed through Norfolk. But the best efforts of the genial doctor failed to make the town an industrial centre. Between 1851 and 1890, its population dropped from 1641 to 1446, and the railroad tracks were eventually sold for scrap iron.

I I I

In 1865 William Wickham put his son through a major emotional crisis. It began inconspicuously, as most crises do. Undoubtedly the boy hardly noticed when his cousin Minnie wrote him on November 25: "Cousin Emily Sedgwick has been staying here for a week but she has just left." Probably he remembered that Emily Sedgwick was a relative of Mrs. John Welch and a sister of the Connecticut general, John Sedgwick. whose impressive funeral he had patriotically attended with many of his schoolmates. Then he thought no more about it.

Another aspect of the evolving drama must, however, have interested him greatly. His grandmother, who had always kept house for his father, became during 1865 so infirm that she was forced to take the dreadful step of resigning from the Sunday School. "The S.S.," she wrote with a resolute hand, "in whose cares I have *deeply* participated and with undiminished (if not increasing) interest *more* than one *third* of my life, is soon to [be] reorganized,—and I find that I cannot anticipate the *event*, but with solemn if not somewhat of *painful* interest. I find to part with its special cares is too nearly akin to parting with those of my own loved Family! But age with its consequent infirmities must be anticipated by me as by others!" Soon the old lady was confined by an illness to an upstairs room, leaving William

Wickham with no loving female to look after his comfort.

A similar drama of loneliness was acting itself out in Cornwall Hollow, the home of Emily Sedgwick. On her mother's death many years before, she had taken over the responsibility for her blind father, to whom she read for hours every day from the Bible, Milton, and Shakespeare. Her military brother, who also had never married, became the centre of her affections; she wrote proudly that after he had spent three weeks with her, recovering from a wound received at the battle of Antietam, "as he took me in his arms for his final embrace he said that the days he had spent with me were the happiest of his life." General Sedgwick was killed at the battle of Spottsylvania. Since her father had also died, Emily enlisted as a nurse, but when the war ended, she was forced to return home to emptiness which she varied by visiting her cousins in Norfolk. There, at the age of forty-six, she became engaged to William Wickham Welch, who was forty-seven.

Late in 1865, William learned that his father was to marry again, that a strange woman was to take the place of his mother, whose memory he had learned to revere. On February 4, 1866, he wrote his sister, who was attending Packer Institute in Brooklyn, a letter full of loathing. "I must tell you what is on my mind viz about Miss Sedgwick (no matter about the spelling) I suppose you know that she has been here about a week. Mrs. Brown says that she has been over all the house from garret to cellar looking into drawers cupboards, suggesting things she would like altered. She thinks it would be so pleasant if there was only a door from the bed-room into the sitting room. One night she sat up for papa until three o'clock and then he did not come. Papa carried her over to Cornwall—Aunt Lib [John Welch's wife] has told Mrs. Brown to clean out the garret as some things would soon be brought over. Old Mrs. Bell says she [Miss Sedgwick] wont work any and that all her dishes are china. I guess they are going to be married about the first of April. I don't know what I am writing about I feel so mad— But I suppose it is all to be expected. But I wish I was here when she went all over the house and you was to see to things.

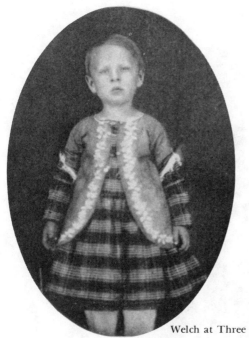

Welch at Three

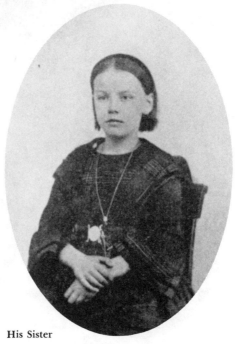

His Sister

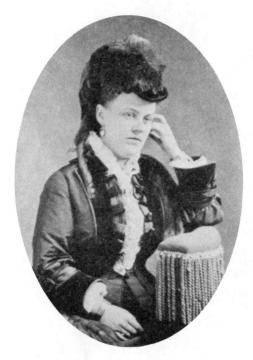

Welch's Sister: Emeline Welch Walcott

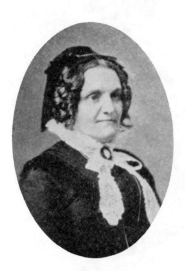

Welch's Stepmother

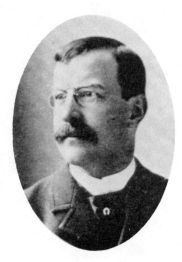

Frederic S. Dennis

But the idea of her looking into the drawers and cupboards. I wish she would keep away I do. I don't see anything attractive about her without it is her eyes and curls which are certainly striking. . . . Oh dear! I wish I could see you to talk with you —I have got so much to tell you."

William must have carried this letter around in his pocket for some time before he mailed it, since Emma's reply is dated February 28. "I received your rather incoherent letter yesterday morning," she wrote, "and I can assure you sympathize most heartily with you in your indignation. I haven't thought of much excepting that since and it has made me terribly blue and disgusted with life generally. It is really rather more than I expected and so soon too its enough to provoke a saint still I suppose its only the beginning of sorrow and we must resign ourselves to submissively pass under the yoke. What makes you think they are to be married in April has papa said any thing to you about it? . . . *I am bound that I won't attend the wedding if I can help it.* . . . When you write do tell me what you are going to call her."

William replied: "I am sorry that I made you 'so terribly blue'—but I can sympathize with you as for a few days past I have had a very hard cold so that I could not go out doors and had nothing to think about except about 'that terrible event' but I guess *terrible* is rather too strong a word—I told you, the simple unvarnished truth. I cant imagine what I shall call her. Do tell me what you are going to. I shall say 'she' whenever I can. One thing is certain. I don't intend to call her mother." William hoped that during their spring vacations Emma would go away somewhere with him, anywhere to flee from Norfolk and impending tragedy.

However, the boy who was to grow into so reticent a man managed to preserve a calm face before the world. "When I was in Winsted," he wrote in a later letter to Emma, "Aunt Lavinia [Mrs. James Welch] was in a great stew to know what you and I thought about papa's being married. I did not commit myself at all."

William, perhaps because of a sense of family propriety, attended the wedding, although his sister stayed away. However, she saw the newly married couple as they passed through New York on their honeymoon. "I had before made up my mind to call her Mother," she wrote William, "but for some cause the Mother was so very faint that I am sure she could not have had the slightest conception of what I intended to say. It was of course very stiff for a few minutes. Very soon Papa went out for the paper and we were left alone. She then took me into the next room and showed me a box of wedding cake which she had brought me she also gave me a beautiful pin it is white onyx with a cross of black onyx and pearls in the center. The setting is of Etruscan gold very handsome indeed. Then of course a terrible pause ensued. She put her arm around me and said she hoped we should be friendly she didn't want me to regard her with any prejudice because she was a stepmother but to feel that she was the best friend I had in the world except my father and Will I couldn't help it I almost loved her then. I do think she is splendid and I mean to be kind to her and do all in my power to make it pleasant. I mean to call her Mother I think we ought and she will of course feel badly if we don't."

The ease with which Emma had been won round seems to have struck William as desertion, and again his control broke. "I am glad you called on father when he was in New York and was so favorably impressed but you say you intend to call her mother but Em I know it is reasonable but I cant do it yet. I cant do it. That name seems to me almost too sacred in its memories to me. I may some time but I dont feel as if I could yet. I have not seen her as you have she indeed spoke very kindly to me at the wedding and I think if we are to have a stepmother she is as good as can be found but I can not bring myself to look at it in the same light you do. I fear I can never look on her as my mother. But I do hope it will all be for the best but I [it?] does look rather dark to me in the future."

It was symbolic of the new regime that the family house, which had been William Wickham's birthplace as well as his son's, was entirely rebuilt, its colonial simplicity giving way to Victorian grandeur. A new wing was added for the doctor's offices, and the ground-floor ceilings raised. Steel engravings of Italian Renaissance paintings appeared on the walls. Gone was the easy carelessness that had characterized William's home since before he could remember; routine entered through the rebuilt portal. Now that there was a woman in the house who was primarily interested in its affairs, meals were ready on time, served piping hot, and if the doctor was late, as he almost always was, he was reproved. Emma's daughter, Mrs. Kellogg, tells us that although Emma and the new Mrs. Welch "always had great respect and affection for each other . . . my mother sometimes felt that the wife was needlessly impatient and sharp with her husband, whom she always called 'Doctor.' Even as a young girl I felt sympathy for the house-keeper who never knew when Doctor Welch would come to his meals, and who was often kept waiting an hour or more. As far as I know my grandfather never lost his even temper and would try to appease the irritation by some pleasant remark or amusing anecdote. Emily Sedgwick was possibly temperamentally unsuited to the type of man she married, but whom she loved, quite passionately perhaps."

There was nothing easy-going about the new Mrs. Welch, and the ambition that burned within her was in the end to be of great encouragement and assistance to William, whose father never yearned for a larger stage than Norfolk or hoped that his son would have a more glorious destiny than following exactly in the footsteps of his ancestors. When the boy wrote him that he would like to study music, William Wickham replied: "I have no objection to your spending a little time, when you have nothing better to do, in practicing on the piano." Emily Sedgwick Welch would have understood the importance of music to a cultivated man.

But for the time being William was more reluctant to accept the marriage than his sister. In his unhappiness, all matters associated with love disgusted him; he wrote Emma: "Last night I went to a sociable at Mr. John McAlpine's, I think it was the best one we have had this winter. All kissing games were dispensed with."

Affairs at school were so absorbing that he was often able to forget his troubles. He was a senior; the following year, he hoped, would find him a lordly student at Yale. For a few dazzling days he had visited his cousin Charles A. Collin at the college, where his ears had been filled with fascinating talk of college customs and the Yale fence. Gravely his cousin told him which clubs to join as they were full of the aristocracy, which to avoid as reeking with rabble. Probably it was William's report of these talks that made his chum Fred Dennis write importantly in his diary: "Never on any account join the Gamanny but if any the Delta Kapps . . . at Yale College."

William spent his last vacation before Yale at Norfolk with his father and stepmother; unhappily, as we gather from a letter to his sister, begging to be allowed to join her in their mother's childhood home, Benton, New York. "Stay! oh stay!" he wrote. "I frantically entreat you to stay! Dont be alarmed at this abrupt manner of commencing my letter. I will come out and meet you if you will only stay. I am afraid you will be gone before this letter reaches you but there is one chance out of ten that you will not and I seize that chance."

CHAPTER IV

Lure of the Classics at Yale

I

WILLIAM'S first reaction to Yale was loneliness; his sister wrote him: "My Poor Darling Homesick Little Brother— I suppose I ought to study every minute this P.M. but considering your most forlorn disconsolate state of mind I am going to write you instead. Really Will I *am* sorry for you and know how to sympathize with you for I have been just so homesick myself. It is lonely enough to feel that you are a stranger in a strange place and haven't any one to whom you can look for comfort or guidance but isn't it a comfort to feel that there is One who is always with us. . . . I thought myself quite seriously of going to N. Haven on the 'night boat' Saturday and if you still continue as homesick may do so some time."

Emma need not have worried; soon William was too absorbed even to read her letters; on November 24 he explained his slowness in answering her last by saying that since it had arrived just before a secret-society meeting, he had put it in his pocket and forgotten it was there. He went on gleefully: "The faculty say that we are the worst class that ever entered college, yet I don't believe that, but I don't think a jollier class ever entered college. I am acquainted with at least half of the class. The temptations here are very numerous and mighty, yet I trust they will only be a means of strengthening my faith instead of weakening it. To God alone I must look for strength to resist. Pray for me as I always do for you."

His letters to Dennis, who was now at Andover Academy, reveal a similar mingling of religion and high spirits. After begging Fred not to "forget me in your prayers as I assure you I do not you," he continued: "The other day as I was coming out of recitation with another fellow, I saw someone directly

in front of me. Supposing it to be a student (it being so dark
that I couldn't recognize him) I said, 'Let's put off his hat and
he will think the Sophs have got it.' Accordingly we grabbed
his hat and run upstairs. He followed and we ran so much the
harder but finally we stopped. He came up and so—who was
it but—a tutor. He asked our names, the usual inquiry on such
occasions, and departed. We of course were utterly thunder-
struck as it would probably end in a public expulsion, so sacred
are the persons of the faculty. . . . We went to him and told
the circumstances of the case and received a lecture on the im-
propriety of stealing hats, etc., but that was all. We were glad
to be let off so easy. The same tutor seems to be subject to all
sorts of calamities. A student ran up to him the other day and
grabbed him about the neck and I was on the point of kicking
him and letting him go upstairs faster when I fortunately discovered who it was.

"Forsake all ideas of my taking such lofty honors as you
speak of. If I can keep in college four years I shall consider myself fortunate."

The last paragraph was inspired by a passage in Dennis's
previous letter in which he said he was sure that Welch would
graduate "either Valedict or some very high honor," and that
Ira Pettibone, the principal of Winchester Institute, agreed.
Indeed, William had left such a reputation behind that his
schoolmates felt he could even protect himself from hazing.
"Do they 'ruff' on you much?" asked Alfred M. Millard. "I
suppose they have their hands full when they undertake it at
all." Although the treatment given freshmen was so rough
that in 1871 the author of *Four Years at Yale* advised them to
keep loaded guns in their rooms with which to frighten away
the sophomores, William did not find the hazing distasteful;
quite the contrary. At the beginning of his sophomore year he
wrote Dennis: "I have been quite busy furnishing my new
room, regulating impudent freshmen, and other things of like
importance."

Wise sophomores, however, avoided molesting his friends.
Frederick Collin, who was a year behind William, tells us that

the day after some of William's classmates had hazed him, they returned to apologize, saying: "We did not know you were Billy Welch's cousin. If we had known you were Billy Welch's cousin we would not have tried the game on you."

William was not impervious to the charms of young ladies; he wrote Emma: "I should be terribly homesick if I had no place to call once in a while. Miss Nelly [Battell] is quite noted among the students as a beauty. . . . All the other unfortunate freshmen quite envy my good fortune in being acquainted with her."

Cupid, however, was preparing another blow for him. His sister's letters had for some time been mentioning one Stuart Walcott with ominous regularity, and on February 17, 1867, she wrote that she had become engaged to him and had left Packer Institute for ever, although if she had stayed a few months longer she would have graduated with high honours. Emma was obviously worried about the way her brother would receive the news: "I hardly need tell you Willie that I am very happy although the joy is strangely mingled with a feeling of regret and sadness at the thought of so soon leaving home and my first thought Willie was for you for I had formed so many plans for the future that I could not and now cannot bear to think that they would never be realized I know of course that I should see very little of you for the next four years and I suppose you will probably be married soon after leaving college still I think we could have been together more than we shall probably now be able to but rest assured my dear Brother my deepest warmest love shall always be yours I do not mean deepest in contrast from my love to of course one other. I shall not leave home certainly before May or June. . . . Write me Willie and tell me just what you think of Stuart and of my plans."

William's answer has been lost, but Emma's reply to it shows that the sister who had been almost a mother to him had been surprised by its moderation. "I feared you would write so differently for I know the change in my plans must be a great disappointment to you as it is to me but Will although our lives will never again be joined as they have been I sincerely hope that our love for each other may deepen and strengthen while life remains. Don't think that my love for you will in the least diminish now that another has gained my affections. I am sure Willie it will grow with my growth and strengthen with my strength for I have only now learned to love."

Welch had by this time become reconciled to his stepmother, even fond of her. As early as November 1866, some seven months after she came into the family, he had broken his bitter resolve by referring to her as "mother" in a letter to Emma; the following spring he stayed with her in Norfolk while his father was away, having "a very pleasant visit." From then on the references to her in his letters were numerous and friendly.

William continued to have a good time at Yale, to be very popular, and at the end of his junior year he was elected a member of the honorary senior society, Skull and Bones, on "scholarship merits," it is true, but over a man who had a higher average than his. He wrote his father that he had pulled no wires to get this distinction. "We have a splendid set of men and the honor is more agreeable to me than any other in College could have been. . . . It is understood to be very literary in its character and has in its possession a very fine library. . . . I have spoken thus at length for when I become a duly initiated member I shall have to adopt the strictest secrecy."

The fifteen members of Bones were chosen not because of social prominence, but because it was felt that they had the most to offer Yale and the world at large. They took this position of leadership very seriously, dedicating themselves in the Bones "temple" to the pursuit of ideals. The rituals of the society were secret—members were supposed to leave the room if Bones was even mentioned by uninitiates—but the entire community of the college was very conscious of which young men had been accorded the honour of membership, an honour universally regarded as the greatest open to an undergraduate. Thus Welch walked the campus, as he had walked the streets of Norfolk, the recognized possessor of a pre-eminent position.

He continued to believe in Bones for the rest of his life. During 1890 he wrote his brother-in-law: "If a boy has no chance of Bones it makes little difference to him comparatively whether he goes to Yale or somewhere else but if he is the right sort of man for B—— then I say Yale over any other college or university in the world."

As William told his father in 1869, "nearly all the members of the faculty are members of this society and keep up their interest in it." The charge was made in articles in the *Nation* and the *Independent* that the secret societies, among which Bones was the leader, controlled the policies of Yale. Be that as it may, Learned's many long letters to Welch show that the management of the college was often a subject of discussion in the windowless, tomb-like temple of Bones; not only the matter of undergraduate offices, although that was important, but also faculty appointments, the nature of the curriculum, the general policy of Yale. As they sat around the fire in their secret home talking college shop by the hour, the members might have been professors. Using his mind with pleasure on matters of academic administration and scholastic policy, Welch joined in the debates with enthusiasm, but, as we learn from one of Learned's letters, he was often "the only one who kept cool."

The members of Bones were not beyond being boys. In a letter to Welch, Learned described how after a long discussion of marriage by the fire, "we sought repose, but found some difficulty in gaining it as McCutcheon insisted on cutting up like a regular devil, and rushed around from one room to another dressed in a flaming red pair of drawers as if he had just come from the infernal regions. McClure hid two shoes in Scutch's bed and Perry stole Jim's nightshirt."

It is interesting to note that in the Bones discussions Welch figured as an opponent of marriage. His clubmate, J. G. K. McClure, wrote him in 1871: "Your discouraging views" of love "have been too much for me and I have decided not to have anything to do with the vanum et mutabile until—I get a good chance. I hear that your opinions on this subject are still the same. . . . I chuckle to myself when I think that some of these days you will confess to the wrong of the past and that a rich experience will reward the faithful as they meet . . . to hear what has happened in a past year."

II

In 1870, the year that Welch graduated, the *Nation* charged: "Yale College has thus far shown, at least as regards its Academical Department, a strong determination to walk in the ancient ways, and, as far as its curriculum is concerned, to yield little, if anything, to what is called the 'spirit of the age.' " A study of the catalogue shows that during William's freshman year the academical department boasted only eight full professors, whose chairs were designated as follows: natural philosophy and astronomy, moral philosophy and metaphysics, geology and mineralogy, Latin language and literature, Greek language and literature, mathematics, rhetoric and English literature, and history. During Welch's sophomore year a radical innovation was made by introducing a course in French, the first modern language ever taught at Yale.

Almost the entire four-year curriculum was made up of required courses; there was virtually no instruction in science, though a course in "natural philosophy" included a smattering of such matters as "mechanics, hydrostatics, pneumatics, acoustics, electricity, magnetism, optics"; and during the senior year a series of afternoon lectures mingled moral philosophy with anatomy, chemistry with "evidences of Christianity."

Welch was later to feel that the instruction to which he had been submitted was very inferior. He made the notation "fine letter" on one he received in 1933 from his classmate Professor E. S. Dana, who wrote as follows: "My thoughts go back to our years of 1866 to 1870, and I am much impressed at the complete change in the intellectual side of the life at Yale. Do you recall 'Pill' Otis, who was our Sophomore Latin tutor? Also 'Nancy' Smith, who commenced 'Natural Philosophy' (Olmstead's) with us in Junior year by telling us frankly that he was not familiar with the subject but would make it as inter-

esting as possible. . . . Sumner began with us in Geometry
and was one of the few who appreciated the difference between
teaching and hearing the boys recite—all that dear old Loomis
[the professor of natural philosophy and astronomy] wanted
was to hear again the exact words in his book—'not a super-
fluous word in the book' was his motto. . . . Certainly we
lived through a strangely stagnant time in Yale's history."

Magazines such as the *Nation* insisted that Yale was under
the domination of the Congregational Church. Indeed, the
president of the college was a minister. The board of trustees was made up of the six senior Senators of Connecticut,
who rarely attended meetings, and ten ministers; although
radicals, banded under the name of "the young Yale," were
agitating for an active lay membership, they did not win until
after Welch's graduation. Thus the atmosphere of Yale was as
ecclesiastical as had been the Welch home and Winchester
Institute. On his arrival at New Haven, Welch had of course
transferred his church membership to that city; he went regularly to worship, joined the Yale Missionary Society, and was
intimate with several undergraduates preparing to join the
ministry.

Although there was no evidence that the professors ever
referred to Darwin, whose *Origin of Species* was published in
1859, some rumblings of the new scientific approach which
was changing men's attitude toward revelation found their way
even into the hushed precincts of Yale. In an essay entitled
The Decay of Faith, which he submitted in a competition,
Welch attempted to reassure those whose belief in religious
revelation had been shaken by scientific fact. "No sadder sight
can there be," he wrote, "than to see a noble soul oppressed
with doubts like these. Have you ever thought, what if this
world were a vast machine unguided by a God of justice or
in the terrible words of one who teaches this system, 'Nature
acts with fearful uniformity; stern as fate, absolute as tyranny,
merciless as death; too vast to praise, too inexplicable to worship, too inexorable to propitiate; it has no ear for prayer, no
heart for sympathy, no arm to save'? Oh is there not bitterness

in such a thought? Does it not make life hopeless and not worth living?"

It is hard to say whether the emotion of this passage was merely the conventional rhetoric of the period, or whether it reflected what William himself felt. In any case, William believed the Gospel was in peril. "There never was an age so profoundly hostile to the supernatural, the essence of all religions. The struggle is no longer about Christian dogmas but about the very foundation of Christianity, faith in the unseen and the eternal." He then attacked the bases of modern unbelief one by one.

The first he defined as pantheism, which found God manifested in all nature, "while the loftier conception of God as a personal being" was rejected. According to this heresy, preached by people such as Emerson, man is a part of God and need not read the Scriptures for revelation; he need merely listen to the promptings of his own soul. However, "if the light in man is the sole light, how feeble and flickering at times it does become. The heathen, who has no other light, oppressed with ignorance and superstition, proves the doctrine a mockery and a lie." Welch argued that although "this dreamy and exaggerated doctrine" might satisfy "the speculative and idealistic cast of the German mind . . . the sturdy English mind demands something more than a poetic rapture for religion."

Welch next turned to those who try to make revelation agree with reason, either by searching for rational explanations of the Gospel or by refusing to believe what cannot be rationally explained. Such heretics forget that "reason teaches that there are truths above reason. Man has within himself ideas and aspirations reaching far beyond this world up to the infinite, the eternal, the inscrutable. These ideas and aspirations are realities and must be acknowledged as such by the mind. But in acknowledging them the reason must stop. If it attempts to raise the veil it finds itself no longer surrounded by the facts and laws of this finite world. Man . . . has come to the boundary of a mysterious world; instinctively he assures himself of

the existence of facts which he can neither grasp nor measure."
God favours him with a "revelation of Himself . . . man could
never discover by the light of his own mind." This revelation is
beyond the power of reason to judge and assay.

Welch then admitted that to keep faith from becoming "an
impotence of the mind" reason must be allowed to judge the
grounds on which faith rests. But having once concluded that
Christianity is the true religion, reason may go no further.
"What more unreasonable than, after acknowledging the authority as Divine, to subject its contents to the arbitration of
human reason! . . . Revelation must either be accepted as a
whole or rejected as a whole."

That the third form of heresy, the conflict between religious
doctrine and scientific law, interested Welch the most is shown
by his making it the subject of the oration his standing as third
in his class entitled him to give at his own graduation. "To the
idea of law," he told his auditors, "science, in its steady march
onward, is giving increasing prominence. Events once deemed
the most abnormal, the most capricious are gradually coming
within the realm of law, so that already science triumphantly
leaps to the grand conclusion, law fixed and universal throughout physical nature. This idea of the government of the world
by laws, immutable, inexorable, has done more than any other
development of science to perplex the faith of many a noble
soul. But when we have reached nature's laws must we really
stop? Is there nothing beyond? 'No,' says rationalism, 'nothing. Law rules and rules alone.' "

Welch, however, felt that he had discovered in the reasoning
of the rationalists a loophole that let all religion in. Admitting
that like causes produce like effects, he insisted that results
could none the less be changed by changing the causes through
the exercise of human or divine will. Then he put forward
three arguments to prove the freedom of the will. First: since
the future course of history cannot be accurately predicted,
the will is obviously free. Second: if there were no free will,
men could not be held responsible for their actions, which is

unthinkable. Third: a man can be demonstrated to have a choice between right and wrong, for if he did not he would either always do right or always do wrong. "As long as the noble nature and the selfish nature are mingled in man, we shall be unable to reduce his actions to a scientific system."

Thus in his youth the future scientist attempted to solve the great philosophical problems that have defeated many a mature philosopher. And thus he reached triumphantly and to the applause of his hearers the conclusion they all desired: "rightly regarded and in its proper sphere" the concept of immutable natural law "has nothing at variance with true faith."

Many years later his roommate, Lauriston L. Scaife, wrote him: "The last few days my mind has kept coming back to the end which crowned our college work,—the Commencement exercises,—and sitting in the old church, with your father's protective arm about my shoulder, while you were proclaiming the 'Reign of Law' . . . and realizing that as your father and I sat together listening to you, I was not only filled with a personal pride in you, but was subconsciously enjoying the affection, however fleeting, of your father, engendered by the complete *rapport* of our feelings for you."

Welch completed his undergraduate days at Yale in a blaze of glory; the veneration some of his friends felt for him may be inferred from another letter from Scaife, this time written shortly after graduation. "Now that we have finally separated I feel that I ought to try to express my great indebtedness for the kindness which you always manifested towards me, the pure example you set me, but more than all, for the patience with which you endured my many annoying practices and habits. Billy, I feel now more deeply than ever the truth of what I often said to others if not to you—that I was utterly unworthy such a chum as yourself. I often pitied you, to think that you were compelled to room with me, your inferior in ability, dignity & every good & noble quality . . . I feel it all; & can say to you on paper what your modesty would never permit you to hear."

III

To be a big man at Yale, a member of Bones, a commencement orator, the admiration of one's friends, and a brilliant student, had been highly gratifying, but now Welch needed to find some place for himself in the world of mature men. The obvious course would have been to follow the importunities of his father and of family tradition by studying medicine. Since William Wickham always needed an assistant, a job would have awaited him the instant he was ready and eventually he would have succeeded to the lucrative family practice. The argument was so complete that it must have amazed the citizens of Norfolk when William adhered to his determination not to be a doctor.

At Yale there had been nothing to make William change his mind about medicine; none of his friends became physicians and, as we have seen, his professors had placed their emphasis not on science, but on God and the humanities. Furthermore, the man who as a member of Bones had become interested in the management of Yale wanted to remain on the campus. "When I was at college," he wrote his niece, "my ambition was to be called back as tutor of Greek, a subject which I think gave me more satisfaction than any other which I studied in college." But there was only one appointment in the classics open, and that went to Learned, who had led the class. Having renounced doctoring, Welch found himself with nothing to look forward to.

He seems never to have considered going into business, or, what is more remarkable, into the law, which was chosen by half the members of Bones and more than half of his eating club. More than a quarter of the Bones men went into the ministry that year, and at least one of them exhorted him to follow, but there is no evidence that he seriously considered the suggestion. He wanted to be a teacher, if not at Yale then in some preparatory school.

No opportunity presented itself. He left his books in New

Haven, hoping he would somehow be able to get back there, and returned to Norfolk, where he spent an uneasy summer. In the middle of August, Learned wrote him: "I am sorry that you are not yet settled"; it seemed almost too late to obtain a school job for the following winter. He was even considering an offer, secured through President Woolsey of Yale, to tutor four boys in elementary subjects when about the middle of September he received a letter from his mathematics professor, H. A. Newton, saying he had recommended Welch to his brother, Isaac S. Newton, who was trying to get together "a select school of say twenty-five pupils" in Norwich, New York. Welch wrote for the position and then in his eagerness telegraphed. Two letters from Isaac S. Newton reached him the same day; the first said that the school, which would have given "a private teacher one thousand dollars and room and fire," was to have been organized as a protest against the management of the Norwich Academy, but that now it was probably too late, since the parents Newton had hoped would dissent had already paid their Academy term bills. The second letter, however, held out hope. "This morning your telegram reached me with no preparation to say, yes come, and yet a wish to that effect. I have today canvassed a little and I find a number ready to join in the matter but not enough to warrant me in saying that we can gather the school, and yet I strongly believe it can be done. If you are at leisure to come here, and make my house your home a week, ready to come if the class be gotten up and to be disappointed if it fails, I cordially bid you come and see us and let us see you."

Welch was in no position to overlook anything; he went to Norwich and made so good an impression that the school was organized in less than a month. He thus described his duties to Fred Dennis: "As you may remember I came here last October to wield the pedagogue's ferule. I found a school of twenty five pupils for me to lead in the thorny paths of knowledge. As the school was of such a mixed character, being of every age from nine to nineteen and of every degree of advancement, it was thought best to add ten more scholars and employ an assistant teacher. Accordingly my labors have been cheered by the co-operation of a maidenly lady of perhaps forty summers, who has taken charge of most of the younger scholars. . . . It has been my embarrassing duty to instruct a class of young ladies of about nineteen or twenty years of age, who are really quite advanced in their studies. With these I have read three German books and some of Cicero's writings that I had never studied before, so that while teaching I have opportunity to learn. Moreover I have found a very pleasant home. Mr. Newton . . . has very kindly taken me into his family. He gives me the use of his library as a sitting room. As he has a miscellaneous library of over one thousand volumes, I have not been in want of companions during the long winter evenings. Thus with a pleasant school and a delightful home I consider my situation quite enviable. Norwich itself is of over five thousand inhabitants and pleasantly situated on the Chenango River. Still, a teacher's life is at times a little bit monotonous and I should think might become exceedingly wearisome in the course of time."

Bored by school teaching, still seeing no chance for an appointment in Greek at Yale, Welch was at loose ends. He comforted himself by exchanging long letters about Yale politics with Learned, who was still in New Haven. For the rest, he taught Sunday School, went on an occasional strawberry festival or picnic, read in his host's library, played with his host's little daughters, and worked very hard. "I don't think," he wrote Emma in June, "there has ever been a school which ran quite as steady as ours has done. We have only had two weeks vacation since we first began last October."

A visit from his parents was the banner occasion of his year, although he complained that Mr. Newton had entertained his parents so well that he had only had an hour apiece alone with them. "I felt rather solemn after they had gone."

Many another young man would have relieved his bored depression by a flirtation, but not Welch. Learned wrote him: "I am glad to hear that you are still free from the fetters" of girls. "I hope you will continue steadfast in your freedom. G.D.M. [George D. Metcalf] and I have about made up our minds that we shall never yield to the fair one."

Although Dennis kept up the Norfolk tradition by occasionally teasing Welch about Alice, the fire seems to have gone out of that childhood romance. His friend Learned, who was closer to him now, since Dennis was separated from him by a gap of two academic years, wrote in March 1871 that he had been to call on Miss Eldridge. "She wanted me to remind you that there was such a person in existence as Alice Eldridge, and send you her love,—or else perhaps it was be remembered to you; it does not make much difference which probably to you."

Welch's reply must have been a stern lecture on flirtation, since several weeks later Learned wrote: "I thank you for your warning in regard to the fair and fickle Goddess, but I think it was not needed. Nothing could exceed my present heroic resolutions on that subject. I have only seen Miss Eldridge once since writing to you, and suppose she is gone now."

As Welch's first year of school teaching drew to a close, it became clear that there would be no further opportunity in Norwich. Planned as a protest, Welch's little school had achieved its purpose; the Norwich Academy was to be reorganized and Welch's pupils returned to it. The young man was again at sea. It was another blow that he could not get away for the Yale commencement, when there would be a delightful reunion at Bones and when he could enjoy again, although for only a day or two, the academic atmosphere he loved. If only there were an opening at Yale as tutor in the classics! Welch's future looked so black and empty that he listened to the proposal he had rejected for so many years: he listened to his father's voice as it urged that he follow the family tradition and go into medicine. At least it was something to do at once, something that offered him the certainty of a livelihood. When he wrote his father that his mind was open to this long-dreaded possibility, it must have been with a heavy heart. But William Wickham was jubilant; at last the boy had seen the light.

CHAPTER V

Convert to Medicine

I

AT the end of his school term in Norwich, William returned home to prepare for medical school by becoming his father's apprentice. Probably this was not a happy period in his life, for during his later years he preferred to pretend that it had never been. As an old man, he said that he had come to the College of Physicians and Surgeons in New York "and attended one lecture by St. John [professor of chemistry] in 1871, and after one lecture I went back to New Haven and spent a year in the study of chemistry in the Sheffield Scientific School." Concerning the one lecture in New York there is no independent evidence, but it is clear from many letters that he did not go to the Sheffield School in 1871, or even discuss the possibility with his intimates at that time; he settled in Norfolk and worked with his father.[1]

Welch, as he himself admitted, disliked writing letters when he was puzzled;[2] it is significant that during his apprenticeship in Norfolk he was a very poor correspondent. In four months he wrote Emma just twice, and he referred to the pursuit of medicine only by giving as a reason for this delinquency the fact that "I have begun the study of the 'human form divine' [anatomy?], a piece of intelligence which mother most unaccountably received with a little shriek of horror. I have not however been able to prosecute the subject with much vigor as my eyes decidedly remonstrated. A succession of sties has rendered me a conspicuous object of beauty to all my friends." For the rest, Welch discussed trivial gossip. The five letters written him by Learned during this period are concerned almost entirely with Yale politics and personalities, giving no indication that in the letters to which they are replies Welch dealt with his introduction to medicine.

It is easy to understand why the young man, who since his childhood had watched his father practise without ever wanting to do the same, found his apprenticeship unpleasant. If only he could return to New Haven, to the world where people lived regular lives, read the classics, and discussed intellectual things! Eventually he decided that, since he knew almost no science, it would be wise to take a course in chemistry at the scientific branch of Yale, the Sheffield School. On January 15, 1872, Learned wrote, obviously in reply to a letter from Welch: "I need hardly say how pleased I was to hear of your idea of coming down here to study. I hope that instead of considering it a wild idea you will proceed to act on it, the sooner the better." But he added that Welch could not count on supporting himself by tutoring undergraduates in the classics.

William had intended for some time to comfort his soul, starved for all cultural activities, by going to Hartford for the performance of an opera; now he extended his trip to New Haven in search of pupils, but he wrote his sister on February 18: "I failed to obtain the object of my search and when I returned home, had about given up the whole affair. Father however thought that a course in chemistry was so desirable that I had better go to New Haven and enter the laboratory, taking the chances of securing any private pupils, the prospect for which being pretty fair, as I had previously ascertained. So here I am in my old haunts. . . .

"I have a sitting room and a bed room adjoining on College St., a few doors from the Scientific School where I am prosecuting my studies. My work consists entirely in laboratory practice under the direction of Prof. [Oscar D.] Allen without recitations. Some previous knowledge of the theory and principles of chemistry is of course required. . . . Each student has a desk assigned him and works mostly by himself, performing the experiments as given in the text book and progressing as slowly or as fast as he is able. . . . Certainly the facilities are excellent, I presume as good as can be found in the country, certainly better than in any Medical School where chemistry as far as I can learn is very much slighted.

"New Haven is not much changed still it seems quite different from college life. To be sure I am not lonely as there are a few friends and class mates here, but I have not that free and easy feeling that belongs to college life. Things look a little more serious and it hardly seems as if I could enjoy the same frolics I delighted in when in college."

On March 30 Welch reported to his sister that he had secured a pupil to prepare for the entrance examinations, who paid him a dollar and a half an hour. "I am much pleased with the study of chemistry and the Professor told me the other day that I was progressing satisfactorily. He gives me all sorts of substances to analyze. I have had bone black and the residue left from electroplating with nickel to analyze, though of course I did not know that these were the substances until after I had completed the analysis as the Professor decidedly objects to furnishing any hints as to the nature of the substance. I am now at work on some alloy in which I have found copper for one thing."

In addition to his work with Allen, Welch sat in on a course given at the Yale Medical School by George Frederick Barker, under whom he mastered, in the original German, Kekulé's epoch-making hypothesis relating to the carbon atoms, the hypothesis which was later to influence Ehrlich in formulating and developing the side-chain theory of immunity.[3]

Welch had gone to the Sheffield School rather than back to the academic department because only there could he find laboratory instruction. When in 1847 the Yale authorities, who were not sympathetic to science, could no longer ignore the trend of the times, they had appointed, not as part of the college but in the graduate school, professors of civil engineering and agricultural chemistry. Although this part of the university was looked down upon as utilitarian rather than intellectual, the scientific faculty grew, was organized into the Sheffield School, and in 1870 began giving a complete course independently of the academic department. The first important executive of this school was Daniel Coit Gilman, who as president of Johns Hopkins University was to play a major part in Welch's career, and one of the first two graduates was T. Mitchell Prudden, who was to be with Welch among the first American prophets of scientific medicine. However, the youthful student, as he pursued his inconspicuous course, met neither of these men.

That Welch felt the need to learn chemistry before beginning the study of medicine is revealing, for he was already highly educated by contemporary standards, which permitted any boy who could read and write to enter medical school. Clearly Welch had an intuition of the role which science was to play in the healing art.

II

In the fall of 1872 Welch left New Haven for the College of Physicians and Surgeons in New York; even Yale College admitted that the Yale Medical School was not first-class. Many years later, when Welch was asked to speak on "The Relation of Yale to Medicine," he wrote that it "is about the most barren theme which I ever tackled. The relation is so slight that I shall have to beat around the bush and talk on side issues. If they had only asked me to talk on the Relation of Yale to Calvinism or Football there would have been something to say."

After his first few weeks in the College of Physicians and Surgeons, Welch confided to Emma: "I am enjoying my studies very much, at least better than I had anticipated. I do not take the entire course. I do not aspire to the intellectual calibre of those who are able to imbibe seven lectures a day. I limit myself to four tickets, those of Anatomy, Physiology, Materia Medica and Theory and Practice. Thus I have on some days four, more commonly three lectures a day." Indeed, Welch was so eager for a thorough medical education that despite his unusually good preparation and his undoubted ability, he spent three years attending courses instead of the required two.

"I believe," he continued to his sister, "I told you what a nice boarding place we have. One fatherly old man at the table, beside whom I sit, is fond of patting me on the shoulder, frequently conducts his conversation with me in Latin, though his horror at my pronunciation is unbounded."

The young man spent what time he could spare from his studies in the opera houses, the concert halls, the art galleries, and the theatres of the city. Music became his principal relaxation; hardly a letter to his sister fails to give sage comments on some performance. He demanded that the young ladies with whom he associated be interested in æsthetic matters. "We certainly have one source of enjoyment in common," he wrote of a Miss Walcott, "viz.: visiting picture galleries and picture stores. Yesterday I was in at Schaus's and had a great treat in seeing the portfolio of their artist's proofs. The great charm of living in New York is really the pleasant way in which you can always spend a leisure hour in looking at pictures, or through Tiffany or Syphers, etc. Have you ever been through Syphers? They have a large stock of antique, richly carved furniture which it is very interesting to see."

In many of his letters he mentioned going to church. He expressed dislike of bombastic sermons—"All the thought was in his text, the rest was mainly declamatory"—but, as the months passed, he increasingly failed to mention the sermons, concentrating his attention on the music: "Today is Easter. I began the day by going to service at seven o'clock. The singing was magnificent, consisting in large measure of selections from the 'Messiah' as you will see by the scheme which I will enclose. The chief soprano alone has a salary of three thousand dollars."

Welch's letters to his father reveal a continual shortage of funds. "My board bill has not been paid for over five weeks. . . . I am now entirely out of money"; this is a perpetual complaint. Twice he writes that he is afraid he will lose a tooth unless costly repairs are immediately made; and his clothes are an unending problem. "My over-coat is not fit to wear any longer; I have worn it now for three winters, it is threadbare and much soiled, so that I am ashamed to appear in it." However, when he bought clothes he bought only the best. Concerning one suit that cost $54, he explained to William Wickham: "If I wear the suit, as I expect to, a year it will after all be more economical than two suits cheaper but of inferior quality." Perhaps the most significant cry that poverty elicited from him is that of November

1875: "My subscription for the Nation expired last month, and I feel quite in the woods without my weekly pabulum. I should like to renew it."

It is improbable that Welch's lack of funds reflected poverty in Norfolk so much as the absent-mindedness of his father; William Wickham, since he never collected bills, was not likely to be impressed by the importance of paying them promptly.[4]

But the young man who had been reluctant to study medicine was soon very happy; his letters reflect unflagging high spirits. "Yesterday," he wrote his sister, "I had a delightful excursion with a classmate up to West Point. We took the boat about nine in the morning and reached New York again in the evening. Nothing could be more charming than the trip up the Hudson, always with the proviso that you have a guide book to tell you what views to admire. We admired the country around West Point and regarded with distant awe the young cadets. As our attempts to pass ourselves off as graduates of the Academy, notwithstanding our martial bearing, were unaccountably failures I cannot give you much idea of the inside workings of the institution.

"The statue of Gen. Sedgwick is very fine and an ornament to the grounds. An old soldier showed with pride the saddle of the General in the museum. About a week ago I sent up to mother a plaster bust taken from the statue, which the Misses Sedgwick have had. The bust and pedestal I think will look very well in the bay window of the parlor. . . .

"I have attended within a few weeks the weddings and receptions of two classmates in Brooklyn. . . . I have recently received the cards of another classmate to be married next week. What a holocaust!

"The only amusement in which I now indulge is the summer night concerts of Thomas orchestra at the Central Park Gardens. They occur every night, the admission fee is quite small and certainly they are a musical feast."

An amazing metamorphosis had taken place in Welch's interests and tastes. Toward the end of his first year in medical school what had been his fondest dream not twelve months before was suddenly realized: he was offered an appointment in Greek at Yale. He turned it down, explaining to his father: "I believe that we have talked it over and agree on the subject. I have chosen my profession, am becoming more and more interested in it, and do not feel at all inclined to relinquish it for any thing else, still less for an interruption which would probably only prove temporary and lead to nothing further in that direction. The duties of a tutor are somewhat arduous so that I should practically have to give up the study of medicine, the salary is not strikingly inviting. I should like to consult you but I doubt not you will consent to my declining the offer considering all the circumstances of the case. The letter is framed in flattering terms but I do not think that means very much."

III

In his later years Welch ascribed the sudden flowering of his interest in medicine not so much to the studies he pursued as to the personality of his teachers. "One can decry the system in those days," he said, ". . . but the results were better than the system. The College of Physicians and Surgeons stood then, as it has always stood, in the front rank of American medical schools. Our teachers were men of fine character, devoted to the duties of their chairs, they inspired us with enthusiasm, interest in our studies and hard work, and they imparted to us sound traditions of our profession; nor did they send us forth so utterly ignorant and unfitted for professional work as those born of the present, greatly improved methods of training and opportunities for practical study are sometimes wont to suppose."

Since, as he tells us, "there were no requirements for admission," Welch was much better trained than most of his fellow-pupils; he found the work very easy. But he judged his achievements according to his own reckoning. During his first year he wrote that Professor Crosby had "praised my recitations more than I deserved. The average medical student is certainly not a very lofty standard of comparison." And after taking the final examination, which determined whether a man might practise on his fellow-creatures, Welch confided to Emma: "To tell the truth it was the easiest examination I ever entered since leaving boarding school."

The students supplemented their lectures by practical experience gained as apprentice to a practising physician; of the required three years of study only two had to be spent in medical school, and the terms each year lasted only six and a half months. The work was not graded, many pupils bought tickets for the entire course every year, and all attended the lectures in whatever order appealed to them. There was only one examination, the final one, which Welch found so extremely easy. Indeed, the professors did not dare fail many of their pupils. Connected only formally with Columbia University and entirely without endowment, the school was supported by tuition fees; after the expenses had been paid, the professors divided among themselves what was left over. At best not well remunerated for their trouble, they feared to raise their standards lest the young men should go elsewhere; every city and many hamlets boasted little groups of doctors who gave instruction, sometimes with a titular university connexion, often with none at all.

Welch's teachers, like the teachers in other medical schools, were the outstanding practitioners in the community, and their object was to pass on to the young the rules and traditions of their art so that their pupils might in turn become successful practitioners. For this purpose they relied on the didactic lecture. Standing confidently on the platform, the professor told exactly what to do for each disease, and his pupils were expected merely to memorize this wisdom. "It was cramming practically every day," Welch remembered.

There was no laboratory instruction of any sort; the young were not encouraged to work things out for themselves. In 1871, Dr. Henry J. Bigelow, the leading spirit of the Harvard Medical School, laid down the following dictum: "In an age of science, like the present, there is more danger that the average medical student will be drawn from what is practical, useful, and even essential, by the well-meant enthusiasm of the votaries of less applicable sciences, than that he will suffer from the want of knowledge of these. . . . The excellence of the practitioner depends far more upon good judgment than upon great learning. . . . We justly honor the patient and learned worker in the remote and exact sciences, but should not for that reason encourage the medical student to while away his time in the labyrinths of Chemistry and Physiology, when he ought to be learning the difference between hernia and hydrocele."

Sometimes, however, the professors whose words were to be memorized possessed excellent scientific training; almost all had rounded out their inferior American medical education with periods in Europe under masters. Alonzo Clark, the professor of practice, had followed Bright and Louis in their hospital rounds. Welch remembered: "He was the one that brought that new French medicine to this country in his early days, and was greatly interested in pathological anatomy." Since Clark's lectures were "supposed to be the embodiment of all the wisdom of the practice of medicine," a set of notes on what he had said was considered the key to professional success; Welch was offered as much as a hundred dollars for the excellent set he had kept.

The lecturers were often great orators, and undoubtedly Welch received much inspiration from them. He remembered till the end of his life as "almost worthy of Huxley" a lecture by Edward Curtis, the professor of materia medica and therapeutics, on the protoplasm theory. "He regards as the physical basis of life in all its manifestations, animal or vegetable, the protoplasm or cell," Welch wrote his father. "The theory was beautifully and eloquently explained." [5]

The lectures were supplemented by clinics, some held in the medical school building, some in Bellevue Hospital. Although many of the students did not bother to attend them, Welch preferred clinics to even the most eloquent pedagogical orations. "After all," he wrote, "the principal thing is the experience in the observation of disease."

His favourite clinic was Dr. Edward C. Seguin's on nervous diseases which he followed during his second year. "I wanted a microscope more than anything else," he remembered, "and Seguin offered a microscope for the best report on his clinical lectures on nervous diseases. Only a handful attended those lectures, because they came in the middle of Saturday afternoon. I regarded them as very remarkable. They were modelled after Charcot. No clinics I have ever attended worked so systematically: we saw hemiplegias, the progressive muscular atrophies, and so forth. They [the patients] would sit in a row, and there was nothing more interesting in those days. . . . We were in the midst of Charcot's best work, and it interested me enormously, and I got that microscope by reporting those lectures. . . . The lenses were extremely good, and it meant a great deal to me because I think it started me along the lines of pathology." Welch fell so much under the influence of Seguin that he decided to specialize in nervous diseases.[6]

The Varick microscope fitted with superior French triplex lenses which Welch had won was more an inspiration than a useful instrument, for, as he admitted to his father, "I can only admire without understanding how to use its apparently complicated mechanism." Although several of his professors were expert microscopists, it never occurred to them to pass their knowledge on to the undergraduates, who should be busy memorizing the symptoms and cures of disease.

Welch stood out in his class, not only 'as a student but as a leader. Toward the end of his first year he wrote William Wickham: "Another fellow has consented to respond to the toast, to my relief. I think I might have accepted it as the committee rather urged it but it seemed very inappropriate that I should. It is to speak for the doctors of the class and there are three or four full fledged M.D.'s in the class while I am only just beginning and I think it would have been in very poor taste if I had accepted."

His old friends helped Welch along whenever they could. Fred Dennis, who was attending the Bellevue Medical College, and another Bones man, John B. Isham, had been assistants to the resident physician of the municipal hospitals; in June 1873 Isham wrote Welch offering to recommend him and some friend of his to succeed them. "We want to keep this fat gift in the Bones family if it is possible to do so," Isham explained. Although he would have received his board, lodging, and washing free, and have gained much practical experience, Welch turned the offer down, perhaps because it would have meant postponing his work in medical school. He was rewarded for this faithfulness to his studies by an appointment, at the beginning of his second year, as a prosector to the professors of anatomy, Thomas T. Sabine and Henry B. Sands; the prosectors prepared the specimens about which the professors lectured.

The story is told that at first Welch could not bear the dissecting room and that the sight of a dead body was long repulsive to him; such weakness, however, bothered him no longer. "We dissected night and day . . ." he remembered. "It seems to me that never were there such dissections! You should have seen our dissections of the radial plexus and the muscles of the back, and so on. It was a work of art, and we had fresh beef blood brought in to smear over the muscles. Then when the lecture came at eleven o'clock Sands would say nice things, and we walked in with the Professor! We sat in front, and the cloth was lifted, and here was this display. I never felt so proud in my life. Now, that was really an education. We were learning Anatomy in the old-fashioned English way. It was the best thing one had for a laboratory subject at that time. That took me away from a good many of the lectures."

Welch's fellow-prosector, E. M. Hegewisch, had studied for five years in Mexico and been in the French army; and his immediate superior, Dr. Charles McBurney, the assistant demonstrator, had just returned from Vienna. "I used to like to talk to McBurney and hear him tell what his experiences in Vienna were, the courses he had taken, his aspirations, and so on. It was a perfectly delightful association that meant a great deal for a young man." Concerning the professor of anatomy, Dr. Sabine, he wrote his father: "We have no more enthusiastic professor and he is very familiar with his subject. His sole aim seems to be to teach and each year he gives more satisfaction."

It was not chance that Welch found his most stimulating contacts in the dissecting room. Anatomy alone of all the subjects he studied offered opportunities for a truly scientific approach.

There was no need, and indeed no place, for guesswork or theorizing; you applied an effective technique directly to the object under scrutiny, achieving results as exact as your ability could make them, results that could be repeated both by yourself and by other investigators. How far superior this was to medical practice, where you dealt with a situation so complex that all its aspects could not be grasped, and where, even when a cure had been effected, you were not sure how it had come about. Welch became passionately interested in pathological anatomy, the study of the physical structure of diseased portions of the body.

On Sabine's advice, he competed during his final year for the thesis prize—"that was *the* prize in those days"—by attempting a résumé of all that had been written about goitre in English, French, and German. "At that time there was little known about it," he remembered. "Extirpation of a goitre was regarded by most as butchery. There was a great deal of interest in the anatomy, physiology, histology, and other lines of treatment, like the ligation of arteries, parenchymatous injection, and the use of iodine."

Welch worked in the library of the New York Hospital, then the second largest medical library in the country, surpassed only by the Surgeon General's in Washington. "I had a key to the library and could go there night and day, whether it was open or closed. That was an extraordinary privilege, and I would stay after twelve o'clock at night. . . . When we consider what the opportunities were, listening to didactic lectures and attending not very stimulating clinics, that library was an education in itself, because you cannot read up on a subject like that without getting interested in all kinds of sidelines, and the English and French journals were very interesting at the time. It was comparatively easy for me to look up a subject after that. I regard that experience as a very important part of my education."

Welch's essay on goitre won the thesis prize and attracted much attention. Since it was the most complete résumé of the literature in English, he was urged to publish it, and Dennis's patron, Dr. James R. Wood, offered to contribute a hundred dollars toward the printing expenses. This was doubly remarkable as Wood was a professor at the Bellevue Hospital Medical College, a most unfriendly rival of the College of Physicians and Surgeons. In his eagerness for knowledge, however, Welch had leaped the barriers between the two schools by attending a summer session at Bellevue College. Indeed, he studied at all three New York schools, having taken Alfred L. Loomis's course in physical diagnosis at the University Medical College.

Welch depreciated his achievement to his sister. "I thank you for your hearty congratulations over my success, but you magnify it out of all proportion. I do not know what more you could have said if I had written Romeo and Juliet or Newton's Principia. Would it not be a fine thing if one's destiny could be decided by mothers and sisters or even by their expectations! It was certainly a great satisfaction to have my patience and industry rewarded, for I have spent a good deal of labor over my thesis during the winter, doing most of my work in the evening at the New York Hospital Library. As I was at the hospital during the day, the two hours work in the evening seemed to amount to very little, but I became very much interested in the subject and persevered."

Welch had not allowed his sister's marriage to impair their intimacy; instead he took his brother-in-law into the family circle. When Stuart came to New York, they enjoyed going to theatres and art sales together. On the birth of his niece, Welch wrote Emma: "I suppose that every uncle and aunt has an inalienable right to suggest names for the little one, so that I shall exercise my privilege. Stuart says you think of Mabel. I don't like it. It has no character and suggests a pretty little girl dressed up like a doll; but this may be an unreasoning prejudice. I am going to add my quota to the list and offer the following:—Mary, Alice, Helen, Elizabeth (Bessie), Agnes, Margaret, Katherine, Grace, Edith, Emily. There is a list from which to select the name of a queen. If I may be so bold, I will also offer another unsolicited suggestion. Do not give the child a middle name. It is unnecessary for a girl and when she is married she will not know what to do with it. But parents are always unmoved by these officious councillors, so that I will refrain from further suggestions." They named her Elisabeth.

In February 1875 Welch was graduated from the College of Physicians and Surgeons, having made a brilliant record. He was somewhat hurt that his father and the stepmother of whom he had become very fond failed to get to the exercises, but it must have been a great pleasure to be a doctor at last.

<h1 style="text-align:center">I V</h1>

At the end of his second year in medical school Welch had entered Dr. Wood's special cram quiz in surgery which prepared applicants for the examinations through which interneships were awarded, but when he heard the rules had been changed so that all internes had to be graduate doctors, he dropped the quiz and spent the summer in Norfolk, having "a good time," as he said. What was his horror when, late in September, a telegram notified him that the rules had been changed back again and that he should present himself for examination. And he had not yet taken any surgery! But the examiner was to be Dr. Wood, so "I thought I would get through because he had always been good to me. However, he was taken ill of summer complaint, and Frank Hamilton was the examiner. I had an extraordinary piece of luck; he asked me about goitre . . . and let me talk on and on." Welch was appointed to Bellevue Hospital six months before his graduation; he tried to make up his deficiency in surgery by beginning on the surgical side. As an old man he said with a chuckle: "I think they decided never to let that happen again."

Welch was delighted to be in a position to see things for himself. "I think I am learning more than I could from attending the lectures which of course I am compelled to neglect as I have to be at the hospital all day." As he explained in another letter, "Bellevue in the number of its patients has an advantage; moreover we have the best visiting physicians and surgeons in the city, we have the advantage of daily clinics and pathological examinations in the Dead House."

At first Welch had to divide his time between the hospital, the medical school, and the preparation of his thesis; not until after his graduation did he live in the hospital. On July 22, 1875, he wrote his father: "I have just finished my two weeks as interne . . . and very busy two weeks they have been. I have had entire charge of our division and the service has been unusually active. The first week I had three poisoning cases, two by arsenic and one by corrosive sublimate. Of these I lost only one case. I have also done my first serious surgical operation, which was laryngotomy [opening the trachea] in a case of bronchocele [a form of goitre which presses on the windpipe]. The operation itself was successful, as I cut down carefully and did not get a single drop of blood into the trachea, but the autopsy proved that no operation could have given relief as both kidneys were in a condition of suppuration. I have been called up a good deal during the night, last week every night but one; so that I feel as if I knew something about the realities of medical life."

To his sister he dwelt on more amusing aspects of hospital life. "I continue to minister to the sick at the hospital daily, breaking, Mr. Olcott says, the commandment 'Thou shalt not kill.' . . . I must tell you of a good story. You remember the old woman in the last ward who had an ovarian tumor. The other morning as the doctors went into the ward, we noticed that she looked smiling and unusually happy. A brown paper bundle lay upon the small table by her bed. We asked her what made her so happy. She said that she had just received a present from her brother-in-law, and wanted us to look at it. We opened the package, and what do you think the gift was? It was her shroud. She said it cost ten dollars and wanted to know how we liked it. Of course we thought it would be very becoming, but told her that she would not have any occasion to use it for a long time we hoped. It seemed to have the most exhilarating influence upon her. She stood well an operation. . . . The tumor has become cancerous and it is wonderful how she holds out. I think I should if my brother-in-law sent me my shroud."

Many years later, Welch wrote: "When I came to Bellevue as an interne I first got to know Abraham Jacobi and he was the one who first directed my attention especially to the great position of German medical science in the world. He used to invite me occasionally to come to his own house, where we would talk over the cases that had interested us in the hospital. . . . It was an inspiration to me."

Jacobi himself remembered that in those days Welch was "never obtrusive, but he would leak [knowledge]. Because he had knowledge, he was modest and gentle . . . gentle to the sick poor and the poor sick. I then felt certain that he would be a great physician or practitioner, whose make-up always requires, though it does not always furnish, head and heart."

Through another one of his hospital superiors, Welch came in further contact with French medicine, which had already been praised to him by Seguin. Francis Delafield, whose elective course in pathological anatomy Welch had taken in medical school, was a disciple of the great pathologist Pierre-Charles-Alexandre Louis. Like his master, who felt that autopsies were the source of most medical knowledge, Delafield studied cadavers by the hundreds and kept elaborate statistical records of what he found. "That is a good paper," he would say. "It is a dead house paper." He made important observations on pneumonia, tuberculosis, tumours, and malaria.

Since it was concrete and practical, Delafield's approach naturally appealed to Welch; it is more remarkable that Welch appealed to Delafield, who was usually distant to his pupils. The young man was allowed to enter the results of his own autopsies in the professor's record books from which his statistical studies were made. In June Welch reported to his father: "Yesterday Dr. Delafield asked me if I would not take his place as curator [of the Wood museum of pathological specimens] and pathologist at the Hospital, for the summer. I accepted of course very gladly, but I fear I shall not be able to do justice to the work. It involves my taking charge of the post mortem examinations two days in the week and recording in a book the pathological appearances. I understand pretty well the lesions visible to the naked eye, but I know nothing about the microscopical appearances. I am sorry I have not yet been able to study with the microscope, but I hope to find opportunity for it some time. It is very important and requires considerable training. It is the position which Dr. Delafield and Dr. Janeway have held as curators at the Bellevue Dead House that has given them their reputations as pathologists, and it is as such that they take rank among the first in the country."

Delafield himself was expert with the microscope, and much of his best work was the result of studying diseased organs through that instrument. For hours each day he sat in his laboratory smoking a long-stemmed meerschaum pipe, cutting sections with the enormous microtome he had built himself, and then slipping the slides under the high-power lenses. Welch was allowed to wander around the laboratory while Delafield worked; he would see the professor's face suddenly fix with interest as he manœuvred the slide; he would see him reach out for his pencil and draw some complicated form. But it never occurred to Delafield to give Welch any instruction in the microscope. Often at night in his room Welch must have stared at the precious instrument he had won for reporting Seguin's lectures; hidden in its mechanism lay the answers to a thousand problems, but Welch was helpless to find them.

He could, however, make his thesis, which he still hoped to publish, as nearly perfect as possible.* During the Christmas vacation of 1875, he journeyed to the Surgeon General's Library in Washington to look up some references he could not find in New York. "I do not know that anything will ever come of my essay on goitre," he wrote his father, "I had not thought anything about it lately. But so long as I have spent so much time in looking up the subject I thought I would not lose so good an opportunity to fill in some gaps which had unavoidably been left and to make some important additions."

Welch stopped off in Baltimore on a mission that was strangely prophetic of his future career; he called on President Gilman of the newly founded Johns Hopkins University. The young man who had never wanted to practise medicine, who had longed

---

* The thesis was never published in complete form, although some use of it was made in St. John, S. B., "Bronchocele," *New York Med. J.*, 1875, *21*, 465.

to remain for ever in the academic halls of Yale, had been fired in the dissecting and autopsy rooms with the desire to become a professor of pathological anatomy, to study and examine for the rest of his life without having to make his living as a practitioner. Although that seemed impossible, since in the United States you could become a professor only by being a successful practitioner first, there was one chance, one wild, almost hopeless chance.

The Johns Hopkins University, for which ample funds had been provided but which was not yet completely organized, had been dedicated to a new idea in American education. It was not to be primarily a training school for undergraduates but a real centre of learning; scholars capable of doing original research were to teach graduate students the arts of scholarship. How excited Welch must have been when he heard that this revolutionary idea was to be carried into the field of medicine; a medical school was to be founded not only to train competent practitioners, but also to further science. As Welch wrote his father, "The university will have a splendid pathological laboratory and will afford great opportunities for original investigations."

And Welch's name had already been called to Gilman's attention! "Fred Dennis," the young man continued, "went over on the steamer to Europe with Gilman and became acquainted with him last summer. Fred praised me very highly to Gilman, with reference to the study of pathological anatomy, so that Fred thinks he may consider my name favorably with reference to filling up the chair of pathology, and I have heard that he has made some inquiries about me in New York; but of course it seems folly for me to aspire to attaining such a position when there are so many distinguished men in the country who have already acquired great reputations as pathologists and whom he could obtain."

Yet Welch decided to do what he could. Dennis accompanied him to Baltimore and, while Welch waited anxiously, called on Gilman to get permission for Welch to call. The permission granted, Welch hurried over to the university offices but found Gilman out. It may be that he tried to calm his nerves by a long walk through the city, for on his return to his room he found that Gilman had dropped in on him during his absence. "I therefore left Baltimore without seeing him," he wrote.

However, the Johns Hopkins remained as a golden aspiration in Welch's mind. In February 1876 he wrote to his father that he had read Gilman's inaugural address in the *Tribune,* and had been delighted to see that the medical school was intended "to be a great advance upon any system of medical instruction in this country." Dennis, Welch continued, had persuaded Dexter, his Greek professor at Yale, to write to Gilman on his behalf. "So far as New Haven influence is concerned I can bring enough of that to bear. But after all I think it will depend upon how much I shall have accomplished in a year or two in the special study in pathological anatomy, and I have a will to devote myself energetically thereto, if I could only have a little encouragement held out to me. If I remain here in the city I must live as cheaply as I can and do all I can to support myself and devote what time I can to the microscope." He recognized that he could not hope for a position at the Hopkins until he understood the microscopical side of pathological anatomy.

In any case, his chances of an appointment were slight; he continued to prepare himself for practice by studying surgery. "I did lithotomy [removing a bladder stone] in Dr. Sabine's class last night," he wrote his father on April 9. "It seemed very simple on the cadaver. When I finished, Dr. S. said that he should call on me if it became necessary to do the operation on him. This class of his is very valuable. I could profit by another course of it, but of course shall not be able to do that. I mean to obtain a subject this summer, and do some of the operations myself, perhaps joining with Andrews or some one else at the hospital."

William Wickham, who hated surgery himself, began to call on his son to do necessary operations in Norfolk; perhaps he hoped that this would gradually get the young man used to the idea of coming home and becoming his assistant. Welch, however, avoided the assignment whenever he could. On one occasion he wrote: "I think it would be in poor taste for me to do the operation, which naturally would fall to Barber [W. L. Barber, William Wickham's pupil-assistant]. If Barber will not perform it, I should like very much to let Fred Dennis do it, as I know he would like to very much. . . . I have every reason for keeping on good terms with Fred as I am at present. He has shown me many favors and has it in his power to be of assistance to me."

On March 9, 1875, Welch wrote his father that Wood and others had advised him to study for a year in Germany, since no American medical school offered a course in histology, as microscopic anatomy was called. He believed such a trip would not cost more than $650 or $700, and he was willing to borrow the difference between this sum and the $300 he had saved from teaching school. "When I returned it would be more probable that I could obtain some position in a medical college, even if I failed of the Johns Hopkins University, and my chances for the latter would certainly be increased." Furthermore, Dennis was planning to go abroad and promised that if Welch accompanied him he would use his father's influence to get Welch passage at half-price; Dennis's father, as president of the New Jersey Railroad and Transportation Company, had an important social and financial position in New York.

William Wickham's answer is lost, but we gather from his son's next letter that it was far from enthusiastic. The successful country practitioner had always regarded his own training as adequate. Having little conception of modern progress in pathological anatomy, he felt that William had already received enough education, more than most successful doctors had received, and that it was time for the young man to get down to work. William's desire to teach rather than to practise medicine must have seemed almost as foolish to his father as William's original determination to stay away from medicine altogether. The old gentleman asked William to find him someone to help with the Norfolk practice, probably more than a hint that the young man should come home and take his rightful place as the next in line of the Welch doctors.

William replied that he would not go abroad "unless you thought it best," but added: "I have said to those who have asked me that it is pretty certain that I shall go and I believe

Fred has told his father to engage passage. . . . The solid advantages to be derived from such a course of study are such as I can not well afford to lose. It may seem egotistical to say that I feel that my success in medicine must depend more upon actual acquirements and merit than upon person, and address, and good luck, which serve many so well.

"I can not be too thankful that you appreciate so fully the benefits of thorough mental discipline and culture and that I have enjoyed, and I know not without personal sacrifices, such educational advantages, to me a far more precious legacy than any fortune could be. But the broadening influence, and culture and knowledge of the world to be derived from a year abroad are not so much to be considered as the actual addition which I think I shall thereby make to my stock in trade, so to speak, so that it will yield a larger return. Even assuming that I do not obtain any position in a medical college, the prestige and knowledge which I should acquire by a year's study in Germany would decidedly increase my chances of success in a large city. The young doctors who are doing well in New York are in a large proportion those who have studied abroad. . . .

"If I had any opening in New York or any immediate prospect of being able to support myself, the matter might not seem so clear, but it will probably cost less for me to spend the year in Germany than in New York. If I remained here I should aim to devote what leisure time I could to the study of pathological anatomy as my chances of a professorship seem to lie in that direction and as I have advantages and taste for the study, but I can certainly pursue the study in Germany to greater advantage and with less expense."

In his sister and brother-in-law Welch found allies; not only were they enthusiastic, but Stuart offered to lend him the $500 that was to make the trip possible. To them he was more frank about his dislike for practice. "If I settle in New York immediately, I must hire a cheap office, and set to work to draw together by hook or by crook a patronage of some kind. Success in this to me distasteful work depends on person, on manner and especially on luck; and, if I may judge from the experience of my friends who are struggling as young doctors in this city, the principal lesson I should learn would be that 'they also serve, who only stand and wait.' Of course it is much finer to hold a chair in a medical college, and to have a salary (for I believe that those with a salary are the most fortunate now-a-days, provided only the salary is large enough) and to be sought by patients instead of seeking them. But I doubt not that the one thousand new fledged doctors this year think the same; and a large proportion probably have similar dreams and reveal their air-castles thus to their sisters. If by absorbing a little German lore I can get a little start of a few thousand rivals and thereby reduce my competitors to a few hundred more or less, it is a good point to tally."

In the end, William Wickham bowed to the inevitable. After a brief visit to Norfolk, Welch sailed the nineteenth of April 1876 on a voyage of exploration that was in its results perhaps the most important ever taken by an American doctor.

CHAPTER VI

The Great Awakening

I

"**I** HAVE not suffered in the least from sea sickness," Welch wrote, "but for all that I am not fascinated with a sea voyage." He was somewhat bothered by the discovery that, instead of getting Welch's passage at half-price as he had said, Dennis's father had made up the full sum. "I disliked to have him pay half. I am rather inclined to think that he was anxious to have me go and expected to pay half all of the time. He seemed glad to do it and it is certainly very kind of him, but if I am able I shall hope to repay him."

On his way to Strasbourg, Welch spent two days in London and several more in Holland and Belgium. The museum in Antwerp, he wrote, "is full of great paintings. . . . I supposed that these pictures, two and three hundred years old, would be so dimmed and faded by time that their enjoyment would require a rather vivid imagination. On the other hand most of them are well preserved; some of Rubens' best pictures look as if they were painted only yesterday."

Welch admired the "canals and high houses with steep gable roofs" in Rotterdam, where he visited Erasmus's house; he went to hear Gounod's *Queen of Sheba* in Brussels, an opera "finer than any I have ever heard"; but all the sights and sounds did not keep him from giving way to a terrible sense of strangeness when, having parted from Dennis, who went to Heidelberg, he arrived at Strasbourg alone. "If I had not so much to occupy me," he wrote his stepmother, "I should feel very homesick. I feel oppressed when I think of the distance which separates us. So far as my surroundings are concerned, the people, the houses, the fields, they seem strange, but after all they do not present such a wonderful change from home scenes, as I had fancied they would."

Since "I find that I can hardly say anything and can understand much less in German," Welch took lodgings with "a good German family where I can hear the language spoken at meals." Then he set out to explore the university and discovered to his amazement that it had no similarity to what he had expected. "In New York," he wrote his sister, "I was told by Dr. Seguin to go to Strassburg, because the Germans had received the university, as it were, full fledged from the French. He is a Frenchman. But there is not a trace of French influence in the University. Everything is German." Indeed, after the victory in 1870 as a result of which they annexed Strasbourg, the Germans had tried to win over the city by sending their most brilliant young men to the university, so that the medical school soon ranked next to Berlin's. This, Welch continued, "has introduced German intellectual life and attracted students from all parts. One can not help contrasting with our unsatisfactory policy of reconstruction in the South, the strong and skillful manner in which the German empire is transforming a region hostile to them for centuries into a friendly one and so acquiring one of their fairest provinces.

"I am therefore fortunate to have hit upon Strassburg," he went on, "for it was really rather a leap in the dark." He found just what he wanted: "laboratories for histology, pathology, physiological chemistry, superintended by the best teachers in Germany, viz., Waldeyer, von Recklinghausen, and Hoppe-Seyler."

Virchow's most brilliant pupil, von Recklinghausen, was, Welch wrote a friend, "perhaps the most celebrated teacher of pathology in Germany," but Welch, who did not know how normal tissues looked under the microscope, could not take his course in pathological histology; he was forced to be satisfied with a demonstration course which "is unsurpassed, but it is in gross pathology of which I have already seen a great deal in New York." He found the post-mortem examinations which the students had to make "thorough beyond anything I have ever seen," and was astonished at the amount of pathological material. However, the professor talked so fast that Welch could hardly catch a word, which must have made him nervous, since "von Recklinghausen does not seem to have much patience with stupidity. Last Monday he almost lost his temper with a stupid fellow who was blundering through an autopsy, but finally his frame of mind changed and he took a jocose view of the matter. I am glad that I was not the victim. The poor fellow fainted."

In order to prepare himself for work in pathological histology with von Recklinghausen the next year, Welch studied normal histology with Waldeyer. The course was not, as it might well have been in America, a series of lectures in which the professor laid down the law. Each student was assigned a microscope; on Mondays the professor gave "minute directions how to prepare the specimens for the week," and after that the student was supposed to come into the laboratory whenever he pleased and work on his own with little or no help from above. Used to American spoon-feeding, Welch was surprised that it was possible to plan out such a course to cover the whole subject in the time allotted, and taken aback at being left so much to his own devices. "At first I made blundering work of it," he admitted.

The interest in chemistry which had taken Welch to the Sheffield Scientific School now prompted him to study physiological chemistry with Hoppe-Seyler, who had been in charge of the chemical division in Virchow's pathological institute and who, as the young man wrote his father, "may almost be said to have founded the science." This was again a laboratory course—Welch was required to make quantitative and qualitative analyses of substances such as urine, bile, and milk—but Hoppe-Seyler, although engaged in original investigations and in writing a book, "found time to visit me (as well as the rest) at my work at least twice daily, always knew what I was working at, and always, before leaving, dropped some suggestive remark. . . . To me he is the most attractive professor whom I have met in Germany."

Aware that he might have to practise on his return to America, Welch also attended von Leyden's lectures on heart disease. However, he discovered that he had undertaken too much work, since German professors required more than Americans, and laboratory courses were more time-consuming than lectures. On June 18 he wrote: "The novelty of my new manner of living has about worn off, and I now feel quite composed and settled here. I am living very quietly, never with less excitement. I find my hands full of work, in fact I can not do justice to both of my laboratory courses, and I think that next winter I shall only take one and that with the microscope. We have nothing in America like these laboratory courses, for example in New York physiology is taught only by lectures, here there is an excellent physiological laboratory where one can do all the experiments and study the subject practically. The idea of the German system of university education is to furnish every facility for study, whether anybody makes use of it or not."

Welch not only admired the university; he became very fond of the city of Strasbourg. He loved the minster, and wrote: "There is something wonderfully grave and canny about these storks as they stand on the top of a chimney over their nests. . . . They seem to have a deeper insight into the philosophy of the unknown than even the German philosophers."

The human inhabitants of the city Welch found less agreeable. Although he considered the German students, with whom he could now converse in their own language, "fine-looking, well-dressed fellows, very polite and obliging," they were fundamentally unfriendly; he associated with other English-speaking students, "to the detriment of our German." With his compatriots he complained of the native food, insisting that all the good was boiled out of the beef, and "I have never seen anything really dainty for dessert." The only meal he considered "delicious" was one the Americans got up for themselves to celebrate the fourth of July; Welch was inspired to the point of singing a solo. "I composed an impromptu over the pleasures of Strassburg and it is unnecessary to add that the melody was marked by even greater originality."

One German social custom gave him an opportunity to tease his stepmother and sister on a subject concerning which a few years before he would never have been flippant. "Yesterday, being Sunday, I made myself notorious by going to church. I could not feel perfectly at my ease as I was the only male among a large number of females. I afterwards saw that there were perhaps half a dozen old men present but they were in a dark and retired corner of the church. I do not think I can stand being stared at so again. In the afternoon I took a walk with one of the young ladies of the household, exclusively to cultivate my German, and found that the beer gardens were a striking contrast to the churches. These gardens abound in the Vorstädte or suburban towns, and are provided with pleasant music. The men with their families sit under the trees, with their beer, enjoy the music and the fresh air. In the evening in most of these gardens there are operettas and light plays. It is certainly a different view of the Sabbath than that which prevails with us; our way of regarding the Sabbath the ordinary German can not comprehend at all."

During a vacation week in June, he walked with some fellow-students in the Vosges mountains. Along with descriptions of the scenery and the ruined castles of robber knights, he gave his step-mother an eloquent description of how the peasant girls, many of whom were very pretty, came back from church with their prayer books in their hands, but dancing in the liveliest manner.

Not till the end of his three months' stay in Strasbourg did Welch have his first really agreeable experience of the social side of German university life; he attended a testimonial dinner to von Leyden, the professor of practice, who had been called to Berlin. It was "an assembly of students and professors to drink beer, make speeches which however must not be too long, give toasts, sing songs and have a good time generally. . . . For convenience instead of paying for each glass of beer separately I did like the rest and bought tickets for so much beer on entering the hall. I was satisfied with a ticket for eight pints, but all were not so readily appeased. In justice to myself I will explain that the pints refer to the glasses which although capacious hold much less than a pint. We Americans all sat together. There were over two hundred students present. It was a good opportunity to see German student customs. The singing of the characteristic student songs was really inspiriting. They have much better songs than we. . . . Of course the most striking feature to the American students was the presence of the professors at what would be considered in New Haven a most disreputable assembly. But here were professors of divinity as venerable as Pres. Woolsey. After the formal exercises the professors came and sat among the students like one of them. Prof Waldeyer, with whom I study microscopy, came and drank my health, as if we were life long friends. I do not think that the professors lost at all in dignity or in the respect of the students by thus mingling with them. The prevailing tone of the occasion was what the Germans call *Gemüthlichkeit,* for which we have no equivalent in English, good nature and jollity come as near to it as anything, but they do not express it."

Welch would have liked to stay in Strasbourg another term, studying microscopic pathology with von Recklinghausen, but the professor accepted only more advanced students; Welch reluctantly searched for another university that would give him the work he needed. He decided on Leipzig.

II

On his way there, Welch took a three weeks' walking tour through Switzerland, northern Italy, and Bavaria, with an Irish medical student named Geoghegan.[1] They climbed the Piz Languard, a mountain of more than 10,000 feet, "without a guide, although one is recommended; but there was very little snow and ice to cross, and the ascent, although toilsome, did not seem dangerous, if one has a steady head." Welch amused himself by pretending he was a Swiss, since Americans were charged four times as much as natives. "They speak such an abominable German dialect in Switzerland that we actually succeeded in making many believe that our native tongue was some other abominable German dialect. After paying our bills it was often great delight to tell the landlord, 'Ich bin ein Amerikaner.' "

"For a person interested in art," he reported, "Munich must be an earthly paradise." He revelled there in the picture galleries, the quaint streets, and the opera. In Nürnberg he enjoyed the sensation of having stepped back many centuries.

When he arrived in Leipzig late in August 1876, he was delighted by the university, "the oldest and largest in Germany," he wrote home, "having been founded in 1409 and now numbering over 3,000 students. . . . There is one part of the city called the medical quarter." And again: "If you could visit the handsome and thoroughly equipped physiological, anatomical, pathological and chemical laboratories and see professors whose fame is already world wide, with their corps of assistants and students hard at work, you would realize how by concentration of labor and devotion to study Germany has outstripped other countries in the science of medicine. There is much less feverish energy and haste and consequent friction, far more repose here than with us in all departments of life. Men do not grow old so soon."

On enrolling in Professor Ernst Wagner's pathological institute, where he studied microscopical anatomy, Welch was pleased to find that the King of Saxony assumed all the expenses of instruction, but he was soon complaining that the professor did not pay enough attention to his pupils, since he "forms an exception to most pathological anatomists in Germany in carrying on a very large practice"; Wagner, indeed, was soon to succeed to the professorship of medicine. Welch considered him much inferior to von Recklinghausen. However, in February Welch reported that he had learned a great deal. "My work this winter in Prof. Wagner's laboratory has been of a general nature, as I thought it best to obtain first a general review of the morbid anatomy of the different tissues and organs, before working upon any special subject. My collection of microscopical sections numbers about five hundred of which over four hundred and fifty are from diseased organs, the remainder (made in Strassburg) from normal anatomy. Most of the specimens, I think, are of considerable value; a pretty good evidence of which being that Prof. Wagner has asked me to give him duplicates of a large number for his own collection. I believe that I can demonstrate from my collection under the microscope most of the pathological changes which occur. . . .

"But what is of greater importance I have acquired a knowledge of methods of preparing and mounting specimens so that I can carry on investigations hereafter wherever I have the material. As you say in your letter," he continued to his father, " 'It is a great thing to accurately interpret what is seen in

the dead body under the microscope.' The science of pathology is still very unsettled and imperfect, but nevertheless without it our knowledge of disease is mostly guess-work. Prof.
Wagner is very kind to me, as in fact are all of the professors whom I meet here. He has given me a case to work up
especially and I shall probably spend the next three or four weeks
on it. It is an extremely interesting case of Lympho-Sarcoma extending by continuity from the glands of the neck into the lung.
He thinks that a careful study and examination of the case may
throw some light upon the very obscure nature of the class of
tumors called Lympho-Sarcoma." Welch's report on the microscopical appearances of these tumours impressed Wagner, who
asked the young man to revise it for publication in one of the
leading medical journals.

In later years Welch was to say that it was not the opportunity
to study with Wagner which had brought him to Leipzig, but
rather his wish, inspired by his admiration for Seguin, to specialize in neurology as soon as he could manage it after his return
to New York; a specialist, he knew, would have more time for
pathology than a practitioner. Johann L. O. Heubner's course in
nervous diseases was the loadstone that attracted him to the Saxon
city. On his arrival, however, he discovered that Heubner was
now giving all his attention to the diseases of children and so, in
order to fill the time left over from his study of histology, Welch
entered the physiological laboratory * of Carl F. W. Ludwig.
Thus another of the major influences of his life, an influence that
may well have changed his whole career, was, as Welch explained
later, a matter of pure chance.[2]

Ludwig, at their first meeting, proved to be "a rather elderly,
formal but very kindly gentleman who took me into his private
room, and asked me what I had studied. When I left him he said,
'If I could only talk English as you can German.' . . . He said
that if I was particularly interested in microscopical work, he
could direct my physiological work in that direction."

Writing his sister a month later, Welch confided that Ludwig

---

* Physiology is the science of the normal functions of living things, as compared with anatomy, which is the science of their structure.

"is my ideal of a scientific man, accepting nothing upon authority, but putting every scientific theory to the severest test. His laboratory is a model of its kind. . . . Only those can work with him who are able to undertake original investigations, he receives no students simply for practice. Consequently the number is always small, and consists almost wholly of doctors. At the end of each year those whose work has resulted in making some contribution to science publish their results in a volume. These 'Contributions from the physiological laboratory in Leipsic' have probably added more to science than any similar work of the present day, and of course the credit is to be divided between Prof. Ludwig and his students. Prof. Ludwig, of course being interested that as many discoveries as possible should be made in his laboratory, gives to each individual's work a great deal of personal advice and supervision. The subject which he has given me to investigate is one which he personally worked up about thirty years ago viz. the microscopical study of the nerves and ganglion cells of the heart, and he thinks that I may be able to find out more than is yet known about the subject by employing new and improved methods. The laboratory is equipped with every appliance necessary for complicated experiments. . . .

"Prof. Ludwig spends the whole day in his laboratory and besides has very competent assistants. Here in Germany it would be considered ridiculous for a man to be at once professor of physiology and at the same time try to keep in practice. With us in America the professor is so poorly paid that he must earn his living by practice; in fact a professorship in a medical college is generally sought as an advertisement in acquiring practice, rather than as an opportunity for study and investigation."

On February 25 Welch reported: "My work with Prof. Ludwig has been very profitable, especially in giving me an insight into the apparatus and methods of modern physiology, which is by far the most exact of any of the branches of medicine, this position of exactness having been obtained more through the efforts of Prof. Ludwig than of any living man. He and the great Frenchman, Claude Bernard, are undoubtedly the two greatest living physiologists. Bernard is a more brilliant genius, but Ludwig sur-

passes him in exactness and really scientific investigation. I hope
I have learned from Prof. Ludwig's precept and practice that most
important lesson for a microscopist, as well as for every man of
science, not to be satisfied with loose thinking and half proofs,
not to speculate and theorize but to observe closely and carefully
facts.

"You inquire as to the results of my observations on the nervous apparatus of the heart. I have not made any very revolutionary discoveries, but I think that I have done about as much as I
could with the means at my disposal. I have made one observation which has never been made before, namely that the processes
of many of the ganglion cells instead of continuing as independent nerve fibres lose themselves in other nerve fibres forming a
T-shaped connection thus [diagram]. Prof. Ludwig considers this
as of importance in reference to the physiological action of these
enigmatical cells. However I do not profess to have completely un-
ravelled all of the mysteries which pertain to the heart. The chief
value of this special work with Prof. Ludwig has been in teaching
me certain important methods of handling fresh tissues, especially
as regards isolating particular elements, while my strictly pathological work has of course been for the most part upon specimens
hardened in alcohol; so that in a certain measure the studies
which I have made in the two laboratories, pathological and
physiological, supplement each other."

It was natural for Ludwig to put Welch to work on a problem
associated with the heart, since his laboratory more than any other
in Europe was engaged in investigating the structure and functions of the organs of circulation. The "new and improved methods" he urged Welch to use were those Cohnheim had worked
out some years earlier in his revealing study of the nerves of the
cornea; the most delicate nerve fibres were made visible under the
microscope by impregnating them with gold chloride. Aided by
this novel technique, Welch made an observation that was original; however, he did not publish it, and the French scientist
Louis-Antoine Ranvier, who brought out a more detailed study
somewhat later, has received credit for the discovery.

In addition to his work with Wagner and Ludwig, Welch attended Rudolf Leuckart's daily lectures on comparative anatomy; studying the relations between the physical structures of man and the lower animals, he was convinced that no sharp line divided the different orders of creation. In confessing to his father that he had embraced Darwinism, that doctrine which had been anathema to the religious teachers of his youth, he adhered to the attitude of his Yale commencement address which had argued that religion and science could be made to agree. "That there is anything irreligious about the doctrine of evolution I can not see," he wrote, but the next two sentences show that basically his point of view had changed. "Just such an uproar was made by the theologians when it was contended that the world is more than 6,000 years old and was not made in six days as described in the first chapter of Genesis, and now no one, not even the theologians believe that Moses wrote all the geology which we are permitted to learn. In the end our preconceived beliefs must change and adapt themselves, the facts of science never will change." No longer did he feel that science must be made to accord with revelation; now it was revelation that had to give way.

His next reference to the subject was less suave and good-humoured, for the theologians had attacked something that was dear to him; the Johns Hopkins had finally opened, and the inaugural address had been delivered by that pernicious Darwinist, Huxley. "I see it said in some of the papers," Welch wrote his sister on October 22, "that inasmuch as the Johns Hopkins University was inaugurated by an atheist instead of with a sermon, the institution should receive no countenance from religious people. Probably those who are so minded will agree with the wise utterances of that ripe fruit of modern scholarship, the great Dr. McClintock, President of Drew Seminary, who says that after much study and experience he has come to the conclusion that only ministers of the gospel should be college professors. I am sorry for those whose faith in God can only stand or fall with the truth or falsity of Darwinism, for it seems to me no longer doubtful but that the theory of evolution will prevail. Those who are best able to judge it, men of science, accept it almost uniformly at the present time. The older men who oppose it, like Agassiz, are passing away, and there are no young men appearing to succeed them in combatting the law of evolution."

A few months later we find Welch teasing his sister by reporting that "there has been recently a series of articles in the leading daily newspapers here, entitled Church-life in America and giving an account in the main true of our churches, Sunday-schools, temperance societies, prayer meetings, etc., institutions which produced such an appalling effect upon the writer's mind that he describes them as one would the diseased religious manifestations of the Chinese."

The completeness of Welch's about-face since the days of his Yale address is shown by a letter in which he denies the doctrine of free will for which he had formerly argued with such passion. "As no human power can change the inevitable succession of events in nature," he wrote his stepmother, "so we are made to be as we are by education, circumstances which surround us, and the evolution of causes over which we have no control."

III

When Welch had moved from Strasbourg to Leipzig he had moved from a recently conquered province to the centre of Germany. On September 16 he wrote: "I observe here more than in Strassburg that self conceit and contempt for the rest of the world which has sprung up in Germany since its victory over France and Austria. I am glad that we are not a military nation and greedy for our neighbors' possessions. I believe that the war of '70 and '71 has greatly benefited France and done no little injury to Germany, and many of the most enlightened Germans do not hesitate to say so themselves."

As the months passed, he became increasingly homesick. "If I were not absorbed in my work," he wrote in January, "I should find my life here in many respects very meagre. I do not have any really very congenial society. . . . The city of Leipsic itself is very uninteresting, its redeeming feature being the good and cheap operas."

The continual criticisms he heard of America irritated Welch.

Professor Wagner, he complained, "said to us when he came into the laboratory that America would have a king yet. Not a few over here believe that our form of government is doomed. On the other hand I think a European form of government would fall under our load of corruption, but it is the strength of our republic that it will come out purified, at least I hope so. . . . A German has recently written a book about the United States in which he has collected with great industry all the facts which bear against us and presents to his countrymen a most deplorable but one-sided view of the effects of a republican government." A planned campaign of vilification against the United States, he explained later, was being conducted by the authorities to discourage Germans from emigrating.

Welch often inveighed against the German undergraduates. "Many of the students seem to be faithful and conscientious workers, but I expect that many, too, lead reckless lives, especially the members of the societies or so-called corps, the almost sole objects of which seem to be to foster beer-drinking and duelling. A corps student usually wears a ridiculous little cap which just covers the top of his head, and a ribbon across his breast; one usually sees several members of the same corps together. . . . Upon the whole, I do not think that I am pleased with the average German student. He is not rude, but his politeness often seems to be formal and on the surface, without an innate regard for others' feelings. There is a peculiar set of expressions and adjectives which the students affect. Everything is 'kolossal' (with a wonderful roll to it) or 'riesig.' His salutation is always 'Mahlzeit.' You never enter a room of students or leave it, unless you scream out 'Mahlzeit' to them. If a thing is indifferent to him, he says 'Es ist mir ganz wurst,' or 'ganz pomade,' etc. In many of the universities the native students do not harmonize well with the English and American students. On the other hand as a rule the professors are rather partial to Americans and English, who, I think, often do the best work."

Alone among the Germans he met Welch liked the advanced scientific students and the professors. Ludwig gave "a very elegant dinner" for those who had been working in his laboratory.

Hugo Kronecker, the assistant professor of physiology, secured Welch's admission to the physiological society, which met once a week to listen to papers, "after the discussion of which the converse becomes more lively although not less instructive in an adjoining beer saloon." At the end of the term, "the society gave a dinner in honor of four of us who leave here at the close of this semester. We, the departing members, were seated in chairs decorated with flowers and were made the subjects of toasts and presents. Among other things I was presented with a large wooden model of a ganglion cell of the heart, which was of course intended to be humorous. I was also given a very pretty beer mug (decorated in the blue which is so much admired now a days) and a photograph of the physiological institute. Three professors were present but were as jolly as any one towards the small hours of the night. A humorous poem was read describing the events at the institute during the winter. The Germans understand how to mingle a little formality and a great deal of joviality on such occasions so as to make it thoroughly enjoyable."

However, even such contacts were not intimate; Welch was glad to visit Dennis, who was studying surgery in near-by Berlin. He went to the opera—"Lohengrin was beyond criticism"—and on his way back pored over the art galleries in Dresden, deciding that Holbein "represents the pinacle of German art, as Raphael does of Italian," and that the Sistine Madonna was the "most sublime and beautiful of paintings." Leipzig seemed even duller on his return.

Always eager to help his friend, Dennis so praised Welch's graduation thesis on goitre to his professor of surgery, Bernhard von Lagenbeck, that the professor asked for a copy to have translated and published in his journal, *Archiv für klinische Chirurgie*. Although Welch considered this "the leading surgical journal in the world," he refused the compliment, since he felt it would be necessary to bring the thesis up to date, "and I can not spare the time for that purpose over here." However, he was grateful to Dennis; "I think," Welch wrote, "that he is a very good friend of mine and will do what he can for me."

Despite his dislike for many aspects of German life, Welch had nothing but enthusiasm for German medical education. "I feel," he wrote his stepmother, "as if I were only just initiated into the great science of medicine. My previous experiences compared with the present are like the difference between reading of a fair country and seeing it with one's own eyes. To live in the atmosphere of these scientific workshops or laboratories, to come into contact with the men who have helped to form and are forming the science of to-day, to have the opportunity of doing a little original investigation myself are all advantages, which, if they do not prove fruitful in my future life, will always be to me a source of pleasure and profit."

In his letters Welch frequently compared the German medical schools with those he had known in America, always to the latter's disadvantage. "I think that the mainspring of German thoroughness lies in their preliminary education. No man can study medicine or any profession who has not gone through a course of study at least equal to a college course at Yale and Harvard." And again: "It seems to me almost our greatest failing in America that we do not appreciate the importance of training. . . . Here in Germany if a man makes himself master of any field of study he knows that he will be recognized, whereas with us it is ten to one if the upstart who cures everything by electricity, or by water, or by sugar pills does not have a larger following than he who has spent years in learning the laws of health and disease."

Welch pointed out that German universities were not dependent for income on the students, but supported by the government; "thus, the great defect of our medical schools is absent; the university does not lower its standard in order to attract students." Adequate financial support made it possible to pay professors salaries large enough to enable them to give up practice and devote their whole time to teaching and scientific work. "The laboratories are richly endowed by the government and are intended to give every encouragement to research. If we only had such laboratories in America I am sure that we should be as productive in scientific discoveries as the Germans, for with such opportunities there would be no lack of patient, conscientious workers. Patience and thoroughness are more the characteristics of German investigators than any peculiar brilliancy."

"I hope," Welch wrote his sister, "that the Johns Hopkins will turn out something better than a second Cornell and that it will be able to introduce German methods of teaching and study, for I believe there are a great many young men in America who are eager for such opportunities of practical study and investigation, especially in physical science, which are at present found only in foreign universities."

Welch's interest in the Hopkins had been greatly stimulated by a chance meeting. One afternoon as he was working quietly in Wagner's laboratory, the professor came in with an American of stiff, military bearing; he introduced John Shaw Billings, librarian of the Surgeon General's Library, "who," Welch wrote his stepmother, "has been appointed to organize the hospital and medical department of the Johns Hopkins University and who is spending a short time in Germany for the purpose of studying the laboratories and methods." Welch accompanied him on a tour through the medical buildings, and met him that night to drink beer at Auerbach's Keller. In the room where Faust was reputed to have met the devil, under sixteenth-century murals depicting this classic rendezvous, the two men, sitting unnoticed by the revellers around them, had an interview that was also to become classic, but in another world across the sea. No siren tale of power that the devil whispered into Faust's ear could have been sweeter than the tale Billings told; he said that the medical department of the Hopkins would not be organized for four years, which gave Welch time to prove himself. "There are to be laboratories like the German," Welch repeated to his stepmother, "and the examinations for admission are to be so severe as to exclude all except those who can appreciate and profit by the instruction given. The classes will therefore necessarily always be small, and it is hoped to attract especially graduates of other colleges, who now go to foreign countries. He said that many of the professorships would have to be filled by young men, who if necessary would be sent to Germany, as there were, for instance, no men in New York whom he would consider competent for the chair of physiology. Of course such young men would at first be taken on trial and not made full professors."

As the steins of beer followed one another to their table, Billings drew Welch out not only about his studies in Germany, although he inquired about these minutely, but also about his attitude toward science and life and many other things. Then he told Welch that he was directing his studies wisely and urged him to spend at least another year in Germany. "He took my name and address and said that he should have to look to such men as we, who were pursuing our studies over here." Although Welch did not ride out of Auerbach's Keller on a giant beer keg as Faust had done, and although it was a stiff military gentleman, not Mephistopheles, who left at his side, Faust could hardly have been more exhilarated than the young man whose dream might be coming true.

Writing to his stepmother in the cold light of morning, Welch restrained his enthusiasm. "My aspirations for obtaining a position in the Johns Hopkins were rather strengthened, still there is nothing solid to build upon. . . . All these hopes seem very airy and egotistical when I think of the numbers of able young men who have been and are over here, some having acquired already some reputation, and who are hoping for the same or similar prospects." Welch did not know that after Billings had returned to his hotel, he said, as he himself remembered, "to Mr. Francis King, the President of the Johns Hopkins Hospital, who was with me in Leipsic, that the young man should be, in my opinion, one of the first men to be secured when the time came to begin the medical school."

On December 18 Welch wrote his father that Billings had convinced him he ought to spend another year in Germany, although of course he lacked the means. He understood the importance of supporting himself as soon as possible, yet if he were ever to be eligible for the Hopkins, he must do some original work in pathology, work for which there were no facilities in New York. "I do not know how you will think it best to do about the money or whether it can be raised or not." He would regard any sum advanced to him as a loan, he insisted, and ended with gratitude for all his parents had already done.

Knowing his father's carelessness, Welch repeated much of this in a letter to his stepmother, but we none the less find him writing after more than two months that he had received no reply. "As the subject is important, I hope that my letter has not miscarried." In ten months he had spent between $550 and $600; he would need at least as much again. His letter of credit, he added significantly, would expire April 18.

Not till the middle of March did he receive a letter from his stepmother saying that his father was arranging for another letter of credit. He waited for it in vain; we can visualize his mounting anxiety as he scanned the post each day. Only three days before his old letter expired was he able to report that he had received the new one.[3]

IV

Welch had already planned his next step. His original intention when he set out for Germany, he was to say years later, had been to study with Virchow, whose demonstration that pathological matter was made up of cells had revolutionized pathology. Ludwig and his assistant Kronecker, however, were less interested in the structural side of pathology than in the determination of how pathological changes influenced the functioning of living organs. They persuaded Welch to go not to Virchow, but to Julius Cohnheim, a German Jew whose brilliant pioneering in the application of physiological methods to pathology had five years before secured him a professorship at Breslau.

After his arrival there in April 1877, Welch explained to his father the difference between Virchowian pathology, as represented by his Leipzig professor Wagner, and Cohnheim's school: "Prof. Cohnheim and Prof. Wagner are in some respects the antipodes of each other. Wagner has perhaps a greater array of facts at his disposal . . . has gone deeper into the microscopic details of a pathological change, but while Wagner is often satisfied with the possession of a bare fact, Cohnheim's interest centres on the explanation of the fact. It is not enough for him to know that congestion of the kidney follows heart disease or that hypertrophy of the heart follows contraction of the kidney, or that atheroma occurs in old age, he is constantly inquiring why does it occur under these circumstances. The result is that Cohnheim has taken for his especial studies such common subjects as inflammation, dropsy, embolism and through his investigations these have become perhaps the only subjects in pathology in which our knowledge approaches in exactness what is known concerning a physical or chemical process.

"Pathology and even practical medicine have entered upon a new era since Cohnheim's discoveries in the process of inflammation for there is hardly a disease of which our conception is not thereby modified. He is almost the founder and certainly the chief representative of the so-called experimental or physiological school of pathology. That is, he occupies himself . . . with the study of the diseased processes induced artificially on animals."

In the manner of many German professors, Cohnheim had adopted one general field of study for his laboratory, assigning single aspects of it to his individual students. During Welch's stay in Breslau, he was working on œdema, trying to explain the excessive passage of the fluid constituents of the blood into the surrounding tissues.* He assigned Welch to study œdema of the lungs.

As he worked on this problem, Welch's primary interest underwent a major change. His entire career had been aimed at Virchowian pathology and his first original investigation, his study of lympho-sarcoma, had been in that field. He had been delighted when Wagner considered it good enough for publication, but after less than six months in Cohnheim's laboratory he wrote his father that he was considering asking Wagner to suppress it. Nor was this a passing whim; the article never appeared.

---

* Some fluid always passes, for it is thus that the tissues are fed, but under normal conditions the excess fluid is returned to the veins through the lymphatic system. In œdema, the fluid moves from the vessels more quickly than the lymphatics can remove it; it stagnates and swells the tissues.

Meanwhile Welch had arrived at important results in his new investigation. He wrote his father: "Oedema of the lungs as you know is the name given to the serous transudation [passage of the watery part of the blood into the surrounding tissues] which occurs acutely in both lungs in the course of the most different diseases and which can lead to death by suffocation in a few minutes. It appears so often during the death agony that it is considered there less a cause than an accompaniment of death. The usual explanation is that any hyperaemia [great increase in the amount of blood in the vessels] of the lungs, when extensive enough, can lead to oedema, but a careful analysis of the different kinds of hyperaemia shows that not one gives a satisfactory explanation. This has led some writers to deny that in the lungs oedema is the result of increased blood pressure when the outflow is obstructed, as is the case everywhere else in the body, but that here peculiar elements are at work of which we know nothing. Prof. Cohnheim himself had come to this conclusion, that the cause must be something else than venous congestion of the lungs. The subject had however not been experimented upon.

"I will not weary you by the details of the experiments which I have made. I proved first that it is possible to produce oedema of the lungs in animals by obstructing the out-flow of blood from the pulmonary veins, either by tying the aorta near the heart or by tying the veins of the lung. But what was of especial interest I found that it was necessary to make the obstruction perfectly enormous, so that for example the out-flow of blood from the left ventricle * must be almost obliterated before any change takes place in the blood pressure in the lungs which I measured with an instrument. While therefore I had proved the possibility of venous congestion in the lungs producing oedema, I had found that this occurs only when the obstruction is so enormous that it was not possible to think of its existing in man.

"I had therefore almost come to the conclusion which Prof.

---

* The left ventricle of the heart propels blood through the body by means of the aorta and inferior arteries. The blood then returns through the veins to the right side of the heart, where the right ventricle propels it to the lungs. Then the blood returns to the left side of the heart and repeats this circulation.

Cohnheim had reached, that oedema of the lungs is essentially different from every other kind of oedema, when I struck upon the following chain of reasoning. Oedema in every other part of the body is due to venous congestion. Venous congestion results because more blood flows into a part than can flow out, owing to some obstruction like a contracted liver (cirrhosis) or pressure on a vein, etc. But my experiments so well as observation on man prove that such mechanical obstructions do not produce oedema of the lungs, until they have reached an enormous grade. Is it possible to think of anything else which will permit more blood to flow into the lungs than can flow out? It occurred to me that if the left ventricle were paralyzed and the right ventricle still retained its power, the latter could continue to pump blood into the lungs while the former had not strength enough to pump it out.

"The idea seemed simple and rational and so soon as I thought of it I wondered why in the thousands of pages which have been written on oedema of the lungs it had occurred to no one. Everybody talked about paralysis of the heart as a cause, but if the right ventricle is paralyzed, it is in the most unfavorable condition to raise the blood pressure in the lungs. Prof. Cohnheim seemed pleased with the idea. The thing was to put it to a proof. How is it possible to paralyze one side of the heart and not the other? We tried different heart poisons but as a rule they weakened both ventricles simultaneously. Finally I hit upon a method which was as simple as the original idea. It was to open the chest [of a dog or rabbit] and expose the heart and to take the left ventricle between my fingers and squeeze it without injuring the right ventricle. To my delight it had the desired effect and the result was oedema of the lungs.

"I could therefore consider it as proven that paralysis of the left side of the heart when the right retains its power does produce oedema of the lungs. It seems to me that this fits very well with clinical experience. I will only give one example. Why is it that oedema of the lungs occurs in the most different kinds of diseases during the last moments of life? The usual answer has been that the heart is weakened, but while it is impossible to explain theoretically how weakness of the heart can increase the blood pressure, the explanation loses all force when we consider that we all die with weakness of the heart but do not all die of oedema of the lungs. But what more natural than that in certain cases the left ventricle should die sooner than the right, that is lose its power quicker, and in these cases oedema appears.

"This is the bare outline of my experimental results. The experiments were unusually difficult as they had to do in great part with the ligature of the large arteries in almost inaccessible places. I do not believe that Roger's ligature of the left subclavian artery on man was much more difficult than I have found it on dogs in some cases."

Welch had cleared up this complicated problem in little more than three months. How much Cohnheim helped him it is impossible to say, but we gather from Welch's statement that the fundamental conception, that of a disproportion between the activity of the left and right ventricles, was Welch's own. Indeed, it went against Cohnheim's general conception of the causes of œdema. He believed that when a congestion in the veins produced this condition, it was because the increased pressure and the slow movement of the blood brought about changes in the walls of the vessels which made them more permeable. This, however, could only happen over a period of time; Welch showed that œdema of the lungs followed almost instantly after the spasm of the left ventricle, much too rapidly for any changes of the vascular wall to have taken place.[4]

At Cohnheim's request Welch wrote in German a forty-page article describing his experiments which appeared in Virchow's *Archiv*. When, however, Cohnheim suggested that he also publish his work in English, he demurred, lest it look "as if I overestimated the importance of my work." In warning his father against putting too broad an interpretation on his findings, he wrote: "I do not believe in considering the results of experiments on animals as proven facts in human pathology, as is too often done, but rather guides to clinical and pathological observations. I only feel justified in stating my conclusions as follows: the current explanations of the cause of oedema of the lungs are unsatisfactory; paralysis of the left ventricle with retained power of the right is capable of causing oedema of the lungs; therefore it is a justifiable and plausible hypothesis that this condition of the heart is the cause of oedema of the lungs in man. But it is only an hypothesis and that is far from saying that it is so. I do not know of any hypothesis other than this which explains the fact, but if there is one pitfall in science more dangerous than another it is that of regarding hypotheses as proven facts and I wish to avoid that error. I do not like to have the matter noised about too much before I have made any publication, for at the best the reports are apt to be misleading and exaggerated."

All the newest medical ideas were being discussed in Breslau, and Welch was taken into the inner circle as he had not been anywhere else in Germany. "There is such freedom in the laboratory," he wrote, "that one has the opportunity of seeing everybody else's work, so that if I did nothing myself, I could not fail to learn a great deal." The Danish pathologist Carl Salomonsen, who was Welch's closest friend, was studying tuberculosis of the eye, and Welch was so enthusiastic when he saw his first example of general tuberculosis in a guinea pig that it evoked hearty laughter from Cohnheim. Welch also became intimate with Carl Weigert, the pathologist who first stained bacteria, and the youthful Ehrlich. Near by was Heidenhain's physiological institute, where Welch listened to brilliant lectures on the physiology of the circulation. And, furthermore, the sky of Breslau was full of signs pointing to the new discovery that was to revolutionize pathology: the definitive proof of the germ origin of disease and the accurate cultivation and identification of the causative bacteria.

The idea that parasitic micro-organisms might cause illness was very old, and the theoretical period may be said to have terminated in 1840 with Jakob Henle's essay, *On Miasmata and Contagia,* in which he outlined with amazing accuracy the germ theory, and even described the type of experiments that would be necessary to verify his postulates. Early in the 1870's various pathologists, including three of Welch's teachers—von Recklinghausen, Waldeyer, and Weigert—had observed through the microscope the presence in pathological tissues of extraneous bodies which they recognized as probably of vegetable or bacterial nature. Efforts at the cultivation and identification of these organisms had been going on in Ferdinand Cohn's laboratory in Breslau, where Welch took a course in "general botany," and in Edwin Klebs's laboratory in Prague. Pollender and Davaine in France had described rod-like bodies in the blood of cattle afflicted with anthrax, while Pasteur, having completed his famous investigation of fermentation and putrefaction, had discovered the bacteria of chicken cholera. Profiting by Pasteur's work, Lister had invented his methods of antiseptic surgery.

In 1876, shortly before Welch sailed for Germany, Robert Koch, a pupil of Henle's who was making his living as a district physician, demonstrated the life history of the anthrax bacillus. Under the microscope he had watched this bacillus change from spore to full vegetable form and back to spore again. He hurried to Breslau to show his work to Cohn, who as early as 1870 had pointed out the vegetable nature of bacteria. Cohnheim and Weigert were present at the demonstration. On returning to his laboratory, Cohnheim cried out to the young men doing experiments there: "Let everything stand and go to Koch! This man has made a great discovery which, in its simplicity and exactitude of method, is the more remarkable as Koch is separated from all scientific associations, and everything which he has done is absolutely complete. Nothing remains to be done. I regard it as the greatest discovery yet made in bacteriology, and I believe Koch will astound and shame us all with discoveries yet to come." [5]

When Welch arrived in Breslau less than two years later, he found that Weigert and Ehrlich were applying aniline dyes to the staining of tissue elements and bacteria, and Weigert had recently completed his study of smallpox, in the course of which he had demonstrated by staining methods the masses of micrococci within the pustules. Ehrlich, that odd genius, wandered around the laboratory with hands covered up to the wrists with dyes of many colours.

During Welch's stay there Koch made another visit to Breslau, this time to demonstrate his anthrax bacillus to a visiting English physiologist, Burdon Sanderson, who, according to Koch's biographer Heymann, was not impressed. As an old man, Welch said with a pardonable twist of memory: "I often recall the fact, which to me was one of the most interesting experiences of my life, that I was a student in Breslau in Cohnheim's laboratory at the time Koch brought down his completed anthrax work to show to Cohnheim. I have never forgotten that he came to that laboratory, passed through the room where we were all working, and spent an hour in Cohnheim's private room, and Cohnheim came through, flushed and realizing the significance of this great work."

Welch added on another occasion, however, that "it was only later, of course, that I myself realized" the significance of Koch's demonstration. In his letters home from Breslau Welch did not mention Koch at all, although he described at length a farewell dinner to Professor Lichtheim at which Koch was present. His correspondence contains no reference to bacteriology until his attention had been called to it again by von Recklinghausen, to whom he returned in Strasbourg; from there he wrote his father that "for the last six or eight years there has been strong and still increasing evidence that infectious diseases are due to the presence in the blood or body of minute microscopical organisms." He added that von Recklinghausen had shown him specimens from the kidney in typhoid fever containing yellowish-white spots in which there were colonies of bacteria and accumulations of pus cells. "This discovery points to the bacteritic nature of typhoid fever, but . . . I do not regard it as proving it."

Welch seems to have been too absorbed in the new techniques he had learned from Cohnheim to be as fascinated with bacteriology as he was to become. In his later years he remembered that at Cohnheim's advice he went to Prague to visit Klebs, who was studying acute endocarditis from the microbiological side, and that Klebs showed him the bacteria in the ulcerative lesions of that disease. He gives that matter only passing mention in his letters home: "The professor received me very kindly and not only showed me over the institute but demonstrated to me many preparations, which were of great interest." Welch was to say that Cohnheim had urged him to study with Klebs, but that prudence had sent him to Vienna, where he might most effectively prepare for the practice of medicine.

It is clear from the correspondence that Welch's parents and sister, although they all helped him with the money that made his German trip possible, felt he was foolish in giving so much time to scientific matters which they considered visionary. His sister argued that pathological anatomy was "impracticable," and his stepmother so lectured him on his lack of patriotism when he praised German education that Welch answered: "I should like so much to be with you now, when I am sure Norfolk must be looking lovely. It is certainly one of the prettiest spots in the world and I have not been spoiled by foreign travel as you seem to insinuate." That William Wickham had no appreciation of German medicine is shown by his making his son promise that if he fell ill he would consult no foreign doctors but call in Dennis, who had the advantage of American training.

Welch did not need any urging from home to make him see that the future of a scientist in America was at best precarious. He had so set his hopes on the Johns Hopkins that he was worried when he learned of another young American studying pathology in Germany. On hearing that Prudden was at work in Arnold's laboratory, Welch wrote Dennis, "I do not know him but undoubtedly he will become a swell at pathology and join the army intending to march on the Johns Hopkins. I expect that he is a pet of Gilman's. Did not Gilman mention his name to you?"

In September Welch received a shock when Dennis wrote him of a rumour, which later proved false, that Gilman had filled the chair of pathology. He replied that if someone with an established reputation like Delafield had been chosen, he would have no reason to complain, but if Gilman had appointed a young man such as Prudden, he would feel "a little sore." He added bravely: "Owing to my innate cheerfulness I do not feel greatly depressed."

He threw himself with increased determination into studies that would prepare him for practice. William Wickham, who still hoped that his son would become his assistant in Norfolk, urged the young man to study the surgery which he himself disliked;

obediently William attended the surgical clinic in Breslau, though he felt he was wasting his time, since he considered German surgery no better than American. He followed a clinic on nervous diseases, the specialty he had chosen to adopt if worst came to worst, and also an eye clinic.[6]

Between periods of worry about the future, Welch enjoyed Breslau. Not only did he discover in Salomonsen and a Dr. Rosenbach "the first really congenial companions whom I have found in Germany . . . with whom I could associate with as much freedom and ease as with college friends," but his professors treated him with great friendliness. The learned excursions to which he was invited were a revelation to Welch because of their gaiety. When the botanical society set out in search of specimens, they picked the most beautiful scenery they could think of, and climbed a mountain followed by "a band of music, which possessed the advantage of always remaining invisible and keeping at such a distance as to 'lend enchantment to its tones.' I think I never saw such a rich Flora, the meadows and groves were full of wild flowers, and presented a lovely spectacle. On the summit of the mountain is a ruin, which gave Prof. Cohn, perhaps the most distinguished living botanist, the opportunity to recite to me the famous lines of Goethe, which translated literally run as follows, 'America, thou hast better than our world, the old, hast no fallen castles, no basalt stones.' The view was lovely, taking in most of the Riesengebirge. In the distance the Schneekoppe, clad with snow, and the more modest peaks of the same mountain chain, around us the hillsides with pine and chestnut groves, at our feet the quiet valley and gay meadows and over all the sky, of an unusually deep blue, and a few fleecy clouds made a picture which I was just in the mood to enjoy to the full. But," he added quickly to placate his stepmother, "thousands of miles away in Litchfield County are just as lovely spots."

Cohnheim, who admired Welch's intellect, was also led to pay him special attention because Welch was the first American to have studied with him. One evening, for instance, Cohnheim invited his young student on a picnic. "The party consisted of five professors with their wives and a very moderate supply of unmarried young ladies and three young doctors including myself. The professors were all quite young and very sociable. Much as I admire German science, I must admit that American ladies are more agreeable and understand how to entertain better than German ladies. My experience is not very great but I rarely see a German professor and his wife without wondering how the professor came to marry her; the wife seems almost always to be inferior to the husband. She is generally well educated but seems to lack that tact and conversational talent which I imagine exists nowhere in a higher degree than in America. I was introduced to a young lady last evening who began the conversation, 'Oh, you are from America. I think English is such an ugly language,' which was certainly not a very soothing way of opening an acquaintance. . . . I am very glad to see something of the social side of German life, but am not so infatuated with it as to care to change my residence from America here. So far as art and music and science are concerned we are very far behind the Germans, farther than is generally believed in America, but as regards the social amenities of life the Germans could take a lesson from us."

It was lucky he found Breslau so agreeable, since Dennis, whose propinquity had been a resource before, was now in London working for the difficult examination for the M.R.C.S. degree of the Royal College of Surgeons. "Studying will never be easy for him," Welch confided to his sister, "but such indomitable energy will carry almost anything before it." To Dennis himself Welch wrote: "I often think that it is a little singular that you in your medical course so far have been led to make trials of your strength in just that direction which I should have predicted in school or college would not have attracted you. I should have anticipated that you would display great aptitude for all that is objective in medicine, especially the clinical side, and would be a very excellent observer, but not that you would go traveling to the four corners of the earth to enter just those contests which seem to require a peculiar devotion to study and retentiveness of mind. After the M.R.C.S. you will be sighing like Alexander the Great that there are 'no more worlds to conquer.' The only thing left which I can think of is a French 'Concours' for a professorship."

Dennis's energy spilled over into many attempts to help his friend. He secured Welch an opportunity to write on German universities for the *Lancet* which Welch refused on the grounds that he did not know enough; he urged Welch to send a copy of his essay on lympho-sarcoma, when published, to Gilman, but Welch thought that would be pushing; he circulated such rumours about Welch's having practically been appointed to the Johns Hopkins that Welch was forced to remonstrate in a letter that was a masterpiece of tact.

On hearing that Dennis had received two positions at the Bellevue Hospital Medical College, where he had many powerful friends, Welch wrote to him: "If you are called upon to teach you will I know aim to build up your reputation by solid work and not by clap-trap. Let people see that you deserve whatever position you attain through accurate and thorough knowledge in your specialties, and that whatever outside influence comes to bear on your success, it is only a recognition of your merits. By keeping up the studies which you have begun over here and constantly widening your knowledge you need not fear any competition which you will find in New York. Pardon this sermon, but you know how ready people are to attribute promotion more to influence than to merit; and you can silence their evil tongues by showing that you have taken back with you from Germany not only German knowledge but German 'Gründlichkeit.' "

Having returned to New York some months before Welch, Dennis rented an expensive office which he asked his friend to share with him. Welch refused, because he felt that he could never pay his half of the rent. He could not, of course, "afford to throw away any opportunities for picking up a case here and there," yet he did not "look forward to obtaining any practice." To Dennis's suggestion that he might be able to get Welch some connexion with the Bellevue Hospital Medical College, Welch replied that he believed he would have more opportunity at the College of Physicians and Surgeons, where Delafield would probably let him get up a class in normal and pathological histology. But he saw there was little hope in either institution, since neither had any microscopes to supply the students or any laboratory in which they could work. Money was the important consideration; he would accept any job that would pay.

He even made arrangement with Cohnheim for securing the rights to translate into English his work on *Allgemeine Pathologie* which was just then being printed in Berlin. "The work of translation is beastly," he confided to Dennis, "but I could defer it until I get back to America. It would of course bring my name somewhat into notice in connection with pathological subjects, but I would not undertake the translation for fame or love alone, unless there was some money in it." Welch began on this task after his return to New York, but soon gave it up as an unendurable bore.[7]

He longed for "some opportunity of following up pathology and at the same time of making a modest livelihood." To his father he listed possible methods other than practice for earning money: he could cram students for their examinations, or get "a position on the health board or as deputy coroner, or as police surgeon and if exceptionally fortunate with an insurance company." Of course, a teaching job would be preferable to any of these, but the chances seemed very remote. Behind all his speculations, although he did not mention it to his father, was the gnawing worry that he might fail to support himself in New York; then he would have to return to Norfolk and the family practice which he had so long struggled to avoid. When this possibility insinuated itself in his mind, he tried to drive it out as quickly as he could.

V

Profoundly concerned about his future, Welch went to Vienna, the conventional Mecca of American practitioners, since a vast number of brief practical courses were given in every specialty, and the amount of pathological material was so great that a man might see in a few weeks as many cases of a disease as he would see in America in years. Arriving there on October 26, Welch was not pleased with what he found. "Vienna is in almost all respects much as I had pictured it in my mind to be and I do not regret that I have not spent more time here," he wrote his sister. "Everything is given up to practical subjects, and the courses are conducted chiefly by young men who have no reputation and whose only aim is to make money." Welch entered upon courses on the skin under Hebra, on neurology and psychiatry under Meynert, on the eye, and on other special subjects.

He was not able, however, to keep his attention entirely on preparation for the practice of medicine. He called on Stricker, but when the professor of general pathology heard that Welch had been working with Cohnheim, whose revolutionary ideas Stricker thought wrong, he was unfriendly and refused to show Welch anything. Then Welch wandered into Schenck's embryological laboratory, where he met Prudden, the rival he had worried about, and was reassured. "He is a very good fellow and I think an excellent microscopist and pathologist. I do not think he has anything to look forward to in America more than I have in a pathological line." Welch had taken some embryology with Waldeyer, and at the end of his month's further study with Schenck he felt that he could carry on investigations in that field after his return to America, where it was almost unknown.

Although he wrote home that Vienna was a charming and gay city, Welch did not enter into the life, partly, we gather, because everything was so expensive. He did find his way to the opera, hearing for the first time the *Walküre,* which had been completed a year before. Much as he liked Wagner's earlier works, "I expected to be bored by his latest production, for I had heard so much of its possessing no melodies or choruses or airs, that I fancied that those who raved over the Walküre did it for affectation, but to my surprise I was perfectly enraptured." He found that the opera is "from beginning to end unending melody." Thus Welch showed himself in advance of the common musical taste, for the critics regularly vilified Wagner.

On December 8, after six weeks in Vienna, Welch travelled back to Strasbourg via Würzburg, Frankfurt, and Heidelberg. "Strassburg appears to me like an old friend again," he wrote his sister. "Whether it is because my first impressions of foreign life were formed here and that they are proverbially the strongest, or whether from other reasons, Strassburg has a peculiar charm for me and still seems as quaint and beautiful as ever; and the old minster is more to me than all of the architectural monuments which I have seen."

Welch had returned to study under von Recklinghausen, whom he had recognized from the first as the outstanding representative of Virchowian pathology, but with whom he had been unable to work, since he lacked normal histology. Now that this requisite had been supplied, he offered himself to the professor and was accepted.

Once von Recklinghausen learned that Welch was fresh from Cohnheim's laboratory, he put him to work on a problem that involved the principal point of controversy between the Virchow and Cohnheim schools. Virchow contended that pus was derived from the multiplication of fixed tissue cells; Cohnheim, correctly, that it was created by the emigration of white corpuscles from the blood vessels. Noting that pus formed in the cornea of the eye where there are no blood vessels, von Recklinghausen thought he saw a hole in Cohnheim's argument; he induced Welch to cause an irritation in a frog's eye with caustic chemicals, and then quickly excise the cornea before pus had formed so that it would be separated from all white corpuscles. The cornea was then immersed in the aqueous humour of a frog or bullock and observed for long hours under the microscope. Welch saw that cells moved toward the injured spot and even multiplied by division. What would have been simpler than to conclude that pus cells were not transplanted white corpuscles? Welch, however, recognized this reasoning as fallacious and reserved judgment, assuming that there must be some other explanation. And he was right, although it required more recently developed scientific techniques to prove him so. We know now that connective tissue cells, among them the corneal corpuscles and the cells of Descemet's membrane, are motile and attracted by certain chemical stimuli. Moreover, we know that these fixed tissue cells can readily multiply in the test tube, and thus we arrive at the conclusion that the chemically altered spot in the cornea attracts toward itself neighbouring uninjured motile corneal and other cells, that these cells gather about the site of the injury and even multiply there, giving the appearance of pus cells although they are something else altogether.

After a month in Strasbourg, Welch made a hurried trip to Paris, where he spent a week or ten days in intensive sightseeing, "working," as he put it, from seven or eight in the morning until twelve or one at night. He spent three days at the Louvre, went to Versailles, and "accomplished nearly all that my Baedeker imposed on me." He did not forget medicine entirely, for he visited hospitals on some mornings and listened to a lecture by Ranvier, the great histologist. It is perhaps natural that his letters make no mention of Pasteur, for, as we have seen, his interest in bacteriology was not yet fully awake and the French scientist had just begun to work specifically on the infectious diseases of animals.

While in Paris, Welch received a letter from Dennis saying that through Dr. Wood's influence he had secured Welch an appointment to demonstrate pathological anatomy during the summer term at the Bellevue Medical College, and that he had also persuaded Dr. Flint, the professor of medicine, to make Welch his assistant. Welch, however, was not as enthusiastic as might have been expected. He felt his future at Bellevue was blocked by Janeway, the pathological anatomist there; he had never met Dr. Flint, though he believed him "a very competent man"; and Dennis had neglected to say whether either position carried a salary. "I shall write to Dr. Wood thanking him cordially," Welch told his stepmother, "but shall express myself with some reserve, until I am back to New York and can personally survey the field and learn what father thinks I had better do." However, he expressed gratitude to Dennis, who he felt had done more for him than most friends would have done.

From Paris Welch went to London. On January 27 he wrote his sister a most unusually emotional letter which may have reflected the tenseness of his nerves now that the time had almost come that would pit him against life no longer as a student but as a professional man in an environment hostile to his ambitions: "If I have had any lingering regrets at leaving Europe they have all disappeared on coming to London. I feel actually homesick in this dull, dreary, doleful, dirty, dismal town. I regret that I left Paris to come here at all, for I do not believe that there exists a city more uninviting to strangers. There may be some comfort in the homes behind these black brick walls, but there is none outside of them. The smallest and most insignificant German nest which I have ever been in is more tolerable, there at least one could find a café where one could sit of an evening and read the papers or write letters or amuse himself by studying the people, but café life is something of which the English know nothing. Today is Sunday and surpasses all which I had even heard of the miseries of a London Sunday. I have taken a bedroom near the University College Hospital and take my meals at a restaurant as convenient. I went out as usual this morning to get my breakfast, but lo, there is not a restaurant, even a baker's shop open. It was really alarming. Finally I saw an eating place with the blinds closed, but the door a little ajar. I dashed in and obtained a piece of meat pie, which I was requested to take with me to eat, as they were not allowed to serve things on Sunday. I went to church and heard a sermon on the reasons why the English nation is so much better than any other nation. Oh you self-satisfied, pietistic Englishman, who only thinks of things material after all, your system breeds more crime and misery and poverty than that of your continental neighbors whom you pray for. I really believe that it is the lager-bier and wine, the cheerful cafés, the open air on Sunday, the good theatres which make the Germans and French so much more temperate, healthy-minded, cheerful and companionable than these Londoners."

On February 6, 1878, Welch sailed for America, a prophet bearing a new revelation that he had learned in a foreign land. He knew that he carried with him a knowledge of scientific medicine, the medicine of the future, the medicine that above all else America needed, but he also knew that America was not conscious of her need. Would he be forced to support himself by uncongenial tasks since no one wanted what he brought? That seemed very likely.

CHAPTER VII

Struggles in New York

I

ON arriving at New York late in February or early in March 1878, Welch lost no time seeking a job, preferably connected with pathology, that would yield him a living. As a stopgap he tutored a young man who was so stupid that Welch was convinced he could never pass the hospital examinations. When he did pass, it probably did not reassure Welch about American standards.

Since the College of Physicians and Surgeons was the leading New York medical school, representing, as Welch later explained, the "Brahmins" of the profession, he began his job-hunt by calling on Delafield there. His former professor offered him an unpaid position as lecturer on pathology during the summer session, but Welch did not accept; he spoke of his greater interest in laboratory courses than in lectures, and asked whether he might not perhaps be allowed to give such a course. In its hundred triumphant years the college had never bothered with laboratories; with a smile Delafield said that if Welch could find an unused room in the building he would let him fix it up. Having walked upstairs and down, having poked about in every corner without finding any space not assigned to other purposes, Welch consulted the Y.M.C.A. across the street, only to learn that they could offer him nothing suitable. When he returned crestfallen, Delafield implied that that closed the matter of a laboratory at the college.

Next Welch went to the Bellevue Hospital Medical College, although it was unheard of that anyone who could secure a connexion with the College of Physicians and Surgeons should bother with the lesser school. After weeks of heart-rending negotiation, arguing with this professor and that, trying to make his scheme fit in with the politics of the college, he at last obtained a laboratory "which I shall have for giving microscopical courses and for teaching." He was pleased with his success and with the political manipulating by which he had achieved it, but the contrast between what he would have and the opportunities young men enjoyed in Germany kept him from being sufficiently elated to suit Dennis. "Fred," he wrote his sister, "is very jubilant and talks about writing you lest I should still misrepresent things to you."

Welch was given three rooms furnished with kitchen tables; as he later said, the college spent "fully twenty-five dollars in equipping the laboratory." Surveying his new domain, devoid of microscopes, devoid of instruments, devoid of specimens with which to work, he became depressed. "I have been trying," he wrote his sister in a letter ungrammatical with emotion, "to get the laboratory in order so as to organize a class this summer, but the material was so scanty that I should have given up the idea of starting anything there this summer, unless those who wish to have their students work there were not so urgent to have me begin. I can get as many students as there are places for, but I can not make much of a success out of the affair at present. I seem to be thrown entirely upon my own resources for equipping the laboratory and do not think that I can accomplish much.

"I sometimes feel rather blue when I look ahead and see that I am not going to be able to realize my aspirations in life. I may be able to make a support in New York, and even if I should succeed in accordance with the hopes of my friends, it would not be the kind of success which I should like. I am not going to have any opportunity for carrying out as I would like the studies and investigations for which I have a taste. There is no opportunity in this country, and it seems improbable that there ever will be. I can quiz students, I can teach microscopy and pathology, perhaps get some practice and make a living after a while, but that is all patchwork and the drudgery of life and what hundreds do. I shall never be independent of these things.

"I was often asked in Germany how it is that no scientific work in medicine is done in this country, how it is that many good men who do well in Germany and show evident talent there are never heard of and never do any good work when they come back here. The answer is that there is no opportunity for, no appreciation of, no demand for that kind of work here. In Germany on the other hand every encouragement is held out to young men with taste for science. I know two young Americans whom I studied with in Germany and who spent most of their time with pathology. They are both here in New York. One told me the other day that there is no use of attempting to do anything here, and he expects to return to Germany and stay there; the other says that if he had any idea he could make a living there he would go. Do not be alarmed. I do not expect to go, but I do think that the condition of medical education here is simply horrible."

Later Welch was to see the picture in exactly opposite colours, and recognize that America's lack of scientific pathology should not have been a cause for depression; it gave him his great chance. In 1927 he said: "Few have been so fortunate in coming, provided with scientific wares from such sources as these [his foreign teachers], upon a scene so ripe for educational and scientific advance, and at a time so pregnant in the history of scientific medicine, and in finding opportunities so favorable, yes, even hungry for disposal of their wares." [1]

Having somehow collected six antique microscopes, Welch put six students to work in May. Since the boys, who were beginners, were not ready to understand pathological specimens from the dead house, he appealed to his sister to comb the marshes of upstate New York for frogs. Dennis's mother also was urged by her son to send the servants out frog-hunting; it was a banner day when the boxes of damp grass arrived croaking with their live cargo, and a great disappointment when "a friend in Bridgeport," not knowing that frogs breathe air, sent ten large specimens in a bucket of water where they were drowned.

When Welch visited his sister, he skipped through the marshes himself, and carried a huge box full of frogs with him on to the New York train. Soon the sleeping car was filled with a mysterious noise, a croaking mad and melancholy as the voice of Pan in the reeds by the river. Gentlemen turned in their seats; timid ladies wondered what could be wrong with the machinery. The young pathologist, who hated to be conspicuous, read his paper stolidly; "I appeared to be as ignorant and much astonished as the other occupants of the sleeping car."

Thus the first laboratory course in pathology ever given in an American medical school got under way, but Welch remained depressed. Teaching the rudiments of microscopy took much time and brought in little money, for he received only the meagre fees paid by his six students. The young man who was eager to do research of his own was forced to spend all his spare time in occupations that would earn his living.

Most helpful to his pocketbook was a partnership with Dr. Henry Goldthwaite in a quiz that prepared medical students for the competitive examinations held for interneships and medical appointments in the army and navy. Since the masters adapted their teachings to the foibles of the various examiners, such quizzes had become a necessity for all candidates; they were an accepted pedagogical method and often highly remunerative. Before he took Welch into partnership, Goldthwaite was already doing well; and with Welch teaching practice and materia medica, he soon forged ahead of all the others; they secured twenty-five pupils who paid $100 each. Welch, however, was not thrilled with this success. He did not enjoy thrusting predigested knowledge into the minds of the young; he was convinced that his pupils were slow-witted, and was usually amazed when they succeeded in the examinations. When, after more than two years, he was able to make enough money by other expedients, he joyfully gave up the quiz, although it was then at the height of its financial success.

Another of Welch's activities was the position as assistant to Dr. Austin Flint, senior, which Dennis had secured for him. This job paid very little, but was considered valuable, since Flint, who was the professor of practice of medicine at Bellevue, was the most important man in that school and also one of the leading consultants in New York City. Rich, socially prominent, and brilliant, Flint was the author of the textbook on the practice of medicine that every progressive physician had to have on his shelves. It was no small thing to work with such a man. Many young doctors streamed through Flint's office, but the great practitioner quickly recognized Welch's unusual ability; as soon as the article on œdema of the lungs, which had been published in the March 1878 issue of Virchow's *Archiv,* arrived in America, Flint did him the honour of reading it with his German teacher. He set Welch to work helping with his lectures and the occasional scientific speeches he delivered before medical associations.

With Lusk and others, Flint threw Welch opportunities to make examinations of pathological specimens for practising doctors, and soon the young man had an experience that did not increase his taste for practice. The wife of a professor at the University Medical College had suddenly collapsed when three months pregnant; the most eminent gynæcologists in the city were called, and a piece of membrane that had passed from her uterus was given to several pathologists for examination. Dr. Seesil, a man of much experience, "reported the membrane to be chorion, in which case of course it would be an abortion and not a tubal pregnancy, and no operation would be indicated. . . . As I found only decidua and no chorion, my opinion was for a tubal pregnancy." The older man's word was taken, no operation was performed, and the woman died. Making the autopsy in the presence of Seesil, Welch demonstrated that he had been right. However, at a medical meeting where the matter was discussed, "Dr. [Emil J.] Noeggerath rose and mentioned my name and said that I had come to his office and examined the specimen and had myself pronounced Seesil's preparation to be chorion. Dr. Thomas [the famous gynæcologist who had referred the case under discussion to Welch] of course was aghast and no one could refute Noeggerath." However, Welch's friends, Sabine and Lusk, called on him immediately and, finding how things stood, promised "to put the matter in a proper light."

A short time later Welch had his revenge. At a meeting of the Gynecological Society Noeggerath presented some microscopical specimens which he said proved "a very great discovery," that ovarian cysts could be developed by a peculiar metamorphosis of the lining of the blood vessels. Then he walked over to Welch "and asked me aloud and in German, if his discovery was not entirely novel. I replied that it was as novel as it was remarkable. . . . I asked him if he had not used chromic acid and alcohol in hardening his specimen. He said he had, which explained the whole thing. What he had supposed to be new cells were nothing but the effects of the reagents on the blood. As Prof. Thomas and several others came and asked my opinion, I think they were rather amused at the exhibition Noeggerath had made."

Welch was beginning to attract attention. His friends saw that his article on œdema was circulated in the right places, although all their urging was unable to make him translate it into English for an American journal.

When his microscopical class ended in May, Welch was induced by eager applicants immediately to start another; young men from all three New York medical schools rushed to Bellevue to take this unusual course which had begun to bridge the gap that separated New York from European scientific developments. Indeed, in three months Welch's work had created such a stir that the alumni association of the College of Physicians and Surgeons contributed the money to set up a pathological laboratory in which every student would be required to work. Delafield, who was made director, promptly offered Welch charge of the histological department, with a salary of $500 the first year and the promise of more to come. "We've got to have you back here," Welch remembered that he said. "We must have pathology here." He had discovered that the ice-cream parlour on the ground floor could be dispensed with to make space for a laboratory.

The leading medical school in the city was offering Welch the opportunity he so greatly desired, but he was trapped. Flint and others said that it would be treachery for him to leave the Bellevue school now; sadly he relinquished what would have been his big chance, and then generously recommended for this opportunity greater than his own Prudden, the man he had most feared as his rival for the position at the Johns Hopkins that was still unfilled. In his letter urging Prudden to accept the position, he said: "Personally I should like to have you here in New York, for I fear I am going to rust out unless I have someone to talk with and help me on concerning the subject in which we are both interested."

Pathology had now been recognized by two of America's leading medical schools as a subject of independent merit that should be taught practically, in the laboratory. And through Welch and Prudden it was at last united with the best sources of inspiration abroad. From now on the need was to widen and deepen this stream and to develop American workers who would contribute their share to the general sum of knowledge. In the accomplishment of these ends Welch's career was to stand pre-eminent.

II

"I first knew him when I was a student at the Bellevue Hospital Medical College during the winters of 1882–3 and 1883–4," Dr. Hugh T. Patrick wrote of Welch. "He was then thirty-two years old, a chubby, round-faced, pink-cheeked, somewhat snub-nosed, quick-moving youngish man. Already a bit bald, with small feet and small adroit hands, he was always nattily dressed, trousers and high-buttoned cutaway coat fitting snugly. Then as now his was a most winning personality. Always he was spoken of by the boys as Billy Welch. He had our unlimited admiration and as much affection as a bunch of medical students has for anyone. To the green student he was kindness itself, ever ready to be helpful."

Dr. Henry C. Coe, who studied with Welch in 1884, tells us that although he did not adequately appreciate his master at the time, "I felt instinctively that he was wasted at Bellevue, and was destined to have a larger circle of hearers. . . . I recall his serious, eager look, his smiling face, his interest in young men which bound them to him. He was always ready to drop any work in which he was engaged and to answer even trivial questions on any subject—in fact, he was never without an answer, for his knowledge was encyclopaedic."

If Welch felt dissatisfaction at being condemned to teach the most elementary subjects when he wanted to do research and establish a laboratory filled with investigators, he was successful in concealing it. Dr. Walter Lester Carr remembers that Welch's bare workrooms were alive with excitement. That pathology was generally considered unimportant in America; that some of the older professors referred to Welch slightingly as "a laboratory man" too incompetent to do anything practical; these things only convinced the young men that they were stepping ahead of their environment.

Microscopical studies were so unusual that the necessary equipment was not for sale. Teasers were made from darning needles or pieces of old wire; sections were cut with razors brought from home. The slides in the few stores that carried such oddities were of varying size and thickness, but you had to take what you could find; word of a new shipment received at one of the optical stores produced a stampede of the young men from Welch's laboratory. Their microscopes were low-powered and imperfect, but the forms seen through the weak lenses on the rickety tables were a vision of a new world. "We had no elaborate laboratory equipment," Carr writes; "there were specimens in jars, rats in cages, and a few tanks with plant growth. . . . You may not appreciate how enthusiastic we were because it is now so easy to get material and equipment in your laboratory courses, but at the time of which I speak everything was new and untried."

Frogs were stared at through the microscope and then "connective tissue from a rat's tail was teased by a student and looked at by Dr. Welch as if he had never seen such a specimen. Sections were hardened, cut, and stained and then examined under the microscope." Eventually students worked up to making slides of simple pathological material from the dead house; more elaborate preparations were made by the professor himself. "I have a box of slides that were made for the course," Welch said in 1930, "and I have recently looked at them. They are just as they would be if made today. I am rather proud of what is exhibited there, but I had an interest in aniline, and I think I traced nearly all of them; some of them were very beautiful. We used gentian violet, haematoxylin, eosin."

Bacteriology was not officially part of the course, although on one occasion it was mentioned in a manner that made a profound impression on the students and, according to Hermann Biggs, determined him to dedicate his life to this fascinating science. In 1882 Koch discovered the tubercle bacillus. Most of the New York medical profession were profoundly unimpressed; had not Dr. Loomis, that pillar of the University Medical College, announced: "The bacterian theory, which so recently has occupied the attention of medical men, especially in Germany, is rapidly being disproved, and consequently is rapidly being abandoned"? Dr. Flint, Welch remembered, was one of the few important practitioners in New York who had any interest in bacteria. One morning as Welch lay in bed after a late evening in the dead house, the door of his room burst open and in came the old gentleman at a run, waving a newspaper in the air. "Welch," he cried, "I knew it, I knew it!" The young man must have blinked in sleepy surprise, but when Flint explained that a dispatch in the paper told of Koch's great triumph, he jumped out of bed as excited as his master. They both set out to wake Dennis.

A short time later Welch demonstrated Koch's discovery before his laboratory class. Biggs writes: "In his most lucid and fascinating manner, he told us of this great work and of its significance to the future development of medicine. He showed us methods of staining sputum and demonstrating the tubercle bacilli. I can now see quite clearly the steam rising from the dish of carbol-fuchsin in the sand-bath containing the sputum while he talked. This served as my first inspiration."

In the lecture rooms of the older professors of all three New York schools the delighted young men repeated what they had seen. Carr tells us that a few days later, as Professor Loomis stood nobly on the lecture platform, he peered into the atmosphere around him and remarked: "People say there are bacteria in the air, but I cannot see them." This witticism brought a burst of applause from the class. When it was repeated to Welch, he said: "That's too bad. Loomis is such a nice man."

Despite Prudden's course at the College of Physicians and Surgeons, students from that school continued to come to Welch. In 1879 he found it necessary to teach two sections, and three years later the parsimonious Bellevue Hospital Medical College had to enlarge his laboratory. Already in 1878, Henry Fairfield Osborn, a rich and prominent Princeton graduate who wanted to study the microscopic anatomy of animals, had come to Welch as a private pupil; Welch wrote home that he was "a most promising young man, the best pupil whom I ever had." When the future palæontologist asked for unusual animals to study, Welch remembered that at a dinner given in Delmonico's by Seguin he had met a thin Canadian with a tremendous moustache who was professor of physiology at the McGill Medical School in Montreal. "I was captivated," Welch wrote years later; the two men promised to correspond. Welch told Osborn that he would ask his acquaintance William Osler to send him some Canadian animals. "We spent hours dissecting strange animals which came to us through Dr. Osler's influence."

Since Osborn had many important connexions in Princeton, his coming brought a little group of students from that college, among them, Welch wrote his sister, "Mr. Libbey, one of the instructors in Princeton College, and a son of a very wealthy man, the partner of A. B. Stewart. It is decidedly for my interest to take him, as he will probably be an influential man at Princeton, and is to take a leading part in the new biological course." Clearly Welch was not overlooking any opportunities to better himself by leaving Bellevue, where he was so busy eking out a livelihood that he had no time for the original work he craved.

During his six years in New York, only one piece of experimental work came from Welch's laboratory. We gather that Dr. S. J. Meltzer, a trained physiologist engaged in the practice of medicine, asked Welch to be allowed to use the facilities of the laboratory to determine how the red blood corpuscles behaved when shaken up with various substances supposed to be chemically inactive. Welch was delighted, and so helpful in working out the problem that Meltzer insisted that Welch write the paper that was signed with both their names. It is indicative of the small means and even smaller space for experimental work in the laboratory that the investigators were forced to borrow the use of a mechanical mixer in the mineral-water factory of Carl H. Schultz.

Most of Welch's time was taken up in multifarious activities associated with making his living. Sharing with Dennis the position of demonstrator of anatomy, Welch supervised the students in the dead house and once a week did an autopsy before the class which was, Dr. Patrick tells us, "a revelation and an inspiration. Most of us came from small cities, towns and villages where autopsies were rare and necessarily Welch first taught us *how* to do an autopsy. I have quite a thrilling recollection of an autopsy I did *à la Welch* during my first vacation. The six or eight country practitioners present stared wide-eyed at the dashing and neat way I went through that cadaver. As I held a kidney in my left hand and went into it with the 'free sweeping strokes' that Welch taught us, they obviously were nervous and one kindly old friend said, 'Look out, Hugh, you'll cut yourself.' But I was there to imitate the master if I died in the attempt. There was nothing flamboyant or oratorical in his teaching but it was crystal clear and left a clean cut impression.

"This weekly demonstration course was given in a large amphitheatre. At the end of the hour the eviscerated cadaver and the specimens Welch had collected during the week were carried into a small anteroom. E. G. Janeway, assuredly one of the greatest internists America has produced, followed Welch and to reach the amphitheatre had to pass this anteroom. But pass it he rarely could without stopping in to see what of unusual interest Welch might have. So the keener of us generally hopped over the railing and hurried to this little room to hear the older and the younger savant comment on the specimens. Janeway . . . had an extensive experience, enormous erudition and photographic memory. This (for us) rich colloquy of him and Welch always made him late for his own lecture."

From the first Welch had delivered some lectures on pathology during the summer term, the traditional time to give young men a chance, as the older men were out of town. "I look back with a great deal of humiliation to my first lecture," Welch said in 1930. "It was the failure known to all young men impressed by what they are trying to do." Not till his fourth year at the Bellevue Medical College was he permitted to lecture during the winter term; Dr. Flint had opened the way by making Janeway associate professor of principles and practice. But Welch was not given the title of professor of pathology that Janeway relinquished; Dennis, whose influence was always greater than Welch's, had just been made adjunct professor of surgery, and the leaders of the school did not dare elevate both young men over the heads of teachers older than they.

Welch outlined his objectives in his opening lecture of the term 1882–83: "I shall make the leading features of the course the demonstration of fresh pathological specimens and the making of post mortem examinations. In doing this I must sacrifice to a considerable extent systematic didactic instruction. I am governed by the fact that it is possible for you to learn from books the didactic part, whereas nothing can replace the careful study of fresh specimens. Pathological histology is a subject which can only be learned by practical work with the microscope in a laboratory."

We can follow in his preserved lecture notes the steps by which Welch acquired the facility that during his Baltimore period permitted him to speak extemporaneously. In New York he worked out minutely on paper even such a subject as inflammation, which, after his Cohnheim period, he must have known by heart. He wrote on the bottom of his pages such comments as: "Only fifteen minutes remained after demonstration of specimens. Work up subject better."

No hesitancy, however, came over to his pupils. "As a lecturer," Coe tells us, "he was earnest and convincing, and presented facts in a lucid, though condensed form. Unlike the popular medical teachers of those days, he avoided clap-trap and never 'played to the galleries.' The students who listened to him were generally of a much lower order of intelligence than those of the present day, few having had more than a common or high school education, hence it was necessary for him to present facts in an elementary form, which must have been irksome to him at times."

Welch, who had been collecting opportunities to dissect in hospitals all over New York, was always able to demonstrate fresh specimens of the same diseases that Flint discussed during the next hour in his lectures on practice. Indeed, the coloured janitor at the Bellevue School, Alexander Dumas Watkins, saw him inject so many cadavers that, until stopped, he mailed handbills to undertakers offering to teach them how to embalm in the manner of Welch.[2]

Welch's connexion with Flint had become increasingly close. For months in 1880 and 1881 he had used every spare moment in helping revise Flint's *Principles and Practice of Medicine,* the most consulted clinical treatise of its day. Although he was paid little and was forced to give up his plan of collaborating with Dennis on a textbook of anatomy, Welch remembered that he "jumped at the chance." The prestige value of working on such a book was tremendous. His name was not mentioned on the title page when the practice was published in 1881, but in the preface Flint gave him credit for contributing "the first seven chapters, embracing the general pathology of the solid tissues and of the blood. He has also revised, and in great part re-written, the descriptions of the anatomical characters of the diseases considered in the rest of the volume." Thus Welch's name was spread to the far corners of the land.

We gather that Welch sometimes assisted the distinguished consultant in his office; he had not forgotten that in America no one lived by scientific medicine alone. On arriving in New York he had hung out his shingle, but since his heart was not in practice, he secured very little. The only patients of whom he talked in his later years were the chief of a dectective agency whom he treated for headaches, and that great theatrical impresario of the Bowery, Tony Pastor. Welch's office was next door to that of the ageing Alonzo Clark, who, confusing Welch with Dennis, sent him surgical cases on which Welch sometimes operated.

Clark's mistake was perhaps natural, for Welch was somewhat under Dennis's shadow. They shared the same rooms on Twenty-First Street, but since he could pay more rent, Dennis had the major share; Welch occupied a bedroom with a Dr. Williams. While Welch walked or rode in the newly constructed elevated railway—which he considered "really elegant" but inexcusably noisy—Dennis visited his patients in a carriage. The rich and socially prominent young man had been generous in using his connexions to further Welch's career, but most of them remained primarily Dennis's connexions. Dennis was able to do things for people that were completely out of Welch's range. When the medical society met in Cleveland, for instance, he sent a group of important colleagues including both Flints out to that city in his father's private railway car, "furnished," Welch wrote his sister, "with kitchen, dining-room, staterooms, balcony and every luxury. They drank champagne, smoked, ate all the delicacies which could be obtained at Delmonico's, and apparently had a delightful time." On another occasion Dennis gave a huge formal dinner for Sir William MacCormac, a visiting English surgeon. Among the guests were Andrew Carnegie and Matthew Arnold, whom Welch considered "the foremost English writer now living." Welch hardly had a chance to speak to the poet, who was seated at Dennis's right.

A surgeon specializing in practice yet well versed in theory, Dennis was striding to worldly success while Welch wandered in the unproductive mazes of pathology, grasping at stop-gaps to make a living. The time soon came, however, when he could have placed his feet on the highroad his friend triumphantly trod. Refusing to believe that so brilliant a young man with so agreeable an address—which could easily be changed into an excellent bedside manner—intended to bury himself in a laboratory, the ageing Flint tried to put Welch in a position to succeed to his own professorship of principles and practice and perhaps eventually to the lucrative practice he himself enjoyed. One day he told Welch that he was going to give him the full professorship of clinical medicine, one of the several positions held by Janeway, who was not a favourite of Flint's. What must have been the distinguished practitioner's amazement when his young protégé refused this magnificent opportunity. Not wishing to offend Flint by admitting his dislike for practice and his determination to be primarily a scientist, Welch explained that he would hate to hurt Janeway's feelings. Then he returned to the weary round of small tasks that gave him little satisfaction.[3]

Welch was too busy to take much part in the life of the city. Concerts and exhibitions hardly ever figure in his letters, and he rarely attended the theatre except when his sister or her husband was in town. He did see Bernhardt act—"there is something strange and wonderful about her personality, a fascination which conquered me completely"—and hurried to inspect the Metropolitan Opera House when it was opened in 1884: "I was disappointed with the house. It is a huge barn-like structure with no architectural effects within or without, and singularly devoid of ornamentation. It is outrageous to build such a pretentious house, which will not compare with any of the great opera-houses in Europe. The singers say that no matter how well they sing they cannot arouse the audience on account of the vast distances and cold interior, and so it appeared." He became an intimate friend of Clarence Olcott, an interior decorator, who joined him in enthusiasm for the Pre-Raphaelites. "Of course," Welch wrote his sister, "anything by Burne Jones must be fine." Welch was to say Olcott taught him "that a gentleman can have taste without being a despised effeminate, and it was a valuable lesson."

Welch occasionally accompanied Dennis to elegant receptions, and he was pleased when the parents of his pupils, "refined and agreeable people" such as the Osborns, invited him to their homes. He used to tell how, when calling on a Vanderbilt, he had inadvertently left a card on the back of which he had jotted down the weights of some organs removed at an autopsy; Mrs. Vanderbilt mailed it back. Yet he usually lacked both the time and the money for society.

As long as he roomed with Dennis, their friendship was a great resource, but in February 1880 Dennis married and moved out. "I feel quite melancholy to have him leave," Welch wrote his sister. Paying the rent became a serious problem; "Fred has rented out his vacant rooms to three fellows, one of whom will occupy the bedroom with me. . . . They are all recent Yale graduates and pleasant fellows."

Welch developed the habit of dining several evenings a week at the University Club; "I always meet some one whom I know and frequently find a dinner-companion. . . . There is an excellent reading-room and library. All the latest magazines, books and papers are here. It makes a bachelor's existence quite tolerable to fall back after dinner into a large easy chair with a cigar and the latest Punch." Welch ate his lunch at some noisy restaurant near the medical school, usually by himself; although he put on no false dignity with his pupils, he did not encourage familiarity. He seems at times to have been so lonely that he regretted he was not married. "No tender hand," he complained to his sister in 1883, ever put his desk to rights.

His own family was a consolation to him. He urged his sister and brother-in-law to visit him in New York, and rushed to Norfolk for brief vacations whenever he could find the time. As his niece remembers, "he filled his bedroom with frogs and other specimens for experimentation and always had his microscope with him. . . . I think he did not play with us very much, but I remember going fishing with him once when I was very young. . . . Later, when I was much older, we went on a longer excursion together to fish for bass. I rowed while my uncle fished." On this occasion Welch went in swimming and when a passer-by asked the little girl as she sat waiting in the boat if she were alone, she called out: "No, my uncle, Professor Welch, is over there having a swim." After Welch had dressed, "he said, 'You must never call me professor. Only dancing-masters are called that.' He said it very gently, but I felt the reproof and have never forgotten my sense of shame." Although he seems not to have known how to talk to them, the welfare of his sister's children was of constant interest to him; he advised on their schooling, and sometimes even wrote them descriptions of the animals in his laboratory.

Welch's associations with his fellow-physicians were pleasant if not very intimate. He remembered, for instance, that he knew his future Hopkins associate William S. Halsted well "in those days of his highest physical and mental vigor, and saw much of him. He sent his students to take courses in histology and pathology in my laboratory . . . He would collect tumors and other specimens from his practice which we would go over together at intervals of two or three weeks, and not infrequently I was a guest at the delightful little dinners where he and Dr. Thomas McBride gathered a few congenial friends at their house on East 25th Street."

Although elected in 1879 to the Academy of Medicine, Welch restricted his activities there. "As I have spoken at the last two

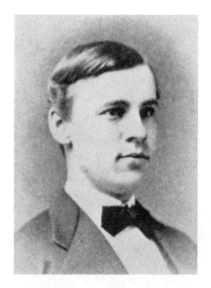

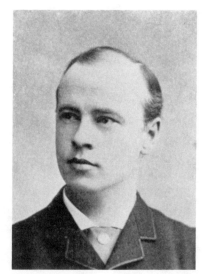

Student at Yale   Teacher at Bellevue

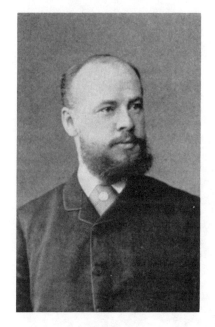

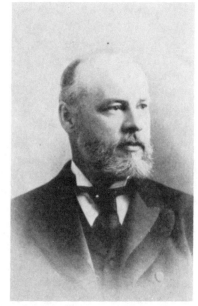

Student of Koch   Teacher in Baltimore

WILLIAM HENRY WELCH

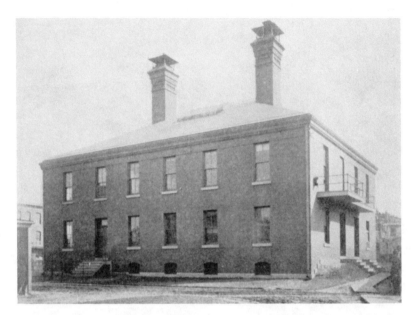

The Beginning: The Old Pathological

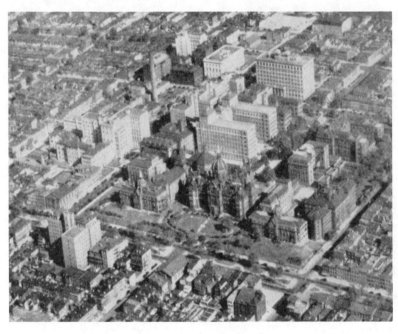

Air View Today

JOHNS HOPKINS MEDICAL SCHOOL AND HOSPITAL

meetings," he wrote his stepmother, "I think it is about time to stop. My wares will become rather too cheap and common. If there is an unenviable reputation in the medical profession it is that of the chronic scribbler in the journals or of the chronic babbler in the societies."

Welch impressed his students with the "almost Spartan simplicity of his life." They felt he was dedicating himself to some high ideal, searching intently in his lodgings for some great discovery. They did not know that this busy and superficially successful young man was really frustrated deep down, since he lacked a chance to do what he longed to do. Would the time never come, he must have asked himself as he hurried from one mechanical job to another, when science would dawn over this clanging city; would none of his colleagues ever see the vision he had seen in Germany of laboratories filled with well-trained young men eager to push back the boundaries of knowledge? Sometimes his German experience must have seemed to him a mirage that had faded now to sober reality.

But one day fate appeared at the door of his workroom in the form of a tall visitor of military bearing. Dr. Billings hoped that Dr. Welch had not forgotten their meeting in Wagner's laboratory; he happened to be in New York, and would Dr. Welch mind if he watched while Dr. Welch taught? The next day the young man was amazed to see his elder in the back of the amphitheatre while he demonstrated an autopsy. When the demonstration was over, Billings engaged Welch in conversation, drawing him out on what he would like to do if adequate facilities were placed at his disposal. The young man's face flushed, his eyes lighted, and he talked of laboratories as he had seen them in Germany, of original research done with his own hands. Billings remembered that Welch told him he had for a long time "been trying to make some original investigations in the causes and pathology of Dysentery" but had lacked the time since he had been forced "to make his living by students' and doctors' fees." The visitor listened to all Welch had to say, asked some searching questions, and then took the train back to Washington.

III

"I saw Dr. Welch," Billings wrote President Gilman of Johns Hopkins on March 1, 1884, "had a long talk with him—heard him lecture—and saw him directing work in his laboratory. He is 33 years old, unmarried, of good personal address—modest, quiet, and a gentleman in every sense so far as I can judge. . . . He is a good lecturer—an excellent laboratory teacher, and has a keen desire for an opportunity to make original investigations, being activated I think by the true scientific spirit. . . . Upon the whole I think he is the best man in this country for the Hopkins. He has not the reputation yet which is possessed by Ponfick or Orth or Weigert or several other Germans who are probably available—but I think he will develop well."

On March 9 Billings added: "I staid with Dr. Flint while in N.Y. He spoke of Welch—said his only fault was a tendency to be a little late always, and that he had to be kept stirred up. I did not give the least hint that you were thinking of him for Baltimore."

The professorship of pathology was about to be filled. Billings called on Welch again and, the younger man wrote his father, "in a very indirect manner sounded me upon the subject. He said that President Gilman wished to have me go down to Baltimore. . . . I went last Sunday night, and Monday morning met President Gilman, who called on me at the Hotel. He showed me over the University, introducing me to the different professors. I was invited to lunch with him, and met Judge Brown and another member of the board of trustees, together with Prof. Remsen (of Chemistry) and Prof. Martin (of Biology). After the lunch President Gilman made me the offer, which I am now considering." Thus was Welch's ambition to be called to the Hopkins realized after years of waiting.

As so often happens with moments that are the turning points in men's lives, Welch's portentous interview with Gilman had a comic side. Suffering from an injured heel, Welch had hobbled into Gilman's office with a shoe on one foot and an arctic on the other. When he rose to go, the university president said with a smile: "Wait a moment, Dr. Welch. The Johns Hopkins does not regard eccentricity as a sign of intelligence."

In a letter unusually disjointed for his orderly mind, Welch wrote his father that the medical school would not be completely organized till the hospital was finished in 1886, but "the idea is to have the more scientific departments in medicine under way when the practical (or clinical) work begins." His would be the first appointment specifically to the medical faculty, although Professors Ira Remsen of chemistry and Newell Martin of biology belonged to it as well as to the philosophical; "these two men, together with Billings and myself, if I accept, will have the responsibility of selecting other men, as well as of organizing the medical department. . . . The aim is not to have a large school. It is to be a faculty of medicine rather than a school. The conditions for admittance will be high, the course of study long and thorough, and a large number of students is not desired and would not come. . . .

"The offer was a great surprise to me, and I do not know how I came to be selected when there are others who have already established excellent reputations in my field, and at the Johns Hopkins they select their men from all countries. I think I owe the appointment to Dr. Billings, but he is anxious that Dr. Flint should not think so."

Later Welch was to find out that many European scientists had been consulted. Willy Kühne, Cohnheim's teacher, had suggested Charles Scott Roy, a young Englishman, and Welch, adding that Cohnheim's opinion should be asked. Cohnheim thereupon wrote Gilman, stating in German that "the person best fitted for the chair of general pathology is Mr. Welch of New York. Welch indeed worked with me for a long time and I regard him as an acute as well as a thoughtful investigator." In announcing the appointment, Gilman was to say: "The trustees had the benefit of many counsellors in the medical profession, among whom it may be proper to name Professor Cohnheim." Welch, however, believed at the end of his life that although Cohnheim and von Recklinghausen had recommended him, his appointment had been really due to Billings.[4]

After his first interview with Gilman, Welch continued to his father: "I have not yet given a definite answer to the proposal, nor have I had time to speak about it to any one. The main attraction at the Johns Hopkins for me is the opportunity it gives me for investigation. It is undoubtedly the best opportunity in this country, with the exception that pathological material can not be abundant there, and certainly before the hospital is organized will be very scanty. I had much rather live in New York than in Baltimore, and from some points of view I am fortunately situated here. The field for teaching is vastly greater here, and perhaps I have been as successful as a teacher as in anything. I do not think that I should better myself pecuniarily by going to Baltimore. I did not learn definitely what the salary is to be . . . but I think probably at first about $3,000.

"But with all the pleasant associations and acquaintances in New York, and notwithstanding the wide circle which I reach in teaching and in my pathological work, I do not feel as if I was accomplishing what I want to do. My energies are split up in too many different directions and are likely to be so long as I remain here. In Baltimore everything would be quieter, more academic; I should be expected to give myself up mostly to original work, to renounce practice altogether. I should be equipped with everything which I want in the way of a laboratory. If I accept the offer I should expect to go abroad this summer and to remain a year preparing myself for the work, taking up especially cultivation of bacteria, comparative and experimental pathology, the fields which it is desired to cultivate especially in Baltimore.

"Somehow or other I feel depressed rather than elated over the prospect. The responsibilities are so great and so many pleasant associations must be broken. I also feel that Baltimore is a good deal farther from home than New York." None the less, Welch wrote, "I think that I shall accept the offer. What do you and mother think about it? What is your advice? I should like to see you and talk over the matter, but I do not see how I can get away just at present."

In a letter to his sister Welch pointed out that, since "the aim is to make the university a centre for research," he would be largely relieved of "the drudgery of teaching. . . . The choice seems to be between an academic, scholar's life with a chance to contribute somewhat to science, and the busy, restless, withal enticing life in New York. I have had a taste of the pleasures and comforts of New York life and they are not easy to relinquish. One who has lived here does not care to live elsewhere. But I suppose that I shall abandon Mammon and go to Baltimore. Still I have not come to a positive decision. I dread the interviews with Dennis and Dr. Flint."

Welch's dread was well founded. Both his friends felt that even to consider such an offer was madness. If only he would stay in New York, Flint gave him to understand, he might eventually succeed to his own position as a consultant; fame and fortune would then be his reward. In Baltimore he would become a mere scholar, rotting away in the provinces.

Dennis, who some ten years before had schemed to get Welch a Hopkins offer, now insisted that to accept it would be treason; he placed their friendship in the balance, saying that if Welch deserted New York and the Bellevue College, Welch would be deserting him in a manner any friend would consider perfidious. Promising that he would find Welch an equal opportunity in New York, Dennis hurried off to Andrew Carnegie and expounded so eloquently the importance of science and the brilliance of Welch that he returned with a promise of $50,000 to build at the Bellevue College a pathological laboratory, the first independent laboratory for medical research in the United States. A few days later the trustees of the college subscribed $45,000 dollars to buy land on which to erect the building.

When William Wickham arrived in town to advise his son, Dennis captured him. Three days after the Baltimore offer was made, the father wrote his son-in-law on Dennis's stationery backing up Dennis's plea that Stuart use his influence to keep Welch in New York. "If he goes," Dennis wrote, "he must sacrifice the friendships of a life and isolate himself in a provincial city among untried and inexperienced persons. . . . Our college has promised him everything, better facilities for teaching, better income, and will relieve him of certain work which he of necessity with others has had to assume. I can not listen a moment to his going and you know I would be the last one to stand in his way. I have been his true friend through thick and thin. . . . He has here a wide field of usefulness, he is here the leading man in New York and hence in America. If he chooses the way all his friends desire for him I know in ten years his income will be twenty thousand dollars and more as contrasted with a salary of ten thousand and then live a life in isolation, seclusion and in fact be a scientific recluse. His ideas imbibed in Germany are impractical in our form of government. He must cut himself aloof from everything in the way of sacred associations and of true friendships and of worldly emoluments for an ideal, which can not ever be realized."

A day later, on March 15, a prominent lawyer, Henry M. Alexander, whose sons had been Welch's pupils, wrote the young man that going to Baltimore "would be the mistake of your life." Having told Welch that his modesty perhaps kept him from recognizing that "it is not in a century that a man of your age has acquired the reputation which you have gained," he held out before Welch a brilliant future in New York, clinching his point by saying that that hard-headed business man, John A. Stewart, the president of the United States Trust Company, had asked him to tell Welch that "however bright the prospect is in Baltimore it is darkness compared with the career which is before him in such a city as New York."

Pressed from every side, Welch laid down conditions that would have to be met if he were to stay. Not only would he need the laboratory which had already been assured, but also the guarantee of a salary of $4000 for himself and of $1000 for an assistant. Since this would require an endowment fund, an unheard-of thing in New York, where medical professors had always been paid by students' fees and the increased practice their prominence brought them, Welch was sure it could not be raised; "pathology has not that importance in the present scheme of medical education in New York. Even if all my conditions are met," he continued, "I never can do the same quality of work here as in Baltimore, still if I can have anything comparable to the opportunities offered in Baltimore I should of course prefer to remain here. I have not been discontented before in New York, partly perhaps because it is not my nature to be, but now that something better presents itself I can not help considering the disadvantages of many of my circumstances of life. Whatever the outcome, at any rate there will be a decided improvement."

Dennis either did not understand Welch's conditions or pretended not to. Where Welch had demanded a salary paid by the college so that he could give all his time to teaching and research, Dennis insisted that Welch's condition was met by the fact that he could certainly earn more than $4000 a year by making pathological examinations for doctors and hospitals, by practising medicine, and taking fees from students. He said that if Welch went now he would be untrue to his word.

On March 28 Alexander wrote him: "I do not see that any alternative is left you. . . . Dr. Dennis is so certain as to what your conditions were—and that they have been fulfilled. I would kindly advise you that if you have any doubts yourself you should before taking any step leave the question to uninterested persons to decide them. It will be a serious matter for you to go from New York with a question like this remaining undecided in some authoritative way."

Meanwhile Welch had received a letter from George H. Williams, the geologist at the Hopkins, which, he wrote his father, "presents the matter in about the light in which I look at it." Williams wrote that although there was undoubtedly more money to be made in New York, "no place in America offers the real opportunity for true scientific work which this does. You have said the same thing to me yourself." Furthermore, as a full professor Welch would have, like the other full professors at the Hopkins, "literally perfect independence and everything for your work that you ask for." He would be able to organize the medical department from the very beginning and to build his laboratory exactly as he wished, thus becoming the founder of a new medical school. "It seems to me," Williams continued, "that it is an opportunity for giving a start and impetus to the spirit of real scientific work which is thus far so sadly lacking on this side of the Atlantic, which can come to a man only once in a lifetime."

With this vision in mind, Welch accepted the professorship on March 31, twenty days after it was offered him.[5] The New York medical profession was aghast; in all the annals of American medicine there had been no instance of so ambitious and able a young man exchanging a brilliant future in practice for an academic professorship in which the rewards were to be like the rewards of a German professor, with the difference of less opportunity for independent work and less remuneration. Welch remembered that some of his friends gave him a farewell dinner, saying: "Well, good-bye. You may become a connoisseur of terrapin and madeira, but as a pathologist, good-bye."

In notifying his father of his decision, Welch wrote that Dennis was insinuating "that my conditions have been complied with and that I do not stand by them." Welch had, however, consulted Alexander and Col. McCook, "two clear-headed lawyers," who had agreed that the necessary guarantee of salaries for himself and an assistant had not been met. "Of course a laboratory larger than the present one without means for running it and without a salary so guaranteed that I should not have to think how my bread and butter is to be earned would make my position worse rather than better than the present modest one. I feel convinced that I have decided for the best. . . .

"I begin with a salary of $4,000—the others mostly began with $3,000—I am the eighth full professor yet appointed in the history of the university. I am to have all of the paid associates and assistants I need, so that I can be the head and not the hands for everything. I do not have to pay the running expenses of the laboratory. I can develop my field in Baltimore unhampered by traditions. The surroundings are scholarly and academic, and of a much higher order than those of Bellevue College in my opinion, where I have never concealed that I did not sympathize with a great deal in the management and associations. The society in Baltimore is said to be very pleasant. It is a mistake to believe that a reputation made there would not equal one made in New York in my line of work. In practice of medicine of course it would not, but the results of research and discovery redound equally to one's reputation whether made in Oshkosh or in New York."

Welch believed that his stepmother, of whom he had so disapproved as a child, had understood his point of view better than other members of his family. To her he wrote: "I felt all of the time that you would have decided as I have done, although you did not even intimate your preference to me. I wish that all of the world were as sensible as you. . . .

"Such great things are expected of the medical faculty at the Johns Hopkins in the way of achievement and of reform of medical education in this country that I feel oppressed by the weight of responsibility. A reputation there will not be so cheaply earned as at Bellevue, but in so far the stimulus to do good work will be the greater. I shall be surrounded by cultivated, refined and distinguished men, who will estimate a man for his intrinsic worth and not for money or glitter.

"My eyes are opened to the fact that in my present position I was not supposed to have the control of my own life in my own hands. I have hardly spoken with Dr. Dennis since I returned from Baltimore. He evidently intends that our intercourse hereafter shall be merely formal. I grieve that a life-long friendship should thus come to an end, but I do not see with what I have to reproach myself, or why I should be preyed upon by remorse. I have no quarrel with him and, perhaps, he may come to take a more reasonable view of it all in the future. I am sure that he is sorely pained, and I am very sorry to make any one unhappy, even if without just cause. It hurts me to have him say that the conditions which I made were fulfilled and that I could not honorably leave, for this is absolutely false and I do not believe that any one who knows me will believe it. . . . It looks almost as if Dr. Dennis thought that he had a lien upon my whole future life. When he appealed to what he had done for me I told him that that was a subject which I would in no way discuss with him, nor did I care to hint that perhaps my association with him may not have been altogether without benefit to him. I hope that I may never ask any one to do anything for me because I have conferred benefits on him, real or imagined."

Welch continued to his father on April 9 that Dennis's behaviour had made it even clearer to him that he should accept the Baltimore offer, which was "something of a deliverance from oppressive and compromising environments here. . . . I doubt not that he intends, if it is in his power, to make me repent my decision." Dennis would make every effort to build up a fine pathological laboratory with the money raised to keep Welch in New York, "and in these respects I certainly hope that his efforts, even if not actuated by the highest motives, will prosper. I am told that both he and Mrs. Dennis say that my success is entirely due to Dr. Dennis, and that now I show a very ungrateful disposition. I do not think that any talk of this kind can harm me in New York, where perhaps the relations between Fred and me have been differently interpreted by medical men. I of course have not mentioned to any one that our relations do not continue cordial."

Five months later Welch received on the steamer that was taking him to Germany for a year's additional study a letter, which Dennis asked him to burn, formally breaking off their friendship. Welch replied: "I reciprocate in every respect your expressions of affection. It can not be other than a source of grief to me that you should deem my course such as to warrant a rupture of the intimate friendly relations which had hitherto existed between us. . . . After all I see at the bottom of our trouble evidence of your affection and this moves me. Will you not believe that I did what seemed to me the best and highest thing to do, even if you consider that I am mistaken? It does not seem to me possible that our friendship is not to be renewed, and I think that I read between the lines of your letter that the same idea is in your mind. It will always be a pleasure to me to hear of your success, of the continuance and increase of which I entertain not the slightest doubt."

Welch was deeply disillusioned by the rift. Never again, never during fifty brilliant years of association with the great of the earth, did he allow any man or woman to get close enough to him to hurt him as Dennis had done. He liked some of his associates better than others, it is true, but it is clear that he never told anyone, except perhaps the immediate members of his family, those intimate secret thoughts whose exchange is the basis of true friendship. Surrounded always with people, popular, adept at swaying men, the bachelor scientist moved on a high plane of loneliness that may have held some of the secret of his power.

Maybe the full force of his disillusionment did not strike Welch till the quiet days of his ocean crossing, for he was so busy in New York that he was forced to put off his sailing again and again. He did some writing for Flint and for William Pepper's *System of Medicine;* [6] he found a partner for his ageing father, after several false starts hitting on his classmate John C. Kendall, who was to stay in Norfolk all his life; he closed up his affairs in New York and sent to Baltimore fourteen boxes of the pathological specimens he had for years been filing away in fruit jars. At Gilman's request he drew up a plan for the new department of pathology in Baltimore, stating that opportunity should be afforded for the study of all branches of the subject, including investigation of the diseases of animals which would be "of interest not only in themselves but also in the light which they shed upon many human diseases." Every facility should be supplied, he continued, for making experimental studies like those of Pasteur and Koch concerning "the share taken by micro-organisms in the causation of diseases. . . . I deem it fortunate that I can devote myself to these researches before beginning active work in the University."

When on September 20 Welch sailed at last for Germany it was the first step in an adventure that was in many ways the realization of his dream.

CHAPTER VIII

The Revelation of Bacteriology

"I AM convinced that for some years the relation of micro-organisms to the causation of disease is to be the most important subject in pathology," Welch wrote Gilman from Leipzig. "I have therefore endeavored to make myself thoroughly familiar with the present methods of investigation in this department, and I hope that we shall be in every way qualified to carry on bacteriological studies successfully at the Johns Hopkins University."

During the half-dozen years Welch had taught in New York, bacteriology under the stimulus of Koch's discoveries had made great advances, yielding knowledge of the causation of such severe diseases as Asiatic cholera, diphtheria, typhoid fever, tetanus, to mention a few examples only. Welch had been forced to stand on the sidelines of this growing movement, since his resources at Bellevue had barely sufficed for the teaching of pathology; bacteriology requires technical equipment far exceeding a few microscopes, a microtome for cutting sections, some staining fluids, and some fruit jars to hold pathological specimens. Once he had begun his studies of micro-organisms in Germany, he did not regret that facilities had previously been denied him. "I am glad," he wrote, "that I did not attempt to dabble at the subject in New York, for I might have made as melancholy a failure of my cultivations and experiments as Formad. The methods can be learned only by personal observation in a laboratory."

When the opportunity had come to him to spend a year abroad before entering on his new duties at Baltimore, Welch had fixed his heart on actually studying with Koch himself in Berlin. The master of the new revelation received him kindly, but explained that his laboratory, which was not really intended for instruction, belonged to the war department; permission to study there must be received from the minister of war. He advised Welch to go to Munich, where one of his pupils, Wilhelm Frobenius, was at that moment concluding the first public course in bacteriology given anywhere in the world. Having written Gilman for an introduction to the American Minister, who he hoped would intercede with the war ministry on his behalf, Welch set out for Munich.

In November he enrolled in Frobenius's second course, but his high expectations were soon cast down. The professor, he wrote, "had rather a narrow horizon. He had evidently taken down practically every word Koch had ever said; and he read them to us and made us do everything precisely as Koch had done it—even to holding the test tube exactly as Koch had held it." Although it covered the ground, this slavish learning by rote failed fully to absorb Welch's active mind.

Throughout his long life Welch was a wanderer into laboratories—a very welcome and inspiring one he was to become; his stay in Munich was no exception. At the pathological laboratory of Otto Bollinger, where Frobenius's course was given, he observed autopsies and other work. He also visited the laboratory of the veterinary school under Theodor Kitt, one of the best in Germany: "The material is so abundant here that in a comparatively short time I have learned a great deal of the diseases of animals, more particularly those which are related to human diseases, such as tuberculosis." Then Welch worked in the famed hygienic laboratory of Max von Pettenkofer and discovered how methods of sanitary reform and purification of soil and water had almost abolished typhoid fever, once very prevalent in Munich; cases had to be imported to show the students. And in the hospital he saw under Hugo Wilhelm von Ziemssen a laboratory for the investigation of disease in the living patient that equalled the laboratories designed to study autopsies and other dead materials. These experiences, as we shall see, were to have a very important influence on his career.

Welch made friends with a brilliant young fellow-student, Angelo Celli, who was later to make important discoveries in connexion with the malarial parasite of Laveran. Together the two young men enjoyed the life of Munich, which Welch considered "one of the pleasantest as it certainly is one of the cheapest of German cities. The opera is produced here with great splendor in the largest opera-house in Germany. . . . The cafés are filled all day and throughout the evening with people who seem to be having a good time. Even the princes here seem to be happy and with modest pretensions. I was introduced the other evening to the nephew of the King, Prince Carl Ludwig, who seemed to be the most unpretentious of mortals. He is a young man about twenty-five years old who amuses himself by studying medicine. He has fitted up in one of the royal palaces a laboratory for studying bacteria."

After less than two months in Munich, Welch travelled to Vienna, Budapest, and Prague, where there were laboratories whose equipment he wished to study. To his delight, he found that the Johns Hopkins was so well known to all the professors that they received him eagerly and helped him whenever they could.

Then Welch settled down in Leipzig to work with Ludwig and with Weigert, Cohnheim's brilliant assistant who had come to Leipzig when Cohnheim was made professor there. "He has given the lectures on pathology since Cohnheim's death," Welch wrote, "and had every reason to expect an appointment as professor, but the nominations of the faculty have just been made and among the three names presented Weigert's is not mentioned. It is a terrible outrage as Weigert is unquestionably one of the leading pathologists living, but he is a Jew and it seems that no Jew is likely to get an appointment in a German university. He speaks some of going to America and inquired what chance there was of his obtaining any place in New York."

Despite his depression, Weigert gave Welch some instruction in staining bacteria. Welch used to tell how on one occasion his teacher asked him to dinner. Finding the fare of a German scientist too frugal, Welch thanked his host for a delightful meal and hurried to a near-by restaurant. No sooner had Welch begun to eat a large steak than Weigert, who liked to read the newspapers over a cup of coffee, walked in.

Welch called on "the widow of my beloved teacher Prof. Cohnheim who died last August. . . . She related to me how often and how pleasantly he had spoken of me even during his last illness, and how while he was very ill and suffering greatly he dictated to her the letter to President Gilman which secured my appointment as professor at the Johns Hopkins University. . . . He would not give up his lectures and it is pitiful to hear how he was carried to the university . . . when every one could see that he was nearly in the grave. . . ." Welch later took advantage of the sale of Cohnheim's library to buy books for the Johns Hopkins.

The strength of Cohnheim's influence on Welch was shown when the American returned to Ludwig's laboratory. During his first period there, nine years before, Welch had asked Ludwig to give him a problem with the microscope, since his major interest had been in the description of dead pathological matter rather than in experimentation concerning the functions of the living body. Now he came to Ludwig because "since Cohnheim's death there is no prominent teacher of general [experimental] pathology in Europe, so that I think that I can profit more by work in physiological laboratories where much experimentation is done than in strictly pathological laboratories. . . . Experimental physiology is the basis of experimental pathology. Cohnheim's superiority as an experimental pathologist was largely due to his training under Ludwig. I feel that I could not find a better opportunity to become familiar with experimental methods and such instruments of precision as I shall need."

Ludwig assigned Welch a problem that grew out of the work on œdema he had done with Cohnheim. The increase in blood pressure in the artery that leads to the lungs had been so instantaneous when Welch paralysed the left ventricle of the heart that Welch had believed the pulmonary arteries differed from the other arteries of the body in that they lacked the vasomotor nerves which modify the blood flow by expanding or contracting the vessels. Doubting this, Ludwig directed him in experiments especially aimed at determining the matter. Welch arrived at no convincing conclusion, and curiously enough the point has remained a debated one. The weight of opinion today, however, is that in the dog the controlling nerves exist in the blood vessels.

Ludwig was pleased with Welch's researches on the problem, as is shown by a note he wrote to Welch on August 5: "One more greeting on European soil. Since your departure I have become lazy and have excised only a few veins and arteries from the lungs of a dog. They are in the glass tube sent herewith—the arteries are on top of the cotton and the veins below. If you make preparations of this material you will be astonished at the wealth of the muscle structure. How grateful I am to you for the elucidation that I have received through your investigations of the lung!"

Success was now dogging the young man's footsteps. Early in January he received from Dr. Loomis, who had so recently derided his interest in bacteriology, an offer of the professorship of anatomy at the University Medical College in New York. "We will add to it that of Pathological Anatomy, with the direction of our new Biological Laboratory. I shall resign my position in Bellevue Hospital within a few years and you shall be my successor. . . . New York is the place for you. I am confident that you will never be happy in the restrictions of such a place as Baltimore. You can now relieve yourself of your obligations to the Johns Hopkins University without discredit."

Welch was not tempted, although he wrote his father: "I suppose that I shall be considered crazy by many in New York for declining such an offer." He knew that hardly a better opportunity could be desired for securing local influence in New York, but his German experiences had shown him that the Hopkins "already has a European reputation while our New York medical schools are not even known by name." Furthermore, "I really prefer the quiet and scholarly surroundings of the Johns Hopkins to the more brilliant but distracting life of a professor in any of the New York medical schools as now organized."

In Leipzig, Welch was happily pursuing a scholarly routine. "One day," he wrote his stepmother, "is about the same as another. After my coffee at half past eight I go to Prof. Ludwig's lecture from nine to ten, then work in the laboratory until one, then go to a rather frugal but substantial dinner and then renew

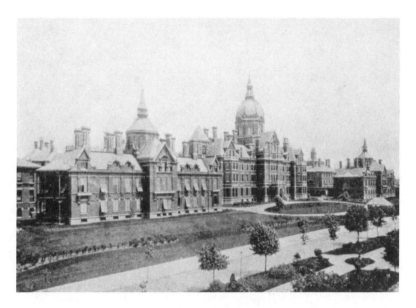

Johns Hopkins Hospital, 1889

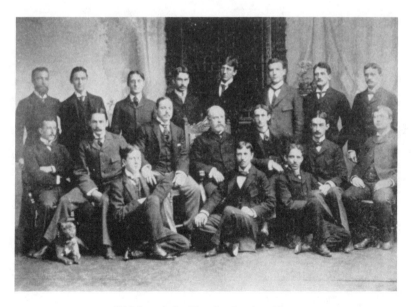

Welch and the First Graduating Class

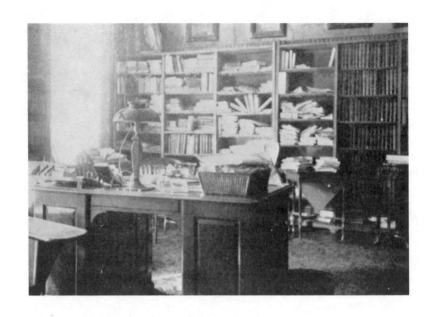

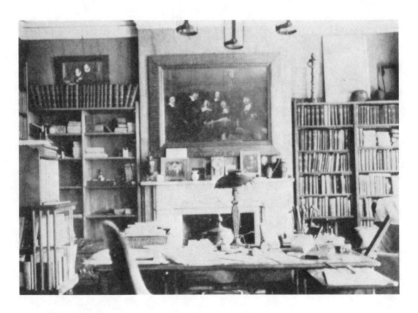

Welch's Rooms

my laboratory work until five when the laboratory closes. I usually then attend a lecture on logic to fill up the hour from five to six. The subject is presented in an entirely new and very interesting manner. In the evening I sometimes go to the theatre or make a call on some American or German friend, rarely the latter as one must be very intimate to call in the evening in Germany, or visit a café and read the newspapers. I take my dinner at the house of two old ladies who are quite delightful. They are very intelligent, and very simple and German in their ways. One is the widow of a German pastor and the other is an old maid. . . .

"During the Messe or Fair which has recently closed I was attracted to a tent over which a large American flag waved. I found that there was there exhibited 'the new American bed.' Among the various contrivances about it were the following: a bell rings by electricity at a given time to wake you up; if you do not get up in a few minutes the room is suddenly illuminated by an electric light and a music box begins to play in the bedstead, then the clothes are pulled off from the bed by electricity and at last you are forcibly thrown out of the bed on the floor if you longer resist. If you have not already heard of the new bed I fear that this account will lead you to invest in several for your family, especially your summer family."

Such light passages, so usual in the letters he wrote during his first German trip, are now rare; Welch concerned himself almost exclusively with serious things. Not only did he carry the responsibility of helping organize America's first scientific medical school, but he was also deeply concerned about his father, who was suffering from glaucoma and was threatened with blindness; everywhere he went, Welch sought out leading oculists, cross-questioned them, and wrote home long, carefully prepared expositions.

Early in February Welch received from Gilman a letter signed by F. T. Frelinghuysen, the Secretary of State, asking the American Minister to help Welch get into Koch's laboratory; Welch hurried to Berlin. Koch, however, told him confidentially: "I shall leave here at the end of this semester. It has not been publicly announced, but I have accepted the professorship of hygiene in the university [of Berlin], and there I shall have my laboratory; the courses will be open to everybody and you would not have to go through all this official formality." He added that the three vacant places in his present work shop had all been promised.

There was nothing for Welch to do but return to Leipzig and wait for the new laboratory to open. But he could not contain his eagerness to learn more bacteriology; during a vacation period he went to Göttingen, where one of Koch's pupils, Karl Flügge, had just opened a course in the new science. Welch remembered that, in contradistinction to Frobenius, Flügge "was a very excellent teacher indeed. He gathered together men from all over the world, and in his laboratory were almost as many foreigners as Germans—names that are very familiar indeed in the bacteriological world." Welch was invited several times to the professor's house and enjoyed studying an exciting subject with excited and brilliant young scientists. "The other evening all of the workers in the laboratory, about twenty, invited Prof. Flügge and his assistants to quite a sumptious dinner in the principal hotel here. I was obliged to make the first speech and to bring the toast to Prof. Flügge. It is sufficiently hard for me to make a speech in English, and as a German orator I should not make much of a living. The party broke up about one o'clock, all able to find their way home."

Returning to Leipzig early in April, Welch hoped to stay only a few weeks, since Koch had said his new laboratory would open in June. As it showed no signs of opening, he posted on May 24 for England to spend some of the $2000 the Hopkins had appropriated for physiological instruments.[1] When a few years before he had been an unknown young student, the coldness of the British had inspired him to one of the few bitter letters of his career; now he was an accredited professor in an exciting new medical school; now everything was changed. He considered the horse-race he saw at Epsom Downs "the greatest sight which I have ever witnessed," and he could "imagine nothing more charming" than Cambridge University, where he was received "with almost embarrassing hospitality" by the professors, among whom was Roy, who had also studied with Cohnheim and been recommended for the Hopkins post. Welch dined at Trinity College at the same table as Prince Albert Victor, "the future king of England," and bought "considerable apparatus" from the Cambridge Scientific Company. "I was never among a more refined and cultivated set of people than those Fellows and Professors at Cambridge," he wrote. "It was 'sweetness and light,' but on the whole sweetness preponderated. The light of science burns more brightly here in Germany."

In his high spirits Welch determined to bring England as well as America more light; with a headlong enthusiasm usually alien to his character he embarked on one of the few impractical adventures of his career. With Roy he prepared the prospectus of a pathological journal to be jointly edited, although neither of the young men had in his own right more than crossed the threshold of the subject, and neither of their countries boasted enough scientific work to fill the pages of the most modest journal. The two enthusiasts even made arrangements with a publisher, but the scheme eventually fell through.

Back in London, Welch had the pleasure of impressing his old superior, Janeway, who was making "his first journey abroad." Welch took him to Oxford, where Professor Burdon Sanderson, whom Ludwig considered the best physiologist in England, "devoted himself to us without interruption throughout our entire stay. . . . I was rather glad for him [Janeway] to see what an introduction it is on this side of the water to be a professor in the Johns Hopkins University. . . . Dr. Janeway quite amuses me with his fresh American way of looking at everything. His constant remark is, 'Well, nobody in America would submit to that.' This applies to everything from the seats the medical students have to sit on over here to the candles in the hotel rooms."

After three delightful weeks in England, Welch returned to Germany. He does not seem to have stopped off in Paris; he wrote to his mother: "There is nothing especial of a scientific nature to lead me there." This is an amazing statement when we remem-

ber that Pasteur was in Paris. Having already developed inoculation for chicken cholera and anthrax, Pasteur was just completing his investigation of rabies. Although the announcement
of his dramatic inoculation of the Alsatian lad Joseph Meister
was not made until Welch had returned to Baltimore, his successful results with dogs had been published early in 1884, and
should have been read by Welch. It is hard to account for the
eager scientist's lack of interest in Pasteur's laboratory, unless it
be that the Frenchman's work was underestimated by Welch's
German teachers for nationalistic reasons. Later, of course,
Welch did full justice to Pasteur's career, and as an old man he
even persuaded himself—though almost certainly without justi-
fication—that he had met the great Frenchman.[2]

The only mention in Welch's letters of a call on Pasteur was
made five years later. In 1890 Welch wrote Mall: "I visited the
Pasteur Institute but everybody was away and no work was being
done except in the rabies vaccinations. Seventy persons were
undergoing the treatment the day I was there. The best part of
the place are the arrangements for keeping animals."

Comparing the contributions to bacteriology of Pasteur and
Koch, Welch said in 1911 that Koch gave the science "its first
exact and fruitful methods of research, and so gave to physicians
and investigators the key to unlock the secrets of the most important diseases of mankind—the infectious diseases. . . . Koch,
then, was the first to demonstrate conclusively that a given micro-
organism is the specific cause of the infectious diseases; and he
was also the first to give conclusive evidence that we can divide
the bacteria into definite species, for he was the first to work out
the complete cyclic life of a bacterial species." Pasteur, having
been concerned with fermentation and the disproof of spontaneous generation, "did not apply himself to the study of infectious
diseases until after Koch did." None the less, Welch admitted
that his was "in some ways a greater name than Koch's. . . .
Pasteur's name will always be identified with the development of
our knowledge of immunity, and particularly with the process
of preventing the spread of infection by inoculation."

Having hurried through Paris, Welch paused to examine

scientific institutions in Strasbourg, Heidelberg, and Frankfurt. Then he waited a few more weeks at Leipzig before the opening of Koch's new laboratory in Berlin enabled him to enrol in the first public course on bacteriology the founder of the science ever gave. It lasted only for the month of July, but remained one of the most cherished memories of his career.

The work itself, as he wrote President Gilman, was largely a repetition of what he had studied with Frobenius and Flügge, but Welch always considered it important for a young man to meet the outstanding personalities of medicine. When in later years his more favoured disciples set out on their *Reisejahre,* he would tell them not to tie themselves down by attempting research in a single laboratory—they could work on problems in America. He would give them letters of introduction and say: "You must get into contact with the great teachers. Then you will have an impression of the men and their work which you will never forget, and every time you read their writings you will remember. Everything will be much more vivid to you."

Welch wrote: "We were, of course, thrown in close daily association with Koch. He was in every way most approachable and affable—indeed in those days he was one of the most simpleminded, unaffected men imaginable. It was a rare opportunity! About once every two weeks he would come and sit with a small group of us about a little table at a restaurant and would join us in refreshment. Indeed, you cannot imagine anyone more approachable in every way. He was not very talkative, but he told a story well and he had a good deal of dry wit and humor. It is said, it is true, that later, in consequence of unfortunate experiences, he became somewhat unapproachable and suspicious of others, but I confess I am very much surprised at this, for I found him unchanged when he came to this country, and only a year before he died when I was in Berlin I spent an hour with him in his laboratory and he was most cordial in his reception. . . . He was a man, I think, of a singularly attractive and agreeable personality, though I cannot claim having had any real intimacy with him."

When Koch discussed the bacillus that causes Asiatic cholera, the young men felt they were taking part in a romantic crusade to save Europe. The disease had started on its fifth recorded migration around the world. It came up from the East, reached Alexandria in Egypt, paused for a moment on the southern shores of the Mediterranean, and leapt to the south of France. In 1883 Koch had met it in Egypt and India, where he had isolated the so-called comma bacillus and determined its mode of origin and transmission. Deeply impressed with the danger of a European epidemic, he did not trust himself to bring with him to Berlin the cultures he had isolated, but preferred to destroy them lest by inadvertence they should gain access to food or water. When, however, cholera appeared in France, the circumstances not only justified but compelled the training of a small army of bacteriologists to recognize the germ so that they could combat the plague. Koch hurried to Toulon, secured the germs from an autopsy, and hid them in a test tube in his pocket. Welch loved to repeat after Koch the story of how he was detained for fumigation at the German border. Koch, according to Welch, "was always much amused at the idea of going through the whole process of fumigation with living cholera germs unsealed in a tube in his pocket."

The dread cultures remained locked up in the innermost recesses of his laboratory, whence only the master brought them with his own hands. Welch, who was making a collection of cultures to take back to the Hopkins, was not cast down when Koch refused to give him any cholera bacilli, for he had already obtained some from Flügge. "Dr. Prudden had them also," he remembered; "and I have often wondered whether Koch suspected us, for one evening when I had been looking at my cultures, Koch as he sat and talked with us remarked that it would be better a man had never been born if he introduced a disease germ into a region where it previously had not existed—suppose they escaped—suppose it could be traced to an accident in the laboratory—better that man had never been born!"

Welch spent a sleepless night. At dawn he rose from bed, unlocked his bureau, and took out the test tube in which was imprisoned the scourge of cholera. Having poured on a solution of bichloride of mercury to kill the germs, he hurried through the silent streets to drop them in the river. At last he reached a bridge; he put his hand into his pocket, but there the hand stopped. A figure with his hat over his eyes and his head down was approaching through the otherwise empty city. Welch stared innocently at the water, but when the footsteps had come so close that he could not resist looking up, he recognized the intruder; it was Prudden engaged on the same errand as his own. Each must have laughed, feeling both foolish and relieved; then both threw their cultures into the Spree. They expected, of course, to see the tubes sink immediately out of sight, instead of which they had the disquieting experience of observing them bobbing up and down as they floated slowly down the stream. The guilty pair hurried away just, it is said, as a large *Schutzman* appeared on the scene. "That," Welch continued, "was long before there was any outbreak of Asiatic cholera in Berlin." [3]

After Koch's course was over, Welch spent a few days in Copenhagen, partly, as he wrote, "by way of sightseeing and partly to visit Dr. Salomonsen, an old Breslau friend." He sailed for New York on August 12, 1885. During the long, monotonous days on shipboard he must often have thought of the contrast between this return to America and his return seven years before. Then he had been girded for battle against an environment hostile to what he wanted to do; now there lay at his feet the greatest opportunity ever enjoyed by an American disciple of scientific medicine. But perhaps this was the more difficult of the homecomings, for the responsibilities were so great. If he failed now, he would have only himself to blame.

CHAPTER IX

Laboratory Years

I

"I AM very sure that I have done wisely in coming to Baltimore and I know that I shall be happy and contented here," Welch wrote his father on October 11, 1885. During his first few weeks at the Hopkins he had seen the two dreams that had successively dominated his ambition merge into one and come true. At Yale he had wanted to be a professor, a power in the quiet and learned halls of academic life. Although in New York he had taught, it had been in a bustling trade school in America's most commercial city. The rumble of traffic, the hoofbeats of horses whipped to go faster than their rivals, were for ever in his ears, and within the walls of the school itself he found the clash of fierce ambitions, struggling for practice, for place, for fame. Now all the noise had died away.

Moving with measured steps in an academic procession, Welch had marched from President Gilman's rooms to the Academy of Music to take part in the opening exercises of the university. As he sat on the stage, scholars not hurried practitioners were grouped around him. Canon Farrar of Westminster Cathedral was the speaker; his address, Welch wrote his stepmother, "proved to be a great treat. It was one of the most eloquent, scholarly and finished speeches to which I have ever listened. His delivery was admirable and his voice rich and sonorous. He treated in a broad way of the subject of education and with such tact as to give equal satisfaction to classical, scientific and religious scholars. Pres. Gilman in his opening remarks referred in a very pleasant way to my appointment and presence."

Thus was the dream of Welch's young manhood realized, the dream of the youth who had wanted to be professor of Greek. But this dream had been superseded by another when failure to get an academic appointment had forced him to follow the hereditary profession of medicine. In foreign universities, he had seen the vision of a scholar's medicine, based on sequestered and rational intellect rather than the bustle of pragmatism and earning a living. Laboratories had become the back-drop of his imaginings, laboratories full of microscopes and instruments of precision and above all of young men eager to advance knowledge. As he sat on the stage and listened to Canon Farrar's address, he knew that this vision too was about to be realized.

"There could hardly be a greater contrast to my life in New York. . . . The university authorities seem to have been afraid to make any arrangements for me before I arrived. They seem willing to do anything which I suggest and leave everything to my discretion. . . . I am expected to give advice and make suggestions as to the whole organization of the medical school, and for the present I seem to be more an advisory than a teaching body." Since his assistant, Dr. William T. Councilman, made many autopsies, "I presume that I shall devote myself in greatest part to experimental pathology and bacteriology."

At thirty-five Welch had found himself a place in the world that was perfect to his needs and desires. For many years a genie confined in a bottle, he rose up, once the cork was pulled, into his true dimensions, and for almost fifty years he was to tower over American medicine, determining, creating, helping change a backward profession into a leading profession of his time. Moving in a highly controversial field toward revolutionary ends, he was always gentle, never raising his voice above the tone of ordinary talk. He won campaign after campaign but never fought a battle; haste was unknown to him, or anger or the exuberant joy of putting an opponent down. He was to win affection and admiration until he became, first to his associates and then to younger scientists everywhere, in common parlance the beloved "Popsy."

I I

When he arrived in Baltimore, Welch found that he had been temporarily assigned three small rooms in Professor Martin's laboratory, but by November 1 a "commodious two-story build-ing," originally designed for a dead house, had been made over according to his specifications. "My quarters," he wrote his sister, "now are certainly a great contrast to my so-called laboratory in New York, and I am sure the laboratory ought to produce some good work." The nature of the equipment that so pleased Welch will seem strange to contemporary scientists who think in terms of tens of thousands of dollars, for by the end of his first academic year in Baltimore Welch had spent for library, apparatus (in-cluding his kymograph), materials, heat, and janitor service, approximately $3000.[1]

Although systematic instruction in pathology did not begin until the following year, Welch and his assistants worked all winter in the laboratory that was being completed around them, and in February Welch began a series of nine public lectures on bacteriology, the first comprehensive ones ever given in this country.[2] They were, he wrote, "quite fully attended, especially by physicians in Baltimore. It is the most intelligent and critical audience which I have ever had to address."

In June he outlined to Gilman his plans for beginning system-atic instruction the following year. He was to teach "pathological histology" in collaboration with Councilman; "demonstrations of gross pathological specimens" and "methods of post-mortem examinations" were to be given by Councilman alone; and he himself was to give "lectures on the general pathology of fever" and a course in bacteriology, concerning which he said: "So far as I know no similar course is given in this country and only three or four in Europe. . . . It may be mentioned that these courses embrace all which it is customary to give, even in German universities, in the department of Pathology, and in fact all which are required for a thorough training in Pathology." Welch was eager to have it made known "that the laboratory is ready for the reception of those who wish to engage in any special re-search in Pathology"; he thought "the bestowal of one or more fellowships" would help, since "a properly selected fellow" would do research "which will be valuable and when published will do much to establish the reputation of the laboratory."

Welch had to return to Germany before this programme could be carried out. In all America, only he and Prudden were working in bacteriology; when some of his cultures died, he appealed to Prudden, who was often in the same dilemma, but Prudden was unable to supply all he needed. Not on this side of the Atlantic could he secure the specimens of bacteria necessary for instruction. After a brief visit to Norfolk, during which he engaged in a highly successful water-lily hunt with his nephew, Welch spent a month in Berlin where, during their master's absence, Koch's assistants gave him the cultures he desired.

In October formal instruction in pathology began at the Hopkins; the following May Welch reported jubilantly that twenty-six medical graduates, all trained in normal histology, had made use of his laboratory, and that eight had undertaken original investigations. Sternberg had studied the thermic death point of bacteria; Booker the bacteriology of the stools in summer diarrhœa of children; Abbott the behaviour of bacteria in drinking water; Councilman the malarial parasite of Laveran; and Herter inflammation of the spinal cord (myelitis) experimentally produced. Coming from New York in December 1886, Halsted had co-operated with Mall, the first fellow, on evolving methods of sewing up wounds in the intestine; Mall, who had studied the structure of the intestinal wall in Ludwig's laboratory, made the important suggestion that the fibrous or submucous coat of the intestine should be used to hold the stitch. Welch himself had begun his work on experimental glomerulonephritis (a pathological condition of the kidney) in Bright's disease, and, in association with Mall, on hæmorrhagic infarction (local death of an organ caused by obstruction of a blood vessel) in the intestine. Walking past eager young men engaged in investigations of their own to the table where his own investigations awaited him, Welch must have felt his heart flood with satisfaction.

Life in Baltimore he also found most agreeable. The Southerners, always hospitable, received him warmly and were charmed in return; soon he was writing his sister: "I accepted five dinner invitations in succession, some being very handsome affairs. I attended recently a beautiful reception at the Bonapartes. This is rather more gayety than I care for." Whenever there was a distinguished visitor to entertain, Baltimoreans almost automatically invited Welch. "I am enjoying immensely the lectures of Prof. Jebb, of Cambridge, England, on Greek poetry. . . . I have been invited four times to meet him at dinner."

Since Welch was a bachelor, the Baltimoreans went out of their way at first to introduce him to their most agreeable young ladies. At the importuning of a mutual friend Welch called during those early days at the stately James mansion, the home of four beautiful daughters. After he had been seated in the front parlour, he was announced in the next room where the charmers sat, all four of them, waiting in their best finery for such callers as fate might bring. On hearing Welch's name they were alarmed; "we were not erudite young ladies," one of them explained, and the professor had the reputation of being so wise. Each told the other it was her duty to go in and entertain him, but all demurred. This caused a dispute; voices grew higher until Welch, sitting alone in the formal front room, could not but have heard. Was he amused or embarrassed or both? We do not know, but we do know that when one of the young ladies was finally pushed through the door by her sisters and came forward armed with her most charming smile, Welch's conversation was a little constrained and he left almost immediately. The belle returned to her sisters and reported that Welch was "stocky in build and not at all handsome."

After this same young lady had reached a riper age and become Mrs. J. Hemsley Johnson, she and Welch grew to admire each other; he sometimes induced her to entertain visiting celebrities whom he wished to impress with Baltimore. Welch preferred the society of women who had reached the age of wisdom to that of even the loveliest young girls. But he never developed the platonic intimacy with a mature married woman that is typical of so many bachelors. In the mass of papers and reminiscences that have come down to us there is no indication that Welch ever permitted any woman outside his immediate family to come closer to him than semi-formal friendship.

From the first, Welch's life in Baltimore was that of a confirmed bachelor who knew how to make himself comfortable. On his arrival he rented for $35 a month two large furnished rooms on the third floor of 20 Cathedral Street. His landlady was Mrs. Thomas Simmons, the widow of a Maryland gentleman farmer and Civil War major who had left her in reduced circumstances. Twice Welch moved with the Simmons family, once to 935 and again to 807 St. Paul Street. When Mrs. Simmons died, her unmarried daughter took over; she was among the few people who dared scold Welch. Before leaving the Maryland Club after a late dinner, Welch once discovered that he had forgotten his key and would have to awaken Miss Simmons to get in. For a moment he was nonplussed; then with a twinkle in his eye he made a bouquet of the flowers that had been a centrepiece on the table. His landlady appeared in her dressing gown in answer to repeated pressure on the bell, but Welch thrust the bouquet under her nose before she had time to open her mouth. This stopped the flow of words long enough for Welch to get to his room unscathed.

No sooner had Welch settled with the Simmons family than he began building a personal library which, although not exclusively medical, soon became the best reference library in Baltimore; a Hopkins student who could not find a book there had to go to the Surgeon General's Library in Washington. When during 1889 Welch's front room caught fire in his absence, "there were," he wrote his father, "1090 books in the room, not including many unbound ones and pamphlets. In the bedroom there were a large number of books and pamphlets not injured." Welch was sorry about the ruined furniture, of course, but what really worried him was that the insurance company might not allow him enough money to rebind the books that had been covered with soot. He carefully picked a representative who "appreciates the value of a good binding."

Welch soon found that the plans for the Hopkins medical school were not popular with the doctors of Baltimore. The avowed intention of importing the best possible medical professors from wherever they could be found ran counter to the long-established American tradition that a medical institution make use of the leading practitioners in its city. The disappointed local profession feared that the competition of the newcomers would reduce their prosperity; they were unable to foresee that the Hopkins would help everyone by making Baltimore a medical centre of the nation.

They did not, however, particularly object to Welch, since he was concerned with the unremunerative field of pathology and showed no desire to practise. Furthermore, Welch's assistant, Councilman, was well known and liked in Baltimore. A graduate of the University of Maryland, he was pathologist to Bay View Hospital, a position which enabled him to secure the pathological material needed for the courses at the Hopkins. Welch remembered that Councilman purchased a tricycle in which to transport the specimens across the city, and that he had "occasional accidents which even got into the newspapers."

In his quiet, unassuming way Welch took advantage of every opportunity to be friendly with the local profession; soon he was able to report: "I have been very pleasantly received by the medical men in Baltimore, a very large number of whom have called on me, and have invited me to their houses." Asked to more medical meetings than he liked to attend, he was continually importuned to make addresses, and in April 1891 he was elected president of the state society, the Medical and Chirurgical Faculty of Maryland. Welch wrote his stepmother that President Gilman was "very much pleased" at this indication that "a certain feeling of jealousy and disappointment on the part of the medical profession of Baltimore . . . is dying out. . . . A banquet was given to me on Thursday evening by the members of the State Society and although I know I do not deserve half that was said I was impressed by the feeling of personal confidence and esteem which is worth having from those with whom your daily life is thrown."

Although serious financial difficulties in the Baltimore and Ohio Railroad, whose stock the university held, had postponed indefinitely the opening of the medical school, a faculty was gradually being built up which occupied itself in giving post-graduate courses to doctors who had studied elsewhere. Osler's appointment as professor of medicine is usually credited to Billings, but Welch said later that Billings had been opposed to the Canadian, whom he regarded as predominantly a laboratory man; Billings wished the appointment to go to the English physician Lauder Brunton,[3] since he was more experienced in the practice of medicine. Welch, however, insisted that physiological and pathological laboratories were the best training ground even for a professor of practice. When his support of Osler finally prevailed, he wrote his sister that the new appointee "is the best man to be found in the country and it is a great acquisition for us to secure him. I know him well and have the highest opinion of him as a scientist and as a man."

The authorities first offered the appointment in surgery to Sir William Macewen of Glasgow, who accepted, but, having no faith in anything American, made it a condition that he might bring his whole staff of nurses with him. When this was refused, the way was opened for Halsted, whom Welch had known well in New York. The last of "the four doctors," the famous first faculty of the Hopkins Medical School, was Howard Atwood Kelly, appointed associate professor of gynæcology and obstetrics in 1889. He was brought by Osler and thus could also be indirectly credited to Welch.

All during Welch's first years in Baltimore, plans were under discussion for organizing the Johns Hopkins Hospital, whose funds were still intact. A memorandum written by Dr. James Carey Thomas, one of the trustees of the university, shows that Welch would have liked Billings to be made director, although he knew that Billings "would expect a salary not only as Director of the Hospital, but as (full) Prof. of Hygiene in the Medical School, and maybe some other paying position." Thomas felt that Welch was too much under Billings's influence. "Dr. W. seemed to give me the impression that it was largely due to Dr. B. the idea of the Medical School as proposed by the University. I, on the contrary, showed Dr. W. that from the first Mr. Gilman and the trustees regarded the Medical School as an ultimate out-growth of the University scheme determined upon. . . .

"As I found that the subject had been discussed between Drs. W. and B.—I took pains to go over the history of the management and how much the good of the whole had been sought and how important it was to avoid cliques or personal preferences. . . . I found also that the general conduct of the University had been discussed and that the question of whether we ought not mainly to develop on the preliminary medical side in order to subordinate the rounded University to the Medical branch. I referred to what we had done—1st for Chemistry, 2nd for Biology and 3rd for Physics. He asked what was the use of teaching Sanscrit. I replied that it was an unoccupied field of great future promise—presided over by an illustrious and able teacher and gave fame and scholars to the University.

"We then spoke of the importance of subordinating everything to the interests of the University and the avoidance of cliques in the selection for the chairs in the Medical department. I found Dr. W. on the whole temperate and fair but largely imbued by Dr. B. with his ideas etc. etc., and I felt the importance of our acting with great caution in the matter or we shall be in the hands of a certain clique which have already divided the Profession in this country." [4]

No other evidence supports Thomas's implication that Welch and Billings formed a clique, although it is clear that Welch greatly valued the opinions of his elder. "I regard it as one of the greatest influences of my life to have known John Shaw Billings," Welch wrote. "Of all the men I have ever known, he was about the wisest. He was a man whose judgment one sought on any difficult subject, and one pinned one's faith to him more than to any man of one's acquaintance." During his last illness Welch told Barker "that he gradually became very intimate with Billings and that next to Weir Mitchell he was probably Billings' closest friend. Billings was a Brahmin; had no especial interest in the general run of people, but picked up a few friends to whom he devoted himself intensely."

The hospital trustees, unable to complete any organization

themselves, appointed Gilman temporary director in February 1889; Welch accompanied him on a trip "inspecting New York hospitals and meeting medical men." On May 7, the hospital opened, and by August Welch was able to write Mall: "The number of patients surpasses all anticipations and Halsted (popularly known in hospital circles as Jack the Ripper) does nothing but operate the whole forenoon and it must be admitted with brilliant results."

The atmosphere in which Welch lived now grew more medical; graduate students came in greater numbers, filling his laboratory. Dr. Loomis of New York, who had once been so outspoken on Welch's idiocy in going to Baltimore, sent his son, and the Surgeon General sent Major Walter Reed, later of yellow fever fame, who studied under Welch and did research on the lymphoid nodules of the liver in typhoid fever. The Hospital Medical Society and the Historical Club began; Welch attended regularly and, with Osler, had a most enlivening effect on the proceedings. Indeed, the first superintendent of the hospital, Dr. Henry M. Hurd,[5] was to say that the tone of Welch's laboratory determined the tone of the whole institution, since it was the nucleus from which the rest grew; because of this influence, "a general spirit of research" characterized the hospital, which developed "a fine esprit de corps. Clinicians and laboratory men were living together under circumstances of delightful intimacy. . . . Each one was interested in all that was going on."

Welch's reputation as a pathologist had already flowed back from the United States to Europe. In the summer of 1890, he attended the International Medical Congress at Berlin, and there, in the capital of the nation where a few years before he had been an inconspicuous medical student, he was chosen an honorary president of the Pathological Section. It was the realization of a dream that had seemed an impossible fancy when he had sailed back to America from his student years, convinced that he would have no opportunities to pursue science but be buried in a hostile environment as he believed so many foreign-trained scientists had been buried before him.

III

That fall, I * came to Baltimore eager to work in Welch's laboratory. A druggist in Louisville, Kentucky, I had studied medicine at an old-fashioned medical school, the University of Louisville. I had not attempted to practise, but had used Delafield and Prudden's book, as well as other simple texts, to teach myself a little pathology. My preparation was thus most rudimentary.

When the registrar introduced me to the professor I had come so far to meet, I saw before me a short, heavy man whose bright blue eyes twinkled over a dark beard; he was well knit, at that time stocky rather than stout, and I noticed that his feet were very small. His clothes were dark and inconspicuous, he had a conventional derby hat in his hand, and his manner was very quiet and comforting; perhaps this impressed me in contrast to my own agitation.

He did not seem particularly interested in my desire to study pathology; what was the culmination of adventure for me was routine for him. He said he did not know whether there would be any class—perhaps not enough students would show up. I had a discouraging wait. Every day I came to the laboratory to inquire, until at last I was told, probably by Welch's laboratory helper Schutz, when the classes would start.

Since Councilman was away, Welch began the course alone. After he had delivered a twenty- or thirty-minute talk on the subject of the day, Schutz would distribute sections to be stained and mounted. These were then studied under the microscope, while Welch went from one man to another, explaining what they saw.

I was enthralled. Welch's introductory talks were such a marvel of lucidity that I never tired of hearing them through all the years I spent in Baltimore. He never used notes, nor did he look up the subject of the lecture beforehand, for his constant and wide reading kept him always up to date; indeed, as I was to dis-

---

* The use of the first person always refers to the senior co-author of this book, Simon Flexner.

cover later, he very often did not know what topic was to be discussed until he entered the classroom. Yet it was always a delight to watch his mind attack the problem under consideration; after a few preliminary words, he would swing into the heart of the matter, and each year the inevitable logic of his thought produced again the same technically perfect structure as in the preceding year; identical words and phrases fell into the same perfect order, but he himself, so he said, was unconscious of the repetition. It was as if the machinery of his intellectual processes could not run otherwise than true.

During my first year of study with him, as always, he began each lecture with a discussion of the normal organ; a few words of description, possibly a hasty sketch on the blackboard, and the class had the necessary background for the pathological description to follow. This he developed clearly, simply, and adequately, with something of the special history of the subject, so that a close student might evaluate present views in relation to the past. The demonstration at the microscope was as illuminating as the lecture. With a few quick shifts of the slide, he would bring out the important points, showing detail under high power and relations under low. The whole proceeding, from the introductory talk to the last field under the microscope, was a fascinating demonstration of Welch's ability.

Attendance at autopsies, of course, was regarded as an important part of the work in pathology. They usually took place in the forenoon in the presence of the chiefs—Osler always, Halsted less often, and Kelly rarely—and the house officers and graduate students. After Councilman's return, Welch seldom did autopsies, but when he did he studied the frozen sections and made bacteriological examinations until late in the afternoon or even into the night, writing detailed descriptions of the findings, pages and pages, which he probably never found the time to reread.

Since I took no courses in medicine or surgery, but spent all my time in the pathological, Welch put me to work studying some tuberculous glands which had been fixed in Müller's fluid. I was to embed and section the glands, stain them, and examine them for tubercle bacilli. Although I knew how the bacilli looked from having examined sputum specimens for Louisville doctors, the work was all new to me, except the section-making. Schutz was doubtless my main teacher, for so far as I recall Welch paid no attention to me whatever, after having set me to work. I suppose that I said to myself that as soon as I found bacilli I might show them to him. Although I struggled with the problem for some time, I found nothing. Then one day a red-faced, rather bluff man, quite large, coatless, with shirt-sleeves rolled up showing red woollen undershirt, came into the laboratory and sat down beside me. He asked what I was doing. When I told him, he said it was all nonsense, that tubercle bacilli could not be stained in Müller's fluid preparations, and it was hopeless anyhow to look for them in caseating lymph glands. He advised me to chuck the whole thing. He asked also, in a surprised way, how I came to enter on such a study, and seemed astonished to learn that Welch had put me to work on it. I had no idea who the man was. Schutz told me it was Councilman, just back from his summer abroad.

During this time, Welch seemed hardly aware of my existence. Although he demonstrated to me in class as he did to the others, he had nothing to say to me outside of class hours; I knew too little to turn up anything new. Doubtless he thought one exercise in pathological histology as good as another for me, if he thought about me at all. He did not even direct me to reading which would make my study more interesting. However, when I consulted him about Osler's advice that I do some clinical work so that I could support myself by practising medicine, he told me to stick to pathology, if that was what I wanted to do.

After a few months I managed without Welch's knowledge to do a piece of work which he considered worthy of publication; instantly his attitude toward me changed. I found the first manifestation of his interest quite dismaying, for when I asked for permission to take the course in bacteriology that came in the second term, he told me not to take it. This was a serious disappointment, since I had planned on my return home to eke out a living from pathology and bacteriology. After several days, I spoke to him again. "There is no occasion to enter the course," he said. "Study a problem."

This most unexpected answer was a shock; I knew little of the literature of bacteriology and had no experience of its technique or in the finding of problems. However, I went to work on recent German articles and dug out a theme to submit to Welch. Looked back on, it seems a most unpromising, not to say impossible, theme for me at the time, although later it might have had some significance. Welch approved it and I began work. It is true that no definite result was obtained; it is also true that I acquired the technique of bacteriology, and perhaps without the interruptions and loss of time inevitable in courses that meet only two or three afternoons a week.

IV

My experiences have been told at some length because they were typical of Welch's method of teaching. He had come to the Hopkins eager to establish the German system of laboratory education there, but the result was very different. In Germany, a laboratory entered on the investigation of a large subject which presented a variety of separate problems that were parcelled out among the advanced students, the professor keeping the many threads in his own hands. The nature and comprehensiveness of the general subject reflected the inventiveness, fertility, and technical skill of the professor, which also determined the results achieved.

This was not Welch's way. He never devoted his laboratory to the investigation of any single subject, nor did he show any special fertility in the choice of problems for himself or others; his own choices, as will appear later, were determined by fortuitous circumstances, not any plan. And he never set a student to work on a concrete problem, seeming rather to avoid any such commitment; he held that men did not work well on assigned tasks.

The secret of Welch's method may perhaps be found in two statements he made many years apart. In 1927 he said: "It should be more widely realized that students in our American medical schools suffer from over-teaching. It is quite as important that educational and scientific institutions should learn how promising investigators may be and often are spoiled, and to protect them as their most precious asset, as it is to provide facilities for research." Twenty-nine years before he had written in a letter to Mall: "After all, if one has enough to subsist, the environment is everything for a scientific man, and environment is our strong point." Welch's success as a teacher depended on that illusive thing, atmosphere. He rarely interfered in what went on around him, yet his example, his intelligence, and his comprehensive knowledge formed the keystone of the arch of scientific medicine in America.

The young men who came to his laboratory, Welch knew, would find themselves surrounded by eager and able scientific workers; experiments would be the talk at the dinner table; new discoveries would be discussed and copies of foreign journals waved by gleeful expositors in excited faces. "In those days," he remembered as an old man, "everything was small; everyone was interested in what was going on in the hospital. Those were very happy days." MacCallum, who visited him constantly during his last illness, tells us: "It seems that his most cherished memories hovered about 'that little group.' He never tired of dwelling on those pleasant days when, fired with his own enthusiasm, those disciples worked at the highest tension and accomplished wonders."

Welch's own part in the development of an investigator was at the outset passive. In the winter months of the rich years of the first Kochian period when discoveries of the causation of infectious diseases followed one another with exhilarating rapidity, Welch gave weekly lectures on pathological and bacteriological subjects of outstanding contemporary interest. One year he covered diphtheria, another cholera, another lobar pneumonia and the pneumococcus. A notion of the stimulating and provocative character of these lectures may be obtained from his published *Papers and Addresses,* some of which, like the Cartwright Lectures on the pathology of fever, are expansions of his weekly talks.

Welch's whole point of view was so positive that it made for an atmosphere of achievement. He criticized only indirectly through suggesting something better. By temperament a realist, he was concerned more with a practical next step than with some distant goal. Although he mentioned them, he did not dwell on the yawning gaps in medical knowledge concerning which no promising leads had been found; he spoke rather of those unsolved questions which were likely to yield to the scientific techniques then available. If a student who listened to him possessed the soul of an investigator, sooner or later some problem would catch his imagination and all by himself he would get down to work. Then Welch would come to his assistance; a lead found, Welch kept the interest at white heat and guided the work into the most rewarding channels. He was alert and helpful, and always encouraging.

This *laissez-faire* method was sometimes hard on timid young men; they had their own inner struggles, as making a false start was far easier than hitting on a rewarding line of work. But so much went on around one, the air was so charged with pathology and bacteriology, the tone of the laboratory was so kindly, that there was a sense of happy adventure, day in and day out.

Welch's system was particularly productive because of the wide range of his interests. In each of the German laboratories where he had worked, one specialty had been taught, but Welch combined the Virchowian pathology of von Recklinghausen with the experimental pathology of Cohnheim, and added to them the bacteriology of Koch, creating a combination that existed perhaps nowhere else in the world in the laboratory of one man.

However, Welch's breadth of mind was not compatible with the rigid routine followed by German professors. Von Recklinghausen, for instance, appeared at his workshop at seven in the morning and did not leave till late in the day. He seemed to have no other life than his laboratory; this was not in Welch's temperament. The American travelled all over the nation as teacher-at-large of scientific medicine; he loved the opera and literature; he was a conversationalist; indeed, he was effective in so many lines, educational and civic, that gradually more and more of his life came to be spent outside the laboratory.

Welch ran his department in the most easy-going manner imaginable. When as fellow in pathology I became a sort of understudy to Councilman, I discovered that there was no real division of duties. After Welch had done what he wished to do, Councilman did as much of what was left as interested him, and I picked up the fragments. There was uncertainty about this loose working scheme, but for me it had educational value, as I learned to do many things. Autopsies fell to me; I did them poorly and slowly at first. Although this must have been trying to Osler and the other clinicians who brought their staffs and graduate students, no one complained to Welch.

When Councilman left in 1892, after I had been at the Hopkins less than two years, my appointment to succeed him put me in a position for which I was not prepared. Yet Welch never spoke to me in any detail about my duties; he left everything to the effects of the system which I had seen operate. Indeed, it is doubtful whether Welch ever discussed the running of the laboratory even with Councilman. The freedom of the place was complete.

Often Welch failed without notice to turn up for his laboratory talks; I had always to be prepared to give them in his stead. If he had not arrived by fifteen minutes after the hour, I would begin, but sometimes after I had got well started I would hear his quick, short steps as he ascended the stairs. I stopped, and, walking to the front of the room, he began the topic all over.

To conclude that Welch was uninterested in teaching or unaware of what was happening in the laboratory would be a major fallacy; he went, for instance, over all the borderline examinations, toning down the excessive severity typical of young instructors. Yet it cannot be denied that his methods of teaching were unconventional. Whether or not a course met on time did not bother him; what if an autopsy or two were imperfect; the important consideration in graduate teaching, he believed, was to give able young men the opportunity and the incentive to work. How far he planned this pedagogical system out in his mind it is impossible to say; probably it was as instinctive as it was personal. Its success depended entirely on one thing: the personality of the teacher.

Everyone agrees that Welch himself was the great attraction at the Pathological. MacCallum tells us that although Welch never gave him a problem to study, he never undertook a problem without asking himself: "What will Dr. Welch think of it?" The desire to be like Welch, the desire to win his approval, these were the principal incentives of the eager young men who crowded his laboratory.

Many things that would have been faults in lesser men were in him a virtue. That he was not always at the Pathological doing routine work invested him with a certain majestic aloofness; by breaking down the walls of academic routine, he had given his personality room to expand into its own individual shape. That he was casual with beginners and did not give them the help that would have at the moment been valuable increased his prestige in the end, for when he finally paid attention to their work they knew they had earned his interest by their own abilities. One unusual feature of Welch's laboratory was the entire lack of distinction between the younger and the more experienced or highly trained men. Opportunity to grasp a theme, opportunities to pursue it, were open equally to both; and the young not infrequently excelled the old.

Welch's interest in his pupils did not end in the laboratory. Indeed, dinner parties at one of his clubs were an important part of his technique both as a teacher and as a medical statesman. Visiting celebrities, even not very important ones, were put into a warm glow of friendship toward the Hopkins by being made guests of honour at banquets to which young workers in the Pathological were invited. Such dinners, and others given solely for members of the hospital staff, are among the rosiest memories of the men who worked under him. After the wholesome but unexciting fare of the hospital, Welch's menu seemed a conglomeration of almost unbelievable delights. Himself a lover of good food and wine and a great believer in their mellowing influence, Welch served the delicacies of the Chesapeake in the most approved manner: diamond-backed terrapin, wild duck, pearly soft-shelled crabs, and of course the prodigious oysters of those celebrated teeming waters. Cocktails, white and red wine, and on gala occasions even champagne, contributed to these festivities.

But strong as were the material attractions, a stronger magnet was Welch himself. To the young men who sat at the table or in the comfortable chairs of some clubroom afterward, the talk of their master, whom they so rarely saw outside of the lecture room or laboratory, was a delight and a fascination. It seemed that his fund of knowledge on every topic was inexhaustible. He could be a good listener, too, but the young men usually preferred to draw him out. Although he never raised his voice or spoke with vehemence, he often became so absorbed that the ash from his perpetual cigar dropped unnoticed onto his swelling waistcoat to join the thick grey powder that was already there. A spell fell over the room as the quiet voice talked on, and the young men, some of them already a little round-shouldered from too much peering into the microscope, felt the richness of the world and resolved not to be dry-as-dust scientists concerned only with the ramifications of one tributary of knowledge. They resolved to go to art galleries, to hear music, to read the masterpieces of literature about which Welch discoursed so excitingly.

When the time came for a young man to leave the Hopkins, Welch would show a deep and intelligent interest in his future. The professor's prestige and the prestige of his laboratory were so great that his pupils and assistants were continually being offered positions elsewhere. As early as 1891 he wrote his sister: "I have now trained three men in the same position [assistant in bacteriology] and after about two years service each has been called to a prominent place." For the rest of his life he continued to have his associates drawn away to rich opportunities. "I have gone through this experience so many times, that I am reconciled," he wrote in 1914; "indeed it is of course a great satisfaction to train up young men for these important posts."

Since Welch was consulted about the filling of medical chairs all over the nation, winning his approval was of great importance to any young man interested in research. And when an offer came, Welch, who had a vast inside knowledge of university conditions and contacts by which he could learn even more, would gladly give disinterested advice about the opportunities at the school in question; he was known to recommend a pupil for a position and later counsel him to refuse it. If there was a choice between immediate financial advantage and laboratory facilities that would make research possible, he never hesitated to advise his disciples to do what he had done and sacrifice Mammon to science. "A good personal salary is not enough," Welch wrote about a chair that had been offered Dr. Eugene L. Opie. "He must be assured of a suitable laboratory, proper equipment and money enough to run it, and also of at least one paid assistant. If they can offer all these things in a definite way so that he can become the head of a really good pathological department in a large city like Cincinnati, then it may be for his interest to accept the offer." Welch, however, never put pressure on young men to make them follow his advice; perhaps he remembered his own troubles with Dennis.

Welch was eager to help his pupils in every professional way. Praise he had for them in abundance; Zinsser, an outside observer, believed that his "urbane benevolence . . . commended them often beyond their deserts." Since he was free of the tendency to criticize, his influence was never destructive. When his associates were out of town, he carried on their work for them, writing them detailed descriptions of what had taken place more as if he were an assistant than the professor in charge. Sometimes he came to their financial aid, too, although in the most delicate manner imaginable. During my early years in Baltimore, when my funds were very scanty, Welch would turn over to me the surgical specimens which the leading New York practitioners continued to send him for diagnosis. After I had sectioned and studied them, Welch himself wrote the very detailed report that went to New York; when the checks came in payment, he would forward them to me without comment.[6]

Welch's interest in the young men around him was professional, not personal. Although he was very approachable, they had the feeling that they must not take up too much of his time, as whatever he was doing was sure to be very important; Welch carried with him the aura of a great man, and this, incidentally, had much to do with his influence. I remember that when there was a craze for posters I borrowed a collection, hung it in a long corridor in the hospital, and invited some of the older staff members to a party of residents and nurses. Osler, who was one of the guests, came up to me and asked: "Where is Welch?" I was taken aback, for, although Welch was my special admiration, it had not occurred to me to ask him to such a gathering.

It was natural for Welch's associates, to whom he often played the part of a father, to make up for him the nickname Popsy; it was also natural that for years they rarely called him Popsy to his face. Only when Welch had become a national figure, and his nickname had spread far beyond his close associates, becoming known all over the world, was he referred to publicly as Popsy. Typically, Welch enjoyed the use of an affectionate name behind his back, and at the same time did not encourage its use in his presence.

Welch never encouraged the young to confide in him their temperamental and nervous difficulties; this aspect of their troubles he preferred to ignore, even as he never repeated to anyone else such personal troubles as he may himself have had. According to Freeman, it was as a defence against his own over-tender heart that Welch "deliberately broke off relationships which seemed to threaten too strong an attachment." Certainly there is reason to believe that his liking for his assistants was greater than his reticence allowed him to show. When Louis E. Livingood was lost at sea, Welch haunted the steamship office until all hope was gone. "I was very fond of him," he wrote, "and intended to make one of the best pathologists in the country out of him. . . . He was a lovable, manly fellow and we are all depressed by the shock."

When Welch's assistants resigned to go to other posts, he sent them letters revealing emotions he suppressed in talk. "We shall miss you greatly here," he wrote to Mall. "I always dislike demonstrative leave-takings and did not express to you the regret which I feel at your departure. I do not expect to become associated with anyone whom I shall find so congenial, helpful and suggestive in the laboratory as you have been."

I shall always cherish the letter Welch wrote me on my leaving the Hopkins in 1899: "I feel unhappy in rushing away just as you are about to depart, but I cannot get out of this trip to New York. I am sure that no words are needed between us to express our mutual feelings in severing relations over which has never come even the shadow of a cloud. These relations have been the closest and the pleasantest which have ever joined me to a colleague. I have no words to express my appreciation of your faithful service. My pride in your good work is so personal that it would be selfish to speak of it. But we will not call this good-bye, for when you return I shall claim an opportunity of a more festal way of bidding you God-speed." He did give me a farewell dinner later that year.

When Schutz, the laboratory helper, became slack, Welch was unwilling to remonstrate with his old servant. Finally the superintendent of the hospital insisted that the helpers be placed in charge of one of the younger men; Welch agreed only on condition that Schutz be not dismissed without his permission. Knowing that this permission would never be given, the young man could do nothing with Schutz, but after repeated warnings he dismissed Schutz's assistant. Popsy promptly interceded for the delinquent, but when the young man was adamant, he sighed and said: "I promised him that I would speak to you, but I also told him I did not think he would be taken back." Schutz went on without reform, became more and more negligent, but held his position under Welch's protection until he died.

Although really intimate with no one, Popsy was continually surrounded by people. At the Maryland Club and later the University Club, which he helped organize in 1887 and of which he was president from 1915 until his death in 1934, he met with the members of "the old gang," as he called it. This was a fluid group consisting roughly during his first years in Baltimore of his colleagues Mall, Osler, and Halsted, and of two bachelors, Francis H. Hambleton, an engineer, and Major Richard M. Venable. Welch was probably closest to Venable, who was famous in Baltimore for his panegyrics on the glories of being a bachelor and for his interest in Higher Criticism, which made him an outstanding agnostic. A leader of the bar, he also played an important role in civic affairs, being considered principally responsible for the Baltimore park system. The *Baltimore Sun* said concerning his membership in the City Council: "Although the Major's constant breaking of the rules by perpetrating jokes upon his fellow councilmen interfered at times with the dignity of the branch, he assisted in accomplishing needed civic improvements."

"The old gang" enjoyed practical jokes. I remember that one afternoon Welch asked me to come with him to dinner at Major Venable's; "The Major," he said, "will be glad to have you." However, when we arrived and found Halsted and Mall already there, the Major looked at me with simulated surprise and disgust. "Who's this?" he asked. As Welch explained that since we had been working late, he had taken the liberty of bringing me along, Venable's frown deepened. "That's all right, I suppose," he said. "I suppose you want him to stay for dinner."

"Yes."

"I suppose it's all right. I suppose there's enough to eat." In the dining room, Venable rang for his maid. "I suppose there's going to be soup enough for one extra. If not, don't give any to Flexner."

There was plenty of food, but at the beginning of each course the Major said: "Serve the rest of us first, and if there's any left give it to Flexner."

I was relieved when dinner was over; Venable had to drop his joke. Soon everyone was telling stories, and as the evening progressed to shouts of laughter I began to feel that I ought to tell a story, too. Finally I launched timidly on a little tale I had brought with me from the provincial city of Louisville. As I progressed, Venable's face assumed a more and more horrified look, and when at last I was silent, he cried: "If I hadn't heard it I wouldn't have believed it possible that anyone would tell that story in my house! Perhaps you do not realize, Flexner, that the date of that story is two thousand years B.C."

After climbing the steps of the Maryland Club, Welch once complained to Halsted of a sharp pain in his heart. Halsted put his ear to Welch's vest, where he felt so herculean a palpitation that it would have made banner headlines in the most conservative medical journal; Welch had concealed a small rubber bulb under his shirt which he made pulsate by squeezing another bulb in his pocket.

He loved to tell stories that would put his friends agreeably in the wrong. Thus he insisted all his life that, on applying from Louisville for a fellowship the year before I actually reached Baltimore, I submitted as examples of my work in pathology slides of insects' eyes and butterfly wings of the type which young ladies make in finishing school; actually I had sent slides of urinary sediments which had illustrated a paper on the subject. When Popsy was poking fun, his eyes, not over-large but startlingly bright under heavy brows, would smile, the rest of his face remaining in repose. Often his fabrications were so plausible that only this twinkle gave them away as humour, and there is at least one case on record of an associate refusing to believe Welch's description of a new discovery, so sure was he that his leg was being pulled.

Welch lost no opportunities to heal, at least superficially, his breach with Dennis. When his old companion's father died in 1890, he sent a letter of condolence, but the wording was formal in the extreme; he signed himself: "Yours most sincerely, William Henry Welch." Five years later, Welch took the time from many pressing duties to prepare a section on the general bacteriology of surgical infection for Dennis's *A System of Surgery*. By 1899 the ice had thawed a little, as is shown by Welch's letter congratulating Dennis on his election to the fellowship of the Royal College of Surgeons; "none of your friends," Welch wrote, "rejoices more in this than I do." The next letter that has come down to us is dated 1910, and from this much of the restraint caused by the old battle is missing. Welch spoke of his pleasure at "the opportunity of seeing you here and recalling the old days when we were so closely associated, an association which has remained dear to me. With advancing years, those old associations seem to grow more vivid and dearer." But even these words, which refer so appreciatively to the past, make it clear that the present was different; Welch enjoyed being able to recall, with agreeable rather than painful sensations, a friendship that was none the less gone.

Welch's only close association that went back into his childhood was his friendship with his sister. The letters he sent her now never rivalled the intimacy of those distant days, but they were the most revealing he wrote. To her he confided his triumphs and occasionally his worries, although always in a factual, unemotional manner, and with an apologetic tone as if it were silly to bother anyone with his personal affairs. He loved to have her visit him in Baltimore. "Everybody asks when my sister is coming. Why can you not spend a few days here? . . . I think that you would have a good time and could enjoy as much of the social gayeties as you like. Now consider this and delight me with a visit. You really ought to come and see my room. How do you know that I am not going into a decline?"

He was greatly interested in the welfare of her children. When he heard a rumour that Fred, then at Yale, might prefer joining Scroll and Key to Skull and Bones, he hurried off a worried letter to Emma saying that the rumour must be scotched if it were untrue. And he did hope it was untrue! "I of course can not judge of the special conditions which may prevail in his class, still I feel very strongly in the matter and shall be disappointed if Fred gives up his chances for Bones. . . . I have known many in his position who have never regretted choosing Bones even when some of their best friends went the other way." That he also wrote the boy on the subject is shown by a letter to Stuart: "I am afraid that I gave Fred more information as to the chances of his election than I ought to have done, but from all I can learn he is universally regarded as a sure man and I wanted to brace him up all I could, but I have no fear that he will not be prudent as to what I wrote him, and of course it was not as if I were writing to a comparative stranger, but rather as a father might to a son."

Welch was delighted when all danger was past and Fred was safely in Bones. Perhaps his conviction of the overwhelming importance of that organization was a little shaken when he went back to Yale a few months later for his twentieth reunion. He wrote Emma that it was "rather curious to note some surprises in the careers of the men. Some who could hardly keep in the class are now distinguished men, and some whom we had expected to lead armies and govern nations are keeping dry goods stores or making coffins in western country towns."

Although closer to his sister, Welch sometimes sided with his stepmother against her; he stood up for the older lady's right to speak publicly on prohibition, telling Emma: "You are evidently an old fogy on woman's function and her silence in matters of public concern. You must become emancipated and try to shake off the shackles of thousands of years of servitude to man. . . . You see I live in an atmosphere in which we spell *The Cause* with capital letters."

When William Wickham had a disagreement with his partner that made the prospect of continuing with him unpleasant, his son offered to pay whatever it would cost to have the partnership dissolved. "Above anything else in the world I want father's old age to be as happy and as free from care as possible." William tried continually to help his parents financially, although this was difficult to do because of their pride; his stepmother had been hurt when, in 1886, he tried to return the money she had lent him to study abroad.

On July 30, 1892, William Wickham Welch died of a cerebral hæmorrhage. "I have felt keenly the loss of my father, as he seemed to be in good health and was actively engaged in the practice of his profession," Welch wrote an associate. "He has left a very pleasant memory to his family." Concerning the estate, Welch told Emma that he wanted his stepmother "to make use of my part as long as she lives and if she has not there enough to live comfortably and without any care I want to contribute enough to accomplish this end. She has done everything for me, with Stuart making it possible for me to complete my studies abroad and this was more than a fortune for me."

According to the Norfolk custom, a memorial was planned to William Wickham Welch; his son offered to contribute a sum sufficient to keep the cost from being an object. And after it had been decided to erect a stone watering trough, Welch asked several of his Hopkins colleagues to help him find a suitable sentiment to be graved on its rim. Professor Gildersleeve suggested "FONS · SUM · SOLATI · TALIS · ET · IPSE · FUIT," which Welch translated: "I am a fountain of solace, such also was he." He thought this sentence, which was finally used, "peculiarly appropriate to father's quality as a physician."

Welch was less efficient in preparing a memorial of his father which his stepmother wished to publish. On November 2, 1892, he wrote her that although he had been delayed, he would complete it "as soon as I can. It is a labor of love and I hope that you will not think that I am neglectful." More than five years later he gave up, sending his sister "the various documents for the memorial," and urging her to co-operate with their stepmother in writing an account of their father's personal characteristics; he would then add "some estimate of father's professional life and character." He enclosed the outline which he had made for himself, and a rough draft of what he had written on the first three points: "ancestry, education, brief description of Norfolk and changes in it during his lifetime." The further points which, despite the usual skill of his pen, he had been unable to clothe in words were: "salient characteristics, physical and mental, purity, temperate, benevolence, equable temper, belief in Christian virtues and their practice, absence of dogmatic positiveness, gentle manners, interest in public affairs, in men, chief events of his career, marriages, political events, last illness, description of funeral." In these matters Welch's emotions were involved, and he always found it almost impossible to express emotion.

V

During his early years in Baltimore Welch was actively engaged on research in pathology and bacteriology. A technical exposition of the problems he studied and the results he achieved will be found in the next chapter. In this place a brief statement only is made to indicate to the general reader the nature and scope of his investigations.[7]

Not determined by any preconceived plan, Welch's choice of problems was due to chance happenings which called promising lines of work to his attention. Thus when Councilman brought to his laboratory a kidney affected in an unusual manner with Bright's disease, he undertook to study it, combining experiments on animals with observations of the natural disease, a device which he was to employ often throughout his research career.

The pathological changes of the kidney in Bright's disease are very various; Welch's work related to those present in the loops of capillaries contained in minute capsules called Malpighian bodies. Since these bodies are of first importance to the function of the kidneys, their impairment involves serious consequences. Welch discovered that in certain cases of Bright's disease the capillaries become obstructed with newly formed cells, and he invented the name "intracapillary glomerulonephritis" to designate the condition. The precise origin of the new cells has remained a subject of investigation and discussion, but the name invented by Welch has endured.

Next Welch devoted his attention to the nature and manner of production of white thrombi, plugs which are formed in the heart and blood vessels by the blood cells and by fibrin, a substance produced when blood coagulates. The subject of thrombosis, as the process is called, was being actively investigated at that time. Again Welch attacked the problem experimentally, and checked his findings with observations on the condition in man. His conclusions on the manner in which the plugs form hold even today, although his views on the origin of the fibrin component have been superseded.

While at Breslau Welch had been greatly impressed with Cohnheim's researches on hæmorrhagic infarction, a condition which arises when a nutrient artery becomes obstructed in such organs as the lung, intestine, etc. In the meantime Cohnheim's views as to the precise origin of the hæmorrhage in the damaged organs had been attacked by Welch's other teacher, von Recklinghausen. With Mall, who had just come to the Pathological from Ludwig's laboratory, Welch set to work to restudy the problem. They chose the intestine of the dog as particularly favourable material on which to work, and the conclusions they reached upheld von Recklinghausen rather than Cohnheim.

These three investigations had belonged in the field of pathology; in 1887 Welch turned to bacteriological studies. As the Johns Hopkins Hospital was still unfinished and his access to human disease limited, Welch chose as a major problem hog cholera, then prevalent in Maryland. Whenever he received word that a fatal illness had broken out on some farm near Baltimore, he hurried to the scene, and he used to love to tell how, on one occasion, he found that the stricken animals had all died and been buried a day or two before. Despite the hot weather, he determined to dig them up for a post-mortem examination and the making of cultures. Two Negroes did the actual exhuming and then drew off to windward. In puzzlement they watched Welch and the veterinarian A. W. Clement leaning over the redolent animals. Finally one Negro turned to the other and remarked: "Ain't it terrible what white men will do for money?"

Welch became quite fond of pigs. He would descant on their wisdom and beauty, calling particular attention to their elegant feet. They could easily enslave the human race, he would say, but fortunately they were too intelligent to take the trouble.

When Welch began his studies on swine diseases great uncertainty and confusion existed regarding them. Their causes were still unestablished, their separation one from another still uneffected, and their nomenclature wholly chaotic. By securing international co-operation he brought order out of the confusion and helped greatly to clarify the situation, although the final word on the causation of hog cholera was to be deferred for another fifteen years until the virus nature of some plant and animal diseases had been discovered.

As soon as the hospital opened, Welch grasped the opportunity to work on human diseases. With Abbott, he investigated the bacteriology of diphtheria; they were the first in this country to confirm Loeffler's work on the diphtheria bacillus.

This period saw a very active investigation of the germ of pneumonia, the pneumococcus. By bringing bacteriology together with an experimental technique and with observations on human disease, Welch was able to contribute essentially to the growing knowledge of the nature and cause of pneumonia in man.

Of all Welch's investigations, probably the most important was the one he undertook when the body of a Negro was brought into the Pathological for autopsy at the end of October 1891. It presented a most remarkable appearance, for everywhere in the blood vessels and in the tissues were bubbles of gas which gave out a crackling sound when handled. A study of the literature revealed that a considerable number of similar cases had been reported in which, as Welch wrote, "gas, which could not be explained as due to ordinary cadaveric decomposition, was found in the blood vessels after death, without any opening through which air could enter the circulation. . . . Some of the older writers and even modern ones have seriously discussed the possibility of the spontaneous generation of air or gas in the circulating blood during life as an explanation of these cases." He pointed out that the condition of such cadavers had induced books on surgery to warn against the danger of letting air enter the veins in certain operations. "Anyone who will examine with critical spirit the reported cases of death from the entrance of air into the vessels will be impressed," Welch continued, "with the unsatisfactory and meagre evidence upon which this conclusion as to the cause of death is based in the majority of the cases. . . . Had there been no bacteriological examination in our case, the evidence in support of the view that air had entered the vessels during life would have been indeed stronger than in most of the reported cases."

Welch made a bacteriological examination in co-operation with Nuttall. He found that the gas was given off by a previously unidentified bacillus, which multiplied rapidly in the blood vessels after the patient's death. He named this new micro-organism *Bacillus ærogenes capsulatus,* or the capsulated gas-producing bacillus, but later writers have preferred to refer to it by Welch's name, calling it *Bacillus welchii* or *Clostridium welchii.* His discovery led to the opening of a new chapter in medicine: pneumopathology.

This most important of Welch's researches was also to be his last, for he was drawn away from the laboratory by the intricate negotiations involved in an attempt to launch the long-delayed Johns Hopkins Medical School. Probably he hoped to return again to the sequestered pursuit of scientific knowledge which had been one of the dreams of his young manhood, but destiny now called on him to play a different role.

CHAPTER X

Research in Medicine

A Technical Chapter

I

AS soon as his temporary laboratory was ready for use, Welch set to work on a research problem. Six years had passed since circumstances favoured a piece of new work with his own hands. He chose a theme in experimental pathology, but one near human disease. Indeed, Welch probably had already discovered that he always needed, in choosing his subjects of experiment, some groundwork in actual experience on which he could tread firmly. None of his investigative undertakings was chosen from the domain of theory.

The first choice was Bright's disease of the kidneys, a common affection, the pathology of which was still surrounded with obscurity and the effects of which were very serious. Welch presented a preliminary report on his studies at the first meeting of the Association of American Physicians. In it he said: "Of the various processes which make up the pathological anatomy of Bright's disease, perhaps the two which at present awaken the greatest interest and the study of which promises the most fruitful results, are the changes which take place in the glomeruli and atrophy and necrosis of the epithelial cells in relation to interstitial changes." Welch chose the former for his especial study. Although unanimity of opinion had not been reached on other fundamental questions relating to the lesions of Bright's disease, the two processes singled out had acquired special prominence through the recognition of their frequency and importance.[1]

The views expressed by different writers concerning glomerulonephritis showed a wide diversity of opinion not only as to the interpretation of the facts observed, but as to the facts themselves.

Therefore Welch concentrated on this condition and, following in the footsteps of earlier investigators, he employed cantharidin as the agent to produce pathological changes in the Malpighian bodies of white rats and rabbits. The effect of the poison was to produce albuminuria with casts, leucocytes, and red blood corpuscles attached. The flow of urine was first diminished and then suppressed altogether. The kidneys removed at autopsy were more succulent than normal, and under the microscope showed some interstitial infiltration, degenerative changes in the epithelium of the tubules, but especially marked changes in the Malpighian bodies. The space between the glomerulus and Bowman's capsule was widened, and in it were cells and granular material arranged in a crescentic mass around the glomerulus, presenting the appearance often seen in glomerulonephritis in man and attributed to swelling and desquamation, possibly even proliferation of either the capsular or the glomerular epithelium. But in these animals the epithelial cells are derived in part from the convoluted tubules in immediate communication with the Malpighian bodies.

Hence Welch saw no propriety in designating as glomerular nephritis the changes just described in the rat's kidney except that the term was used with much latitude of significance, and embraced nearly all the changes observed in acute nephritis in the Malpighian bodies and many of those found in chronic nephritis as well. In the acute cantharidin nephritis of rabbits, the capsular spaces also contained granular material and cells of uncertain origin. But Welch noticed for the first time in the rabbits necrosis of the epithelial cells in tubes occupying the boundary zone of the pyramid and medullary rays.

One of the objects in making the experiments on cantharidin nephritis was to determine whether accumulations of cells were produced in the glomerular capillaries such as had been described in acute and chronic nephritis, cells regarded as proliferated endothelium. No changes comparable to those found in the human cases were observed in the animals. On the other hand, Welch had seen such accumulations of cells in the glomerular capillaries not only in scarlatinal nephritis, but in the nephritis complicating typhoid fever in man.

He reported a case of acute nephritis attending malaria to illustrate this condition. The patient was the subject of anasarca for two months, and death resulted from uræmic convulsions. At autopsy the kidneys were large, the surface smooth, the capsule non-adherent, and the cortex swollen. The Malpighian bodies were large and pale. The microscope showed little abnormality except in the Malpighian bodies, which were rich in cells. The glomeruli completely filled Bowman's capsule. "The case seemed a puzzling one, until after the examination of very thin sections it was found that almost everywhere the glomerular capillaries were dilated, and contained a large number of cells, partly resembling white blood corpuscles, but mostly larger, and of an endotheloid type." Aside from the changes in the Malpighian bodies, no other lesions existed in the kidneys adequate to explain the symptoms. Welch emphasized the importance which attached to the lesions of the glomerular capillaries described in consideration of their physiological function.

For the lesions of the glomerulus Welch proposed two names: the form characterized by an accumulation of cells between the glomerulus and Bowman's capsule he would call *desquamative glomerulitis,* and the form characterized by an accumulation of cells, or other changes in the interior of the capillaries, he would call *intracapillary glomerulitis,* "and this without prejudging the question as to the propriety of considering all of these changes as inflammatory."

The term "intracapillary glomerulitis" has endured, but discussion has continued as to whether the cells called endotheloid actually are derived from endothelial cells which line the glomerular capillaries. MacCallum, especially, has recently restudied the pathology of so-called intracapillary glomerulitis and has come to the conclusion that the new cells are outside (inter), not inside (intra), the capillaries, and arise from connective tissue elements in the tufts of the glomerulus and not from cells within the capillaries themselves.

II

Before a year had passed, Welch reported his work on the structure of white thrombi to the Pathological Society of Philadelphia. "While all that pertains to the subject of thrombosis is of importance," he said, "recent investigations have lent special interest to the study of the minute structure and the mode of formation of white thrombi." He reminded his audience that since Virchow's studies forty years earlier, it had been generally believed that a thrombus is essentially a blood coagulum, differing from an ordinary post-mortem clot only in its arrangement and the relative proportion of the constituent histological elements, which he explained by the slow formation of the thrombi from the circulating blood, in contrast with the rapid coagulation of the blood at rest, and by secondary changes in the thrombus.

But in the middle eighties, the problem of thrombus formation and structure had taken on a different aspect; there were under discussion the parts played in thrombus formation by the leucocytes, by fibrin, and especially by blood platelets. Welch came into the controversy after Eberth and Schimmelbusch in 1885 published their thorough study, in which (1) they confirmed the existence of blood plates in the normal circulation by direct observation of them in the circulating mesenteric vessels of dogs and rabbits; (2) they denied that the plates have any share in the coagulation of fibrin; and (3) they observed the accumulation of platelets in the living mesenteric vessels of the dog subjected to injury. The platelets adhering one to another and to the vessel wall in consequence of a change which they called "viscous metamorphosis" (conglutination) formed plugs which constituted the beginning thrombus. Red and white corpuscles may be included in the mass of plates, but their presence is purely accidental and they are not to be regarded as an essential constituent of the primary thrombus.

Welch said that he was led to repeat the work on the structure of white thrombi by the fundamental importance of the question whether fibrin and leucocytes are or are not essential constituents of the thrombi, and because it is necessary to demonstrate, before drawing far-reaching conclusions, that the process of thrombosis is identical in human beings and in experimental animals. He started out, therefore, with a study of human thrombi under a wide variety of conditions and he reached the conclusion that any satisfactory explanation of the process of thrombosis must account for the presence of blood plates, of fibrin, and of leucocytes, for these are the essential constituents of thrombi.

The experimental part of Welch's study was carried out chiefly on dogs. The femoral artery, the femoral vein, or the jugular vein was injured mechanically or chemically, or foreign bodies were introduced within them. At intervals the injured parts of the vessels were enclosed in ligatures and removed, slit open, examined, hardened, and eventually sectioned and stained with hæmatoxylin and eosin. He described in detail the fresh appearance of the experimental thrombi and the microscopical findings of the plugs in the fresh state. The thrombic process, as observed by Welch, was as follows: "Given suitable conditions, such as alteration of the vessel wall, slowing and irregularity of the circulation, the first constituents of the thrombus to accumulate are the blood plates. But although the plates collect at first in larger number and more rapidly, the leucocytes do not long remain absent, and in the course of time they are present in such quantity that they must be considered an essential constituent of the completed thrombus. At first the conditions for the coagulation of fibrin are not present, but with the increasing accumulation of leucocytes these conditions appear and fibrillated fibrin is deposited. It is in harmony with the current ideas concerning the cause of the coagulation of fibrin, to suppose that at first the fibrin ferment is absent, and that this is subsequently furnished by the leucocytes. The absence of fibrin in the early thrombi composed wholly of plates, is an argument additional to the evidence brought forward by Löwit and others, that the plates do not furnish the fibrin ferment. It is apparently only after the leucocytes have been included for a time in the thrombus that they die or undergo some alteration in their constitution which leads to the formation of fibrin ferment. The final result is a plug composed of plates, leucocytes, and fibrin, and included red blood corpuscles." [2]

Welch regarded it as an error to base the conception of the thrombus exclusively upon the constitution of the thrombus at its inception. "Our ideas," he said, "as to the constitution of thrombi are based upon the examinations of the completed plugs which contain fibrin and leucocytes as well as plates." On the other hand, the study of experimental thrombi enables us to form a clearer conception of the mode of formation of the thrombus. It does not necessitate any radical change in our ideas of what constitutes a thrombus.

There was one more point of interest in Welch's observations, namely, that he agreed with the pathologists, including von Recklinghausen, who held that Cohnheim's views on the relation between changes in the walls of the vessels and thrombosis were too exclusive.

Two facts may be noted especially regarding Welch's address: first, he checked the experimental observations with findings in human cases of thrombosis; and second, the address was responsible for the comprehensive articles on thrombosis and embolism that he contributed to Allbutt's *Practice*.

III

Mall came to the Pathological as fellow in pathology directly from Ludwig's laboratory in 1886 and brought with him high technical skill in physiological and anatomical methods of experiment. Welch, influenced perhaps by this circumstance, chose as a theme for a joint piece of research that of hæmorrhagic infarction. In 1877 Welch had written his father from Breslau that Cohnheim had succeeded beyond his predecessors in clearing up the complex problem of infarction. Cohnheim had studied microscopically, in the tongues of curarized frogs, the process of formation of hæmorrhagic infarctions produced by artificial emboli which, after introduction into the aorta, lodged in branches of the lingual arteries. He reached the conclusions

that the blood which produces the infarction is derived by regurgitant flow from the veins, that the hæmorrhage occurs by
diapedesis, and that the diapedesis is the result of some molecular
alteration in the vascular walls deprived of their normal circulation.

This explanation, however, was soon challenged from von
Recklinghausen's laboratory, where different conclusions were
reached on the basis of experiment, the main ones being that
the blood which produces the hæmorrhage after the obstruction
of an artery comes from the collateral vessels and not by reflux
from the veins, and that the hæmorrhage is at least quite as much
the result of stasis in the capillaries, and consequently increased
pressure, as of changes in the vascular walls.

These two opposed views, with still other minor divergences,
continued to prevail, so that Welch, who reviewed the history,
could say that there was still much to explain in the causation of
infarction, and that there was abundant opportunity for further
experimental work.

Two papers came from the Pathological on this subject, one
by Welch alone, the other a joint paper by Welch and Mall not
published until 1920.

The intestine was chosen as the organ on which to experiment
because it was easy to produce infarction in this situation while
it was difficult to produce hæmorrhagic infarction of the lungs
artificially. The occlusion of the mesenteric artery in man is followed by hæmorrhagic infarction extending throughout nearly
the whole length of the small intestine and even into the upper
part of the large intestine. In the dog, the animal chosen for the
experiments, the branches of the superior mesenteric artery anas-
tomose freely, forming only one row of arches from the sum-
mits of which branches are given off which enter the walls of the
intestine. It is possible to convert any one of these main arteries
into a terminal artery, and the collateral circulation can be limited to any extent.

The experimental methods employed were described in detail in the second paper, on the basis of which certain conclusions
were reached. Hence it was thought desirable to observe directly

under the microscope the circulation in the mesentery while the infarction process was taking place. "Immediately after the occlusion of the superior mesenteric artery the circulation ceases in the veins, arteries, and capillaries of the mesentery. In a very short time the circulation returns and has the following characters. The arteries contain a much smaller quantity of blood than normal, and they appear contracted. The blood flows in the arteries with considerable, although much diminished, rapidity and without distinct pulsation. The movement of blood in the veins and capillaries is sluggish and irregular. In some of the veins the direction of the current is normal; in others it is backward, but we were not able to trace the regurgitant flow into the capillaries. In many of the veins and capillaries there is entire cessation of the current. Frequently the circulation becomes reestablished in vessels where it had previously ceased, and in other vessels stasis occurs. The distinction between axial and plasmatic current is obliterated. Gradually the veins become more and more distended with blood, and these as well as many of the capillaries become filled with homogeneous red cylinders of blood. Sometimes the red corpuscles become clumped together, and such clumps can be seen moving in the veins. We also noticed frequently clumps of white corpuscles in the circulation. The extravasations of blood took place chiefly from the small and medium sized veins, but also from the capillaries, and at least, in part, by the process of diapedesis. The microscopical appearances in the veins and capillaries resembled those seen in passive congestion resulting from venous obstruction, and yet we were unable to discover coagula in the larger veins."

As a result of the experimental studies, Welch reached the following conclusions:

"1. The blood which produces hemorrhagic infarction comes from the collateral circulation and not by reflux from the veins.

"2. The blood pressure is very low in the region where hemorrhagic infarction is taking place in consequence of the occlusion of the main artery.

"3. If the force of the arterial and capillary circulation sinks below a certain point, no hemorrhagic infarction occurs.

"4. There is no evidence that changes in the vascular walls are concerned in the production of hemorrhagic infarction.

"5. Where hemorrhagic infarction, resulting from arterial obstruction, is taking place, the large and small veins are distended with blood, and the arteries contain less blood than normal. The circulation is sluggish and irregular in the veins and capillaries, in many of which stasis and probably physical alterations in the red corpuscles occur.

"6. The hemorrhage occurs by diapedesis."

Welch made a final comment on these conclusions to the effect that, under the conditions described, the consequences were due simply to mechanical alterations of the circulation, although, he said, it was not easy to give an entirely satisfactory mechanical explanation of all the phenomena. However, the knowledge of the dynamics of the circulation of the blood was still imperfect, and the circulation was influenced by complicated physiological conditions, and by a fluid containing solid particles of complicated physical properties.

IV

The premier lectureship at the College of Physicians and Surgeons in New York was the Cartwright Lectures. Welch was invited to deliver them in the spring of 1888. He chose for his theme the general pathology of fever, a wide subject, appealing both to the practising physician and to the theoretical man, based so directly on physiology that its presentation gave wide scope to the lecturer and yet permitted of an experimental approach which Welch could employ.[3]

"There is no subject in medicine," said Welch, "of more general and varied interest than fever. The practitioner in every department of medicine, the pathologist and the physiologist are equally interested in the investigation of the nature and effects of fever. Even the physicist and chemist, who are not directly concerned with medical science, have lent their aid to the study of animal heat and its disorders. The history of opinion regarding fever is in great part the history of medicine itself, for no feature of the great systems of medicine from Hippocrates and Galen to the present century so characterizes these systems as the views held concerning the nature of fever. In consequence of the importance of the subject and of the number and ability of those engaged in its investigation, it might be supposed that no chapter in medical science would be better understood than that pertaining to fever. That such is not the case is due to the fact which is becoming more and more evident that the reaction of the animal system which we call fever is dependent upon the most fundamental and essential properties of protoplasm and of nerve energy. In proportion as our knowledge of these properties increases and becomes more accurate, we gain a clearer insight into the complicated processes involved in the production of fever." And Welch continued: "I should hardly have selected . . . a subject where so many problems remain unsolved and which must necessarily be presented in so fragmentary a form, were it not that in all ages the opinions held concerning the nature of fever have controlled measures employed in its treatment. . . . In our own time the treatment of fever is intimately connected with the answers variously given to such questions as whether fever aids in the elimination or destruction of infectious agents concerned in its production; whether increased waste of tissue is a constant condition and a source of danger in fever; what part is played by infection and what part by elevation of temperature in causing the grave symptoms of fever; what in addition to lowering of temperature are the effects of so-called anti-pyretic treatment?"

Welch gave three lectures, called respectively: "The Nature of Fever," "The Effects of Increased Temperature of the Body," and "The Etiology of Fever." The collation of the mass of material from the literature must have been arduous and time-consuming, but the actual preparation of the lectures was done, we know, under pressure. Welch was eager to have his father attend at least one of the lectures. He wrote his sister: "As I shall have to prepare the lectures during the weeks of their delivery [March 29, April 5 and 12] I shall spend probably only one night in New York at the time of the first and second lectures."

Welch dealt with fever as a condition common to all febrile diseases, and the increased temperature as the essential factor of fever, upon which all the discussions of the nature of fever centre. He brought forward two agencies as affecting the febrile rise in temperature: (1) disturbance or direct injury of the central nervous system, and (2) the effects of pyrogenic (fever-producing) substances. The factors which co-operate to preserve a nearly constant temperature in health in the warm-blooded animals are: (1) the production of heat within the body, (2) the loss of heat from the body, and (3) the regulating mechanism by which the varying heat production and heat loss are so balanced that the internal temperature remains practically constant. Theoretically, the rise of temperature in fever may be due to any one of these three factors.

As Ott had done before him, Welch approached the subject from the experimental side and found that the pyrexia induced by puncture of the caudate nucleus in the rabbit could be regularly obtained. He summed up the existing data on this point by stating that the chemical processes resulting in the production of heat energy are under direct control of the nervous system and "possibly of nerves distinct from those now recognized as motor or secretory," and that there are regions in the central nervous system in some way connected with these nerves through which control of the chemical processes resulting in heat is secured. The pyrexia produced by puncture of the caudate nucleus possessed all the essential properties of fever regarded as an abnormal elevation of temperature, namely, increased production and dissipation of heat, excessive elimination of urea and carbonic acid, and excessive absorption of oxygen. The breathing and pulse rate were increased in frequency. As no observations on regulation of heat in these animals existed, Welch placed rabbits in which puncture of the caudate nucleus had been made in a cold environment and in a box heated to various temperatures, and he found that their powers of temperature regulation were less than those of normal animals. Welch believed, therefore, that fever of purely nervous origin might arise in the absence of any pyrogenic agent in the blood.

Welch made an experiment to ascertain whether the shutting off of all impulses to the muscles, the great heat producers, would prevent a rise of temperature. It was known that thoroughly curarized animals do not respond to pyrogenic agents, and Welch found that after section of the spinal cord in the lower cervical region, the injection of pyrogenic agents neither produces rise of temperature nor checks its fall.[4]

A second series of experiments, the main ones which Welch carried out, related to the effects of increased temperature of the body. In order not to be disturbed by the presence of the other factors, such as infection, he raised the internal temperature by external application of heat. Following Naunyn's example, Welch had constructed a suitable double-walled wooden box in which rabbits could be placed and the temperature elevated at will and kept sufficiently even. In such a box rabbits could be kept for two or three weeks, the average rectal temperatures fluctuating between 105.5° F. (40.8° C.) and 108° F. (42.2° C.). They took their food greedily and did not appear ill. After removal from the box, the animals remained well. When sacrificed, they presented marked fatty degeneration of the heart, liver, and kidneys. Different rabbits reacted to the elevated heat differently; some animals have less power of temperature regulation than others; failure of this power may lead to a sudden rise of internal temperature which may quickly attain a point (111° F. [43.9° C.] to 113° F. [45° C.]) incompatible with life. Rabbits rendered anæmic by bleeding were found less resistant to high temperatures.

Welch confirmed Newell Martin's experiments showing that the isolated mammalian heart beats quicker when supplied with warmed blood. In Welch's own tests on the isolated cat's heart, the heart beat regularly and more and more rapidly as the blood was gradually raised to 111.2° F. (44° C.), when the beats became irregular, but were restored to their normal rhythm when cooler blood was supplied. At 122° F. (50° C.) the heart's action ceased, but the heart was made to beat again by supplying it with cooler blood, showing that the cessation was not due to heat rigor. The inference drawn was that the increased frequency of the pulse in fever was referable to direct action of the warmer blood on the nervo-muscular substance of the heart itself. But clinical observations of cases of fever indicated that still other circumstances influenced the rapidity of the heart's pulsations.

The question which Welch put to himself was whether the hearts of rabbits subjected to high internal temperatures with resulting marked fatty degeneration of the muscle were impaired physiologically. In three instances rabbits were removed from the box at the end of ten days to two weeks and their blood pressure measured by a mercury manometer attached to Ludwig's kymograph. In no instance was the blood pressure found to be lower than that normally present in rabbits. Immediately after the measurement of the blood pressure, the animals were sacrificed and marked fatty degeneration of the muscle fibres was found. The conclusion Welch reached was that the experiments, as well as careful pathological and clinical observations, necessitated some revision of the current opinions concerning the significance of fatty degeneration of the heart in fever.

In the third lecture, on the ætiology of fever, Welch asked: "What is the significance of fever, is a question which thrusts itself upon us no less than it has upon physicians in all ages. Unfortunately, we cannot today, any more than could our predecessors, give other than a speculative answer to this question. There have been in all ages enlightened physicians who have held the opinion that fever is a process which aids in the elimination or destruction of injurious substances which gain access to the body. Under the influence of ideas which sought in increased temperature the origin of the grave symptoms of fever, we have in recent times in great part lost sight of the doctrine once prevalent, that there may be in fever a conservative element. There is much which speaks in favor of this doctrine. The real enemy in most fevers, is the noxious substance which invades the body, and there is nothing to prevent us from believing that fever is a weapon employed by nature to combat the assaults of this enemy. The doctrine of evolution indicates that a process which characterizes the reaction of all warm-blooded animals against the invasion of a host of harmful substances, has not been developed to so wide an extent, and is not retained with such pertinacity without subserving some useful purpose. This is a point of view from which many pathological processes can be regarded with advantage. . . . It is impossible, with our present knowledge, to say in exactly what way fever accomplishes a useful purpose. There are facts which suggest that in some cases of fever the increased temperature as such may impair the vitality or check the virulence of pathogenic microorganisms." [5]

V

From 1887 onward, Welch's research was predominantly in the field of the bacteriology of the infectious diseases. It may excite surprise that the beginning was with a disease of animals rather than of man, but a sufficient explanation is afforded by the fact that the Johns Hopkins Hospital was not yet completed and hence access to cases of human infection was not conveniently obtained. Welch's natural wish was to study bacteriologically not isolated cases of infection, but rather a prevalent infectious disease. Then the problems of infectious diseases in animals have all the intrinsic interest of those in man, and for the pathologist they have the added value that they can be studied far more completely than can diseases in human beings. The whole biological history of a disease of animals stands ready to be unfolded, for in the instance of an inoculable, transmissible disease every stage from the very inception to the final termination in death or recovery can be explored.

The immediate opportunity to investigate diseases of animals was provided by the occurrence of epizootic diseases of swine in the neighbourhood of Baltimore. The diseases from which these animals suffered were hog cholera and swine plague. As subsequent events were to prove, the two diseases prevailed either singly or in combination one with the other. The problem from the strictly bacteriological point of view was complex and from the point of view of nomenclature very confusing. To the disentanglement of the bacteriological problem Welch was to devote himself either altogether or along with other bacteriological studies for several years.

He reported on hog cholera and swine plague in 1889 and in 1894. The first report was of a preliminary nature, but the second, a comprehensive one, was made before the First International Veterinary Congress of America and dealt with both the American and European investigations on swine diseases and with the general literature of the subject.

Welch's studies were preceded by the studies of Salmon and Theobald Smith at the Bureau of Animal Industry in Washington, the results of which were published in the reports of the bureau for the years 1885 and 1886. Welch found, as did the earlier investigators, two species of bacteria associated so constantly with the epizootics as to suggest ætiological relationships of the two diseases, one, first described by Theobald Smith, the hog cholera, and the other the swine plague bacillus. Welch's purpose was to make as complete a study of both the pathology and the bacteriology of the diseases as possible, to produce infection with pure cultures, and to identify if possible the experimentally induced diseases with those occurring naturally. Then as the work developed, he undertook to correlate the American epizootics with similar outbreaks reported from Europe.

The need for this proceeding grew out of the highly confused state of the nomenclature of the epizootic diseases of swine. "In each country where hog cholera occurs different names are used for it. In England it is generally called swine fever . . . in Denmark and Sweden, swine pest and swine diphtheritis, and in France, pneumo-enteritis of swine, and lately the American name, hog cholera, has also been used in France. Some confusion, particularly in the minds of some German writers, and excusably so, has resulted from the fact that the disease called hog cholera by the Bureau of Animal Industry and by veterinarians in this country, is called by F. Billings swine plague. . . . The disentanglement of the two diseases, hog cholera and swine plague, and still more of the two microorganisms, the hog-cholera bacillus and the swine-plague bacillus, as regards their relations to each other and to the bacteria isolated from swine epizootics in Europe, and even as to their relation to swine diseases in this country, has been rendered difficult partly in consequence of difficulties inherent in the bacteriological study of these diseases, but largely from imperfections in these bacteriological studies, both in this country and in Europe, and also from ill-considered and confusing writings by more than one contributor to the literature of these subjects."

In his first paper Welch devoted himself chiefly to an account of his observations on hog cholera, for there existed for that disease a pathological criterion which he regarded as of the first importance. While the possible anatomical lesions met with were so manifold as to require a large experience to render one practically familiar with them, he pointed out that there was one lesion, the so-called "buttons" of the intestine, which was as characteristic of hog cholera as the typhoid ulcers of the intestine were of typhoid fever. Moreover, lesions similar to the "buttons" may occur in various parts of the body besides the intestine and stomach: on the pharynx, tonsils, tongue, lips, nasal membrane, gall bladder, etc. Then Welch observed "an interesting change, hitherto overlooked," in the occurrence of hyaline thrombosis of the renal capillaries, both glomerular and intertubular. He found that when this condition was marked it was impossible to force more than a minimal amount of injecting fluid into the renal vessels, and that the Weigert fibrin stain gave to sections the appearance of blood vessels injected with Berlin blue.

The hog cholera bacilli were obtained without special difficulty in pure culture from the blood, intestine, and other organs, although the distribution in the body may be less wide. But even in the first paper Welch was puzzled by the fact that the bacilli were missed in a number of cases of hog cholera. He ventured on explanations of this failure, but it is clear that his own reasons did not satisfy, since he found in several instances that rabbits inoculated with typical "buttons" survived. Salmon and Smith had encountered the same difficulty and were inclined to believe that the bacilli may disappear in the later stages of the disease. While thinking this explanation probable, Welch could not "distinguish anatomically cases in which hog-cholera bacilli could not be detected from some of those in which they were present." But the real test of the specific nature of the hog cholera bacilli was the test of inoculation. Every precaution to avoid error in the experiments was adopted by Welch. The experimental pigs were drawn from places where the disease was not known to occur and from persons who had raised their own pigs. Clean stables were used, in which no pigs had ever been kept. In the same way precaution was exercised against accidental infection, as in feeding, etc. The results were that, "by inoculation of pure cultures of the hog-cholera bacillus," he had succeeded in "reproducing experimentally in pigs every lesion of the natural disease, including necrotic buttons in the intestine and in all of the other situations mentioned above. . . . By simply rubbing the lips of pigs with potato cultures we have produced the disease in fatal form." And after recording the variety of successful inoculations, Welch concluded that "the evidence is now complete, more so than in any previous experiments, that the hog-cholera bacillus is the cause of hog cholera in swine."

Welch asked the question whether the hog cholera bacilli are identical with any of the bacteria which had been found in Europe in diseases of swine. "The only bacteria which come into question are the bacillus of swine fever or pneumo-enteritis in England, the bacillus of Scandinavian swine pest, and that of the French pneumo-enteritis of swine." From the anatomical descriptions alone, Welch concluded that those diseases corresponded with American hog cholera, and cultures subsequently obtained by him from England and Scandinavia confirmed this belief.

Finally he directed attention to the swine plague bacillus, concerning which he stated that no evidence existed to prove that the bacillus could produce intestinal lesions characteristic of hog cholera. On the other hand, the bacillus was capable of producing general infection and more especially local infections characterized by pneumonia and fibrinous inflammation of the serous membranes.

This was in essence the knowledge of the subject of hog cholera at the end of the nineteenth century. In the meantime a new chapter in the pathology of the infectious diseases had been opened. The first virus disease discovered was that of mosaic of tobacco in 1892, the second that of hoof-and-mouth disease of cattle in 1898; and in 1903–04 a group of investigators at the Bureau of Animal Industry found that hog cholera also was a virus disease.

In the light of the new knowledge derived from the study of virus hog cholera we can now explain the discrepancies which so puzzled Welch and Theobald Smith. Their main difficulty arose from the facts that they both worked with pigs which had succumbed to the disease, and that they depended largely upon the "buttons" to establish diagnosis. It is now known that the "buttons" are chiefly due to secondary invading bacteria, such as the hog cholera bacillus, which multiply in the ulcers produced in the intestinal mucous membrane by the hog cholera virus. When the sick pigs are killed early, after fever has developed, they rarely show the hog cholera bacilli; and in clean surroundings the virus-injected pigs may even die of the disease without the bacilli's being present in them. It is worth mentioning that Smith, as early as 1887, noted the absence of bacilli from swine killed early in the disease, but he drew the wrong inference from the important observation: that only in the later stages do the bacilli appear in sufficient numbers to be detected in cultures.

Today there is little interest in the hog cholera bacillus, since it is looked upon merely as an unimportant complicating factor in the pathology of hog cholera. And yet as both Welch and Smith showed half a century ago, the bacilli are capable alone of producing a severe intestinal disease in pigs sometimes still confused with the true, or virus-induced, hog cholera.

VI

The Johns Hopkins Hospital was opened to patients in May 1889, and in February 1890 Welch reported on ten cases of pneumonia from which he had isolated the pneumococcus.[6] At the time of the opening of the hospital Welch had two choices of a theme in prevalent bacteriological disease to investigate: (1) typhoid fever, always endemic in Baltimore, and (2) pneumonia, a common infection then as now. He set his pupil Blachstein to work on typhoid fever, and two important observations came from this study: the discovery of the chronic carrier of typhoid bacilli because of their survival in the biliary passages, and the relationship between typhoid infection of the gall bladder and the formation of gall-stones. For himself, Welch divided his working time between the studies on the pneumococcus and his investigations on the gas bacillus during the last two years of his investigative period. The bacteriology of pneumococcus pneumonia was still under discussion. The disease itself was often severe and the mortality rate high. And yet it was known that the saliva carries regularly a pneumococcus-like organism.[7] This seemed a singular paradox. In his class lectures Welch used to dramatize the sudden onset of pneumonia in the drunken vagabond lying all night in the gutter and found next day a victim of the disease. The constant presence of the pneumococcus in the healthy person offered a ready explanation of the phenomenon. There were still other uncertainties calling for clarification —for example, the Friedlander bacillus, the account of which in 1883 caused no little sensation.[8]

The questions which were uppermost in the early nineties, now that Fränkel's and Weichselbaum's pneumococcus was accepted as the bacterial cause of lobar pneumonia, related to the distribution of the micro-organism in the blood and tissues: the part it took in the production of associated inflammations, as in the pleura, joints, meninges, etc.; the degree and variation of virulence in the pneumococcus as ascertained by the inoculation of laboratory animals—rabbits and mice especially; its capacity for survival in the infected body and in artificial cultures; the relation of the periods of survival to virulence; and the dependence of the severity of the attack of the disease on virulence— whether, for example, in the diseased lung the pneumococcus is ever attenuated, etc. Among other highly important questions of the time was the existence of distinguishable varieties, or types, of pneumococci which determined the precise character of the pathological processes found at autopsies in human cases of disease and in animals experimentally inoculated.

It was not long before the fate of the pneumococcus in the diseased so-called hepatized lungs was investigated and it was found that progressive diminution of virulence could sometimes be detected as the duration of the disease lengthened and in the older or resolving parts of the lung compared with the more recent or advancing part of the pathological process. The capsules which surround the small lancet-shaped double cocci (diplococci) early claimed attention. That they are more evident in animal tissues than in artificial cultures could be quickly ascertained. Welch was early among those who found the cocci sometimes fragmented and disappearing, leaving the capsules largely empty. Vast numbers of such empty capsules could be discovered by suitable staining methods, and Welch perfected one of the best of these stains by proceeding on the assumption that the capsules contained mucin and making use of chemicals which would fix and stain this substance. Certain properties of the inflammatory material (exudate) poured out in the diseased body were attributed to the capsules, among them the glutinous quality of the fluid which sometimes accumulated in the pleural cavity producing so-called empyæma which occasionally attended the pneumonia.[9]

The pneumococcus was found to be a fastidious body in its artificial culture requirements and a fragile micro-organism as measured by its survival power, both inside and outside the body. Great attention was paid its characteristics in cultures in solid and fluid media. Welch noted that "the variability in the properties of this coccus is manifested not less in its behavior in culture media than in other respects. . . . Important modifications in the culture characters, particularly as to the luxuriance of the growth and the capacity of development at low temperatures, can often be brought about by artificial cultivation. Abundant growth at low temperatures is generally associated with loss of virulence and is often observed in late generations of artificial cultures of primarily virulent pneumococci."

Many difficulties were encountered in the course of experiment because of sudden diminution or loss of virulence. Then there was the intricate question of varieties of the pneumococcus, to which Welch gave much attention.

"The attempt has been made to establish distinct varieties of *Micrococcus lanceolatus* on the basis of . . . diverse pathological effects. . . . Those who attempt to distinguish distinct biological varieties of the lanceolate coccus do not agree with each other in their classification. . . . I am not able to draw the lines of separation . . . sharply . . . as in my experience types with inconstant or mixed characters are common. . . . We must recognize, therefore, varieties of *Micrococcus lanceolatus* with different biological attributes. I have also obtained from single colonies pure cultures which produced" a variety of pathological effects. . . . "I have repeatedly found that cultures or direct inoculations from a rabbit dead of one type of septicaemia produced in a second rabbit the other type of septicaemia. . . .

"The question as to how far we are justified in recognizing distinct varieties of *Diplococcus pneumoniæ* [the pneumococcus] will be answered differently by different bacteriologists, according to one's conception of the meaning in biological classification of the term variety. Those who insist that in order to justify the designation variety there should be a considerable degree of fixity and transmissibility of distinctive characters will find it difficult to establish well defined varieties of this organism. It seems to me, however, that we must give a somewhat looser meaning to the term variety in the classification of bacteria, and that we cannot conveniently dispense with this word in speaking of the different modifications of *Micrococcus lanceolatus*. These modifications are endowed, as we have seen, with very diverse pathogenic attributes." To present-day bacteriologists who base the concept of variety, or type, of bacteria on immunological properties, this measured statement will serve to show how great has been the advance accomplished in the definition of bacterial varieties.

After the discovery of diphtheria antitoxin in 1890–91, it was natural to study the pneumococcus infections in the light of the new and exciting knowledge of immunity. Welch took only a small part in these investigations. He was, however, impressed with the humoral as opposed to the tissue types of immunity and expressed the opinion that it was in the former that hope for a useful mode of treatment lay. Time has confirmed this foresight. He saw also that pneumococci produced their injurious effects through toxic action, that is, they give off soluble poisons which injure the cells of the body. He drew attention especially and for the first time to the small areas of cell death—necroses—in the liver, visible to the naked eye, similar to those he had previously seen in hog cholera, typhoid fever, and diphtheria.

But what is especially apparent is that Welch viewed the manifold problems presented by pneumococcus infection in man and laboratory animals as a human pathologist. He possessed in this respect a great advantage over many of his contemporary students of the subject. When he found that experimenters were being led far astray, as in the belief that they actually reproduced in laboratory animals acute lobar pneumonia, he reminded them that "acute lobar pneumonia as it occurs in human beings is a very definite and well characterized affection both anatomically and clinically. So far as is known, the domestic animals are not subject to a form of pneumonia . . . identical with croupous pneumonia of man. Bacteriologists are not always pathologists, and the bare statement that the pneumonia produced experimentally is in all respects identical with acute lobar pneumonia in human beings should be received with caution."

In 1892, when Welch's last published paper appeared, the ætiological relation of the pneumococcus to lobar pneumonia was not yet accepted everywhere. He therefore expressed the opinion based on his own studies, and on the work of others which he had passed in review, that the evidence of this relationship rested upon many points which, he said, would seem incontrovertible.

VII

It seems singular to us, considering the importance of the disease, that although Loeffler discovered the diphtheria bacillus in 1884, no attempt to confirm his finding in this country was made until 1889, the year Prudden published a series of cases tending to refute Loeffler's observations. Prudden's conclusions were based on the bacteriological examination of twenty-four cases in hospitals and asylums in New York. In no single case did he find the Loeffler bacillus. This failure, and especially Loeffler's comment on it, stirred Welch and Abbott to make their bacteriological study, published in 1890. Loeffler's comment on Prudden's paper was: "I do not believe that in North America a form of diphtheria prevails different from that with us. With us the bacilli are found regularly by every investigator. . . . Further investigations must and will clear up this contradiction."

The discrepancy between Prudden's results and those of European investigators was quickly resolved by Welch and Abbott's studies. They examined only cases of primary diphtheria, so diagnosed by competent clinicians, and found the Loeffler bacillus [10] in all of them. Prudden's cases had attended measles, scarlet fever, and some other diseases, and belonged to the miscellaneous class of pseudomembranous angina in which the common microorganism met with is the streptococcus. Once Welch and Abbott's paper based on Baltimore cases appeared, Prudden studied cases of primary diphtheria in New York and now found no difficulty in obtaining Loeffler's bacillus from them.

Welch reviewed the entire subject of diphtheria in his winter lectures at the Johns Hopkins Hospital in 1890–91, and he used the same material for an annual address before the Medical and Chirurgical Faculty of Maryland in April of 1891. This was a usual method with him: having prepared the comprehensive lectures on the pathology of fever for the Cartwright Lectures, he gave them over again at the Hopkins Hospital, and so with the lectures on *Micrococcus lanceolatus,* which he used at the Hopkins Hospital and for his presidential address before the Medical and Chirurgical Faculty.

Welch told the Medical and Chirurgical Faculty that the devastating nature of diphtheria had led to widely divergent views concerning it and to modes of treatment based on these conflicting views. In the later printed address, Welch said: "The history of our knowledge of diphtheria illustrates the difficulties which we encounter in endeavoring to reach a full understanding of a disease upon the basis of its symptomatology and pathological anatomy alone. Consider for a moment what are some of the uncertain and still much disputed questions concerning this disease." He then listed a series of questions to which it was hoped that a knowledge of the causation of the disease might give "clear and certain answers."

1. Is diphtheria primarily constitutional or local in origin?

2. Are all pseudomembranous inflammations of the throat, not directly referable to caustic irritants, diphtheria?

3. Is there a purely local, non-contagious pseudomembranous laryngitis called croup distinguishable from diphtheria?

4. Are the pseudomembranous anginas secondary to scarlet fever, and less frequently measles and other infectious diseases, diphtheria?

5. Is there any relation between follicular tonsilitis and diphtheria?

6. May diphtheria occur in a mild form as a simple catarrhal inflammation of the throat?

7. Are pneumonia, acute nephritis, suppuration of the glands in the neck, etc., referable to the diphtheric virus?

Having explained how the discovery of the Loeffler bacillus was serving to give answers to this formidable list of questions, Welch could say that "with the exception of tuberculosis, no disease has had greater light shed upon it than diphtheria by the study of its specific cause."

Welch's own contributions consisted, first, of the demonstration that diphtheria as it occurs in America conforms with that occurring in Europe. But there was one important question which had not yet been satisfactorily answered. Loeffler had stated that among the obstacles to the establishment of the bacillus isolated by him as the definitive cause of diphtheria in man was his failure to find in inoculated animals the characteristic lesions described by Oertel in human diphtheria. Now this failure bears directly on the long mooted question as to the primarily local or constitutional nature of diphtheria. It had been surmised that the grave constitutional symptoms arise from a poison produced in the local inflammatory false membrane in the throat which enters and diffuses widely in the body, carrying cell injury and death with it. The lesions of Oertel are the visible signs of that cell injury. Their absence in the guinea pigs inoculated with the cultures and in which a corresponding false membrane occurred was therefore a defect in the chain of events uniting the identity of the natural and the experimental pathological processes.

This problem was attacked by Welch and Flexner, the latter making the actual experiments. Guinea pigs were inoculated in the usual way in a pocket in the skin. The lymphoid glands and other organs were submitted to minute microscopical study and it was found that, as a matter of fact, pathological changes, of course on a correspondingly small scale, comparable to those occurring in cases of diphtheria in children existed in the fatal cases of the inoculated disease.

We can now reconstruct the pathological phenomena. In man and in the laboratory animal the bacilli develop only at the point of infection, in the former usually in the throat, in the latter in the skin. They do not invade the body, and are not found in the blood or tissues. They develop locally, induce a false membrane, and produce a poison—toxin—which, passing into the body, brings about the organic lesions.

"Diphtheria," said Welch, "is without a doubt local in its origin. . . . This settlement of the controversy as to the local or constitutional origin of diphtheria is one of the most important outcomes of the bacteriological study of this affection. Nevertheless, from the point of view from which this controversy has been waged, the triumph is, in my opinion, only a partial one for the localists, for, as will be shown later, I believe that

there are reasons as strong as ever for the employment of constitutional measures of treatment in combination with local ones."
The discovery of diphtheria antitoxin made between 1890 and
1892 confirmed the correctness of this point of view.

Welch had become the spokesman for this country on the subject of diphtheria. In 1894 he reported on behalf of the American Committee on Diphtheria to the Eighth International Congress on Hygiene and Demography held in Budapest. His report
summarized the work on the bacteriology of diphtheria carried
out in America between his and Abbott's publication in 1891
and the spring and summer of 1894. A highly creditable series
of papers could be assembled, all confirming Loeffler's work.
Publication of this informative review had important educational value. It brought the present knowledge of diphtheria
within the range of the practising physician and it served to remove scepticism and doubt as to the bacterial nature of diphtheria. It constituted, therefore, a timely preparation for the
wider introduction of the antitoxin treatment of the disease, then
at its beginning.

But a more onerous and taxing responsibility was to be imposed on Welch. He was selected to make the opening address
on the treatment of diphtheria by antitoxin before the Association of American Physicians in Washington in 1895. Although
Behring's discovery of antitoxin had been made in 1891 and the
first trials in human diphtheria in 1891 and 1892, no real test of
a potent serum had been made before the serum prepared at the
Höchst factory became available in August 1894. Welch's statistical review therefore covers the first year of antitoxin treatment
and is based on 7000 recorded cases so treated and about 100,000
injections. The world literature is minutely examined, classified,
tabulated, and analysed. The practical conclusions drawn from
the study and based on the data presented are: "that our study of
the results of the treatment of over seven thousand cases of diphtheria by antitoxin demonstrate beyond all reasonable doubt
that anti-diphtheria serum is a specific curative agent for diphtheria, surpassing in its efficacy all other known methods of

treatment for this disease" and that "it is the duty of the physician to use it." To this he adds that "the later reports show in general a decided improvement in the results of the treatment over the earlier ones, and there is every reason to believe that the results of the second year's employment of the new treatment will make a much more favorable showing than those of the first year. The discovery of the healing serum is entirely the result of laboratory work. It is an outcome of the studies of immunity. In no sense was the discovery an accidental one. Every step leading to it can be traced, and every step was taken with a definite purpose and to solve a definite problem. These studies and the resulting discoveries mark an epoch in the history of medicine."

VIII

There came to autopsy in October 1891 a mulatto who had been admitted to Osler's ward suffering from aneurysm of the aorta. The large sac had pressed both on the bony structures of the chest, wearing them away, and on the skin, causing ulcerations. From the ulcers several hæmorrhages had occurred, followed finally by sudden death.

Welch performed the autopsy, his attention having been arrested by a peculiar swelling of the skin over the neck, arms, and chest and other regions which on pressure emitted a crackling sound. The veins of the skin could be followed by the naked eye and seen to contain gas. The body showed no signs of putrefactive changes; the peculiar appearances therefore were not to be explained by decomposition. Welch exposed some of the veins, nicked them, held a lighted match to the escaping gas, which ignited with a slight explosion and burned with a pale bluish flame. The gas was obviously not air.

Of course Welch thought at once of the many cases in the medical literature in which the blood vessels after death contained air or gas which did not seem attributable to post-mortem decomposition and for which many explanations had been offered. Hence he said that "the observation to be here reported is calculated to shed light upon some of these mysterious cases."

Immediate examination of the blood from the heart and vessels showed for the first time numerous short bacilli, and similar bacilli were found in the laminated clot lining the aneurysm, in the liver, spleen, and kidneys. The bacilli were in pure culture, they stained readily with aniline dyes, and they were surrounded by a capsule. They grew readily in cultures under ordinary anærobic conditions, and they did not contain spores.

A striking appearance was presented by frozen sections of the liver and heart muscles. To the naked eye they showed small cavities, and sections of the alcohol-hardened organs stained with aniline dyes revealed masses of the bacilli in the tissues about the cavities.

The bacilli proved non-pathogenic for rabbits; but when the animals injected intravenously with the bacilli were killed, the micro-organisms quickly developed in the blood vessels and organs, reproducing the appearances observed at the human autopsy. The growth of the bacilli was many times more rapid at higher temperatures than at 20° C. In one instance only did a rabbit—a pregnant one—succumb after an intravenous injection of a culture. It seemed probable from the autopsy that two of the embryos in the uterus were already dead when the injection was made, and that in these embryos and the part of the uterus containing them the bacilli were able to develop. Welch regarded this case as "especially suggestive in view of the number of cases which have been reported of death from supposed entrance of air into the uterine veins after abortions and injections into the uterine cavity."

It was Welch's opinion that the bacilli entered the aneurysmal sac through the external openings in the chest wall, developed in the thick clots in the sac, and were carried into the circulating blood and distributed in the body before death. He thought it was not impossible that the entrance of gas and of bacilli into the circulation may have been concerned with the sudden death of the patient.

Welch's review of the literature on the reported cases of death from the entrance of air into the vessels impressed him with the unsatisfactory and meagre evidence upon which this conclusion as to the cause of death was based, in the majority of the cases. He expressed surprise that no previous attempt had been made to determine by bacteriological examination whether or not what was taken to be atmospheric air might not have been generated by the growth of micro-organisms. "Hereafter," he said, "in all similar cases a careful bacteriological examination, including anærobic cultures, must be made before it can be admitted that the gas in the vessels has not been generated by microorganisms."

Two years after Welch's original report of the isolation of the gas bacillus, E. Fränkel published his monograph on gas phlegmons in which he described a bacillus which he had obtained from four cases of gas gangrene.[11] Welch suspected this bacillus of being identical with *Bacillus ærogenes capsulatus* and later proved it to be so by comparing cultures sent him by Fränkel and also by the effects of inoculation of the two micro-organisms in animals. The surmise made by Welch that those cases in which entrance of "air" into the uterine veins was reported were explained by the presence of gas-producing micro-organisms was, in the same year (1893), borne out by observed instances.

The first number of the *Journal of Experimental Medicine* appeared in January 1896, and the first article in it was on the gas bacillus.[12] In that paper Welch reported that the bacillus had been isolated at the Pathological from patients in the Johns Hopkins Hospital suffering from gas gangrene, perforative peritonitis, morbid conditions of the urinary tract, hæmorrhagic infarction of the lung, gas cysts of the intestine, and biliary infection.[13] Five years later (1900) in the Shattuck lecture, Welch surveyed the rapidly growing literature in what he termed "pneumatology . . . fields comparatively new and little trodden," and he published in the same year a note on the normal habitat of the bacillus, which had been found at the Pathological to be the intestines of man and animals, and the soil.

The common occurrence of gas-producing bacilli in cultivated land was to have a sinister significance during the World War and to give rise to wide prevalence of gas gangrene. Bull studied the Welch bacillus after America's entrance into the war, for toxin production. He secured an exotoxin with which he produced an antitoxin in horses that was employed on the western front in combating gas gangrene. Recently, since the discovery of the chemotherapeutic action of sulfanilamide and sulfapyridine in gas bacillus infections, the combined use of antitoxin and chemicals has been studied and the combined action found to be greater than that of drugs or antitoxin alone.

Welch was to make another contribution to the treatment of wound infection by distinguishing the bacterium *Staphylococcus epidermidis albus* from the *Staphylococcus pyogenes albus*. The presence of the *epidermidis albus* in the deeper layers of the skin, of which it is a regular inhabitant, withdraws it from the restraining influence of chemical disinfectants. The microorganism was found in wounds where every possible antiseptic precaution had been taken, and regularly in the sterile silk used for stitches, often in considerable numbers, and sometimes enclosed in leucocytes, notably where stitch abscesses had formed, but also where there was not a trace of suppuration. Besides being the most frequent cause of stitch abscess, it was found to grow along drainage tubes introduced into the body cavity and to set up inflammation in the tract.

In reporting his findings, Welch said: "I hardly need to say that these observations on the bacteria of the normal skin, and the depth to which they penetrate, indicate that the skin of the patient may be a source of wound infection and that the surgeon should take greater precautions than has hitherto been customary to guard against this danger. Dr. Halsted, in view of our results on cutaneous disinfection, has discarded for the most part the use of cutaneous suture, and is very well satisfied with the results obtained by bringing the edges of wounds together by subcutaneous sutures."

CHAPTER XI

The Johns Hopkins Medical School

I

"WHERE is the man to endow the Medical School?" Francis T. King, president of the trustees of the Johns Hopkins Hospital, wrote Gilman in June 1889. This had become a burning question since the long delay in starting the school had developed strains that threatened to make impossible the advanced institution with which the partisans of scientific medicine had hoped to inaugurate a new era.

Speaking in 1886, at the tenth anniversary of the founding of the university, Welch outlined the way it was hoped the school would be organized. The first necessity was an organic connexion with the university. This, he said, "conduces to greater solidity, to a more elevated tone, and to a broader and more enlightened system of medical education," particularly since certain branches of scientific medicine lie on the borderline between the medical and philosophical faculties.

It is indicative of the continued opposition with which the plans for the medical school were faced that before he proceeded Welch felt it necessary to defend scientific medicine from the charge of being impractical. Dwelling on the many contributions made by the laboratory to the treatment of specific diseases, he showed how the changes thus produced in the practice of medicine necessitated changes in the education of the practitioner. Then he argued that the didactic lecture, based as it was on traditional rather than experimental medicine, must make way for the laboratory instruction that was demanded by the trend of the times. Of special importance were "hygienic laboratories, in which are investigated the causation of diseases, the laws governing the origin and the spread of epidemics, the principles of ventilation, of heating, of sewerage, the influence of the air, of the ground, of the water in the production of certain diseases, in a word, all that pertains to the preservation of the health of communities and the warding off of preventable disease." But laboratories were so expensive that a medical school could not rely on the earnings from students' fees to provide them; an endowment was necessary.

Welch welcomed the new changes. "The attractions of study and the pursuit of medicine," he said, "have been greatly increased. . . . Many departments of medicine now possess the interest and the attractions of a natural science. Here will be found problems of absorbing interest, some of which call into requisition powers of acute observation, some demand for their solution ingenuity in the device of new methods and of apparatus, others require a profound knowledge of physics, or of chemistry, or of mathematics, and others call especially for well developed faculties of logical inference and of wide generalization." [1]

Such was the conception of medical education which was about to be put into practice when the financial difficulties of the Baltimore and Ohio Railroad deprived the university of the necessary funds. As delay followed delay, discontent and disillusionment mounted even in the minds of the individuals to whom the carrying out of the plan had been entrusted. The hospital trustees, forced to take over the expenses of such medical departments as were already under way, opposed this use of funds which exhausted their entire surplus, "leaving little or nothing for things yet unprovided." And some of the professors also became restive; where was the medical school in whose name they had deserted excellent positions elsewhere; where were the classes they had expected to teach? Osler, who at McGill and Pennsylvania had become used to the excitements of undergraduate lecturing, complained bitterly of "the dry bones of postgraduate teaching," and intimated to Dr. Henry M. Thomas that "unless something were done he might be forced to go where there were some real medical students." Although Welch, preferring to work with graduate students and happy in his laboratory, was probably the least dissatisfied of the whole medical faculty, the growing tension must have affected him too, since he must have been aware that the Baltimore experiment to which he had dedicated his career was in danger of collapse.

Gilman, worn out by the labour of getting the hospital started, was about to sail for Europe for a year's rest when the opening gun was fired in a campaign to substitute for the advanced medical school that had so long been planned a more backward institution; in October 1889 the hospital trustees "without any reference to the President, Professors or Trustees of the University requested the Superintendent of the Hospital together with the members of the Medical and Surgical Staff of the Hospital, to prepare a plan for medical lectures to be given this winter." Although this proposal was put forward merely as a stop-gap until the university school could be founded, in it lay the seeds of an institution only superficially linked to the university, and supported, as was frankly the intention, by the students' fees. Since there would be no endowment to pay for laboratories, and since the financial need of a large enrolment would necessarily keep entrance requirements down, the school would have resembled the other medical schools in the nation; clinical instruction would be given in the wards, the professors would deliver lectures, anatomy would be taught by dissection, but the only laboratory would be Welch's. Undoubtedly seeing in this scheme the overthrow of all his plans for remaking American medical education, Welch refused to associate himself with it.[2]

Gilman promptly wrote King, the president of the hospital trustees, a letter in which he threatened to fight the issue out in public if his board did not reconsider their action. "Johns Hopkins," he continued, "in his mandatory letter said: 'Bear constantly in mind that it is my wish and purpose that the Hospital shall ultimately form a part of the Medical School of that University, for which I have made ample provision by my Will.' Clearer language could hardly be employed to show that he expected the medical school to belong to the University, and that the Hospital when completed was to afford the requisite facilities for observing the treatment of injuries and disease." Pointing out that for fifteen years the university had drawn up plans for an advanced medical school, founded laboratories, paid professors, Gilman insisted that the action of the hospital trustees placed the whole scheme in "imminent danger."

He asked who were included in "the medical and surgical staff of the Hospital," the body supposed to organize medical lectures, and said he presumed that the trustees meant "the senior salaried gentlemen. . . . One of this number, Dr. Welch, informs me that according to the usage of hospitals, the Pathologist is not regarded as a member of the medical and surgical staff. The other persons are Drs. Hurd, Osler, Kelly and Halsted, all of whom are men of the highest professional standing, whose counsel and co-operation must of course be secured in the development of our plans. For this reason they have all been appointed Professors in the University. I submit, however, to your attention this fact, that not one of them has been six months in the service of the Johns Hopkins foundations, and not one of them has had the opportunity, except informally, to become acquainted with the methods of the University or with all that has been done in preparation for medical instruction. . . .

"The experience of this entire country has shown that a faculty or school of medicine should not be merely in the hands of the Professors, but should be in close and intimate relations with the other chairs or faculties of a university. On this point no one has spoken more clearly than the Pathologist of the Hospital, Dr. Welch.

"It is difficult to foretell what complications will arise unless the action of the Hospital is re-considered. The public, which for fifteen years has looked forward to the beginning of our medical course as to an epoch in medical education, will unquestionably hold us all to a strict accountability in this matter."

Gilman never mailed the letter from which we have quoted, since after "a long and earnest conversation" which must have followed much the same lines King assured him that the matter would be dropped. However, it was agreed that the hospital might try to raise funds by charging admission to a series of special lectures given by members of the staff. The general uneasiness was heightened when they were a failure, "hardly half a dozen persons" coming to hear the outsiders whose importation were resented by the Baltimore profession.

Gilman sailed for his holiday at last, but he was allowed no peace, for letters followed him which reflected heated conferences in Baltimore. On one hand, it was urged that the university itself should start a school without waiting for an endowment. Acting President Ira Remsen wrote: "Hurd thinks the school could be opened next Fall with a slight effort, and that the expense would be offset by the fees." It seemed certain, he added, that a majority of the university trustees would favour such action. "The more I think of it, the simpler the problem appears. We have nearly everything we need now." But he added reassuringly: "You need not fear that any step will be taken without your distinct approval." George W. Brown wrote in another letter: "Dr. Welch, as Dr. Hurd informs me, says that on the ground bought for the University there are two small houses standing together which with some alterations, would be sufficient for dissecting purposes, and Dr. Welch thinks that the buildings on the Hospital [grounds] would furnish the rest." This scheme quickly proved impractical and was dropped.

A possibility soon arose for securing the necessary endowment, but to Gilman this cure seemed worse than the disease. Dr. James Carey Thomas wrote him: "I think our lady friends might be good for $200,000 should the necessary balance be raised—provided we would give women an entrance."

Baltimore, and the Thomas household in particular, had long been a center of agitation for better educational opportunities for women. Miss M. Carey Thomas, the trustee's daughter, was one of a group of intelligent and active women including Miss Mary Garrett, inheritor of a large fortune from a former president of the Baltimore and Ohio Railroad; Miss Elizabeth King, daughter of the hospital president; and Miss Mary Gwinn, whose father was a trustee of the university. These women had organized the Bryn Mawr School, to give girls college preparatory training equal to that of men, and Miss Thomas herself, as dean of the newly founded Bryn Mawr College, had used her influence to establish there a curriculum based on the undergraduate and graduate departments of the Hopkins. Searching for new worlds to conquer, they saw in the troubles of the medical school an opportunity to secure for women the most advanced medical education to be offered in America.

The Hopkins authorities, long citizens of a man's world, received the intervention of the ladies with reluctance and scepticism. George W. Dobbin confided to Gilman that it was only to please Francis King that he and another trustee, Francis White, met with Miss Thomas and Miss King. "We listened patiently to what they said (and they stated their case with great eloquence) and we told them in reply that with whatever favor we might look upon this enterprise in the future, the University was not now in a condition to commence the school, especially in your absence, and that we could not even talk about it for the present. It was the opinion of both Mr. White and myself that the ladies deceive themselves in assuming their ability to raise the large sum of money [$200,000] they talk so freely about."

Not discouraged, the ladies organized on a national scale "The Women's Fund for the Higher Medical Education of Women"; Miss Garrett opened the subscription with $10,000, and in an amazingly short time, by October 1890, they were able to offer $100,000 to the trustees on condition that women be admitted to the medical school.[3]

Gilman had been back from Europe for some months. Although an intellectual radical who had played a major part in reforming American higher education, he was a social conservative. Determined there should be no coeducation at the Hopkins, he engaged in a heroic battle with the ladies. On one side stood the stiff university president, his handsome, grave face framed in the whiskers that proclaimed him a gentleman of the old school. Opposed to him were the group of eager women, marriageable all of them, but unmarried; most of them still in their thirties, but concerned with reform, not men. In his dealings with the sex, Gilman had always resorted to rigid courtliness, but these strange women repudiated courtly evasions; they were determined to discuss affairs as man to man and no ingratiating words would turn them from their purpose. What the president thought of the ladies we may only speculate, for he was too polite to say, but Miss Thomas has told us what the ladies thought of him. She wrote: "Mr. Gilman, although he had approved of our attempting to raise the money when we consulted him before hand, used every unfair device—and he had many in his bag of tricks—to persuade the trustees to refuse this $100,000 and would finally have defeated us had it not been that two of our fathers, mine and Mamie Gwinn's, were on the board and another father, Francis T. King, was president of the hospital board." As it was, the trustees made their acceptance depend on the ladies' raising the full sum of $500,000, "sufficient for the establishment and maintenance of a medical school worthy of the reputation of this university." Only then would the condition that women be admitted become operative.

The trustees adopted a conciliatory minute which, however, made it clear that they held no elevated views concerning the medical opportunities open to women. "This board is satisfied," they wrote, "that in hospital practice among women, in penal institutions in which women are prisoners, in charitable institutions in which women are cared for, and in private life when women are to be attended, there is a need and place for learned and capable women physicians." Gilman himself tried to calm the heated passions by publicly congratulating the ladies on their "intelligent and persistent enthusiasms." Insisting that their conditions had been accepted with "no dissent," he swallowed the bitter pill bravely. "It is but right," he wrote, "that those women who wish to study and practice the healing arts should have, if properly prepared, the highest opportunities that can be afforded."

Although Welch took no active part in the negotiations, it had been clear that he was on Gilman's side; the bachelor professor, we gather from a statement he made much later, was embarrassed by the idea of having women in his classes, where he had to explain indelicate things. From the letter urging acceptance of the women's fund signed by Osler, Hurd, and Kelly, his signature is missing. He wrote his sister that he was unable to pay her a visit because of "the receptions at the hospital in the afternoon and at Miss Garrett's in the evening of the ladies who are interested in raising the money for admission of women to the Medical School at the University. Mrs. President Harrison and a crowd of women from Washington, Philadelphia, and New York are to be here and there is to be high jinks I suppose. As I have hitherto held aloof from the movement and have refused to sign the papers which the rest of the hospital staff have signed recommending the Trustees to accept the money, I think that my absence would be conspicuous. I do not like coeducation in medicine and they know it, but now that the Trustees have decided to accept the money ($100,000) raised by the women, I do not wish to be regarded as an obstructionist or standing in the way of the success of a movement which has been decided upon."

Continuing their campaign in the hope of raising the entire $500,000 demanded, the women set out to convince the public that ladies might be doctors without upsetting the laws of the universe. Open letters were published in the *Century* for February 1891. Cardinal Gibbons stated that "there is no obstacle in ecclesiastical or canon law to the education of women for the medical profession." Women in the past had been influential in medicine, he pointed out; during the Middle Ages midwifery had been exclusively in their hands, and there had been women professors in some of the oldest Italian universities. Finally, he decried the prejudice that allowed women to be nurses but excluded them from the practice of medicine. Also contributing to the forum, Osler reported enthusiastically on Swiss and French medical schools, where complete coeducation existed. He gave his full approval to the proposal, adding impishly that he did not think "the women students themselves would object to it." [4]

Yet Welch wrote Mall in November: "Pres. Gilman and some of the trustees really do not want (sub rosa) the women to succeed, for they do not like the idea of co-sexual medical education. I do not myself hanker after it, but I do not see how they can refuse such a large sum of money."

Indeed, it was becoming increasingly clear that a medical school must be secured at once lest the faculty be dissipated, for other institutions were fishing in the troubled waters. There was agitation to call both Welch and Osler to the University of Pennsylvania; Hurd wrote Gilman: "Mr. King had a feeling that this item of news might impress upon you more deeply the necessity of a strong effort to get a Medical School." Then Harvard tried to lure Osler and Welch to Cambridge to help inaugurate "a four years' graded course"; the two Hopkins professors declined. Writing the Harvard authorities that he was contented where he was, Welch secured the appointment for his associate Councilman, who stated many years later: "My leaving for Boston had some connection with the opening of the medical school which I have never seen referred to. Both Welch and Osler had become very restive under the delay in opening the school. The position here was offered to Welch, and he was able to use the offer to accelerate the formation of the Baltimore school."

In the fall of 1892 the faculty was still intact, but it was none the less clear that Osler would be lost unless something were done; his alma mater, McGill, was dangling before him a $1,000,-000 gift to secure his return, and he was greatly tempted. As Cushing comments in his life of Osler, "there was certainly need for expedition" in beginning undergraduate teaching.

Again the women stepped into the breach, but again in a manner that raised in Gilman's mind more fears than hopes. In December 1892 Miss Garrett added to the sum collected by the Women's Committee a personal gift of $306,977, making up the $500,000 necessary for the opening of the school, but added further conditions which were received with amazement and dismay. Most important for the future of American medical education was her insistence that no students be accepted who had not satisfied the requirements for admission to the graduate schools of the university (an A.B. degree or its equivalent); and that in addition applicants must possess a knowledge of French, German, and certain pre-medical studies. Although such requirements had long been an ideal in the minds of the leaders of the Hopkins experiment, it had been planned to achieve them gradually. When Billings had suggested much the same thing in 1878, Gilman had written: "If the question be asked why not insist that every one shall come up to this standard, the answer may be made that in the present condition of the country, it would be useless for this University to exact as introductory to three years of merely preparatory work, higher qualifications than are now called for in the highest schools of medicine in this country, and especially, when youths who cannot even enter this preliminary course, may be admitted to a professional school and graduate Doctors of Medicine before their more educated comrades have completed our introductory studies."

Writing to Cushing in 1922, Welch said: "The terms of admission to the medical school were not the invention of Miss Garrett or Miss Thomas, but years before I had set them down in a document which Mr. Gilman and the Trustees asked me to prepare soon after I came to Baltimore. Miss Garrett got this document through her lawyer, Mr. Gwinn, who was an influential trustee of the university. She naturally supposed that this was exactly what we wanted. It is one thing to build an educational castle in the air at your library table, and another to face its actual appearance under the existing circumstances." [5]

Miss Thomas remembers: "When it came to laying down requirements our fathers deserted us and joined the trustees in begging Mary [Garrett] not to insist. My father almost wept and told me it was incredible that two young women should take such a position. The trustees called on us separately and together (I was always present) but at the last critical moment Dr. Welch saved the situation." The high entrance requirements were agreed to, although Osler expressed the general feeling when he said: "Welch, we are lucky to get in as professors, for I am sure that neither you nor I could ever get in as students."

Welch had been opposed to another of Miss Garrett's conditions; he wrote many years later: "One little epithet seems now very trifling to have caused so much controversy—namely, that women should be admitted on *the same* terms as men. It was thought at the time that it might be wiser to use the word 'equal' rather than 'the same,' but Miss Garrett, with the characteristic determination which always distinguished her when once she had made up her mind on grounds based on knowledge and experience, was unwilling to make this change and we do not now regret that we are giving *the same* medical teaching to women as to men."

Several of Miss Garrett's stipulations were accepted without question: that not more than $50,000 be used to erect the so-named "Women's Fund Memorial Building"; that the school should be an integral part of the university; and that it was to provide a four-year course leading to the degree of doctor of medicine.*

The difficulties of the negotiations led Miss Garrett to make it a condition of her gift that the entire sum revert to her estate "in the event of any violation of any or all of the aforesaid stipulations." And she provided for a self-perpetuating committee of six women appointed by herself who were charged with making sure that women were treated on the same terms as men in every particular of the school's operation. On December 24, 1892, the trustees accepted this stipulation with the rest. After further disagreements had been ironed out, plans were speeded for opening the Johns Hopkins Medical School in the autumn of 1893.

Devoting his 1893 Commemoration Day address to the medical school, Gilman undertook to give "the evolution of a great idea." The end in view, he recalled, "was the establishment in close connection with an endowed university and an endowed hospital, of an endowed medical school fitted to give instruction of the best and highest character to students especially prepared to receive it by the previous study of modern languages, the natural sciences, and other liberal arts." The germs of this conception had been planted twenty years before when Mr. Hopkins had provided that the hospital should form part of the medical school of the university. Then Gilman reminded his audience

---

* Northwestern University had been the pioneer in lengthening the curriculum, having established a three-year graded course in medicine in 1859. When the Hopkins Medical School opened in 1893, Harvard, the University of Pennsylvania, and the University of Michigan had just gone on the four-year plan of instruction, with a school year of eight months, although Provost Pepper of Pennsylvania was very apprehensive about the change. The College of Physicians and Surgeons had come under the control of Columbia University in 1892, but the lengthening and grading of the curriculum had not yet followed.

that in adding pre-clinical courses to the curriculum the Hopkins had followed in the footsteps of the Sheffield Scientific School at New Haven, but he did not say that he was secretary of that school when the first pre-medical course in this country was there introduced.

The words "biological sciences," Gilman recalled, had once raised spectres in the minds of the citizens of Baltimore. "It was like a ghost, alarming enough to those who were timid or who dwelt in the dark." But intelligent people quickly discovered that "the biological sciences were only their old familiar friends —anatomy and physiology, botany and zoology,—sporting under a new name, employing modern methods and making free use of modern instruments of precision." When the psychological laboratory was opened under Stanley Hall, again apprehensions were aroused. "It seemed as if mind was to be treated like matter, as if the human eye was trying to penetrate with profane curiosity the sacred mysteries of the soul." Here again intelligence came to the rescue and it was discovered that "every investigation that throws light upon the healthy or the diseased action of the brain . . . would promote and not hinder the development of man's noblest faculty. So experimental psychology assumed an honorable place among the sciences relating to medicine."

At the end of his speech, Gilman said: "To me and to almost every one of my colleagues the letter of Miss Garrett came as a great surprise. We could hardly believe it possible that the uncertainties and disappointments which had delayed the opening of our school of medicine were gone and that one benefactor had rendered the service which many had been invited to undertake."

The announcement of the revolutionary plan of the medical school was left to Welch, who made it at the commencement exercises that June. He began by discussing requirements of admission, "the most perplexing problem concerning medical education, especially in this country." To make the difficulties clear, he pointed out that "at present in this country no medical school requires for admission knowledge approaching that necessary for entrance into the freshman class of a respectable college; many schools demand only the most elementary education, and

some require no evidence of any preliminary education whatever."

So far as the Hopkins requirements were concerned, Welch
believed that "only experience can determine whether or not the
plan which we have adopted is the best one for our purpose."
But he was pleased with escaping "the reproach most frequently
brought against American medical schools, viz.: a low standard
of admission—for our standard is not only vastly higher than has
ever before been attempted in this country, but it is not surpassed in any medical school in the world.*

"The aim of the school," he added, "will be primarily to train
practitioners of medicine and surgery. . . . We hold that the
medical art should rest upon a thorough training in the medical
sciences, and that, other things being equal, he is the best practitioner who has that thorough training. . . . It is not only or
chiefly the quantity of knowledge which the student takes with
him from the school which will help him in his future work; it
is also the quality of mind, the methods of work, the disciplined
habit of correct reasoning, the way of looking at medical problems. In order to cultivate in the student this habit of thought,
this method of work, I believe that there is no one thing so essential as that the teacher be also an investigator and should be
capable of imparting something of the spirit of investigation to
the student. The medical school should be a place where medicine is not only taught but also studied. It should do its part to
advance medical science and art by encouraging original work,
and by selecting as its teachers those who have the training and
capacity for such work."

We now feel Welch's heart expanding as he makes the next
pronouncement, already used more than once in his educational
addresses: "In no other department of natural science are to be

---

* The entrance requirements of the better American schools were gradually
rising; some science was being demanded, although it was usually taught from
books, not in a laboratory. The University of Michigan had gone further than
any Eastern school except of course the Hopkins in raising entrance requirements.
Harvard was still discussing whether medicine was to be regarded as a full university department or a technological school; Councilman in 1892 was the first
medical professor called from outside.

found problems awaiting solution more attractive, more significant, than those in medicine; and certainly these problems do
not lose in dignity because they relate to the physical well-being
of mankind."

II

As first dean of the medical school, Welch helped Gilman
complete the faculty in time for the opening that autumn. The
major clinical chairs, of course, were functioning actively, but
professors were needed in the pre-clinical branches of anatomy,
physiology, and physiological chemistry and pharmacology.

The choice in physiology was W. H. Howell, a pupil of Martin's, who had taken his doctor of philosophy degree in that subject, after which he had been successively associate professor of
physiology at the Hopkins, professor of physiology and histology
at the University of Michigan, and had just become associate
professor of physiology at Harvard. Gilman himself went to Boston to interview Howell and quickly arranged for his return to
Baltimore.

Welch had kept in close touch with Mall, who had been his
first fellow in pathology. Trained in embryology under His,
Mall had spent one year studying physiology with Ludwig, a
superior combination for an anatomist; that it would have sufficed also in physiology was only a stronger recommendation to
Welch. And best of all, in the two years that Mall had been attached to the Pathological, he had shown unusual gifts as an investigator, joined with a strong and winning personality.

From Baltimore, Mall had gone to Clark University and
thence to the University of Chicago, where he became professor
of anatomy. Now Welch wrote him, asking if he would consider
the professorship of that subject at the Hopkins. Pointing out
that the intention was to have an anatomical department "which
should develop co-ordinately with the other great scientific departments of the University such as physics, chemistry, and biology," Welch reminded Mall that Baltimore was congenial to
"good, quiet scientific work" and assured him that the medical

school would be just as much a part of the university as the philosophical department.

Mall's situation in Chicago, however, had become so important that he found himself in a dilemma. In his element in those rapidly moving days, he had, as he confided to Welch, "formulated the biological department and practically planned its building," and was "stirring up the medical men and have them all on our side." By bringing together anatomy, physiology, botany, zoology, etc., a preliminary course covering two and a half years could be organized, besides which a large institute of "experimental diseases" in which should be housed all pathology, bacteriology, and sanitary science was being projected; in it the clinical subjects were to be taught by experiment as well as observation.

If this programme, which required a minimum of $4,000,000, sounds extravagant for its day, it could not have seemed so at Chicago at the time and it did not seem so to Mall, whose imagination was vivid but not uncontrolled. He was really looking ahead logically, the logic of the situation being the union of the fundamental or pre-clinical sciences with the clinical sciences in a co-ordinate whole in which both teaching and research should go on hand in hand. But he wrote at the end of his letter that Baltimore "has already solved most of these problems" and that he regarded the opportunity there as magnificent. "I consider you the greatest attraction," he wrote. "You make the opportunities. . . . So you see I am between two fires."

Mall hoped that Welch, who had been offered a professorship at Chicago with a considerable increase in salary, would himself become head of the institute. Welch, however, refused the offer and invited Mall to come to Baltimore for a conference. "The scheme which you outline for medical education in Chicago is a grand one," he told his former assistant, "but how coolly you talk about millions." Knowing that the income from the Women's Fund, a mere $20,000 yearly, would seem small compared to what was projected in Chicago, he added in his next letter: "I can think of but one motive which might influence you to come here with us and that is the desire to live here and a belief in our ideals and our future. I have confidence in our ideals as to medical education. . . . Whether with any amount of money you can attain them in Chicago is a question. They will not appeal to the mass of the public, not even to the medical public, for a considerable time. What we shall consider success, the mass of doctors will not consider success."

Mall's expected visit raised great hopes in Baltimore, but Welch was apprehensive. "It is amusing to see the assurance with which Halsted and Booker speak of your accepting our offer. I have not thought it proper to emphasize unduly this matter of our personal attachment to you, for after all the first considera- tion is where you will find the best opportunity for your life work, the most congenial surroundings for this work, the highest incentive not to fall short of your ideal."

There was great rejoicing when Mall telegraphed: "Shall cast my lot with Johns Hopkins." After his departure, the plans for a richly endowed institute at Chicago lapsed.

The third pre-clinical chair at the Hopkins, that of pharmacol- ogy and chemistry, was filled by calling John J. Abel from the University of Michigan.[6] He had studied at seven foreign uni- versities, taking his doctor's degree under the great Schmiede- berg at Strasbourg. Perhaps more deeply grounded in chemistry than in pharmacology, Abel was to make his most important con- tributions in that field.

The three additions to the faculty followed the Gilman tradi- tion of selecting young men for teachers. The ages of the medical professors at the time of their appointments were: Welch, thirty- four; Osler, forty; Halsted, thirty-seven; Kelly, thirty-one; How- ell, thirty-three; Abel, thirty-six; Mall, thirty-one. In this respect at least the university was repeating history, for its original ap- pointees to the philosophical faculty included Remsen at thirty, and Martin and Rowland each at twenty-eight. It is a remark- able fact that Welch, Mall, and Abel had all worked with Ludwig in Leipzig; and that Howell, Abel, and Mall had all been gradu- ate students at the Hopkins.[7]

In later years, Welch drew attention to the accident that had enabled the school to start with a faculty so well suited to its particular purpose. For had the school and hospital opened in 1886, as originally planned, they would have missed Osler, Halsted, and Mall. How serious a loss this would have been calls for no emphasis. And it may be added that Matthew Hay instead of Abel might have filled the chair of pharmacology, which would have been at severe cost to the strength of the school.[8]

III

Although nowhere else in this country had so specially and highly trained a group of teachers been assembled in an attempt to place medical education on a plane as high as existed anywhere in Europe, the school's success was by no means assured; Welch admitted later that all formalities were dispensed with at the opening in the fall of 1893 for fear that there would be no students. The severe entrance requirements might easily prove a fatal barrier, especially as only half the faculty were well known to the medical profession as a whole. The clinical group, and particularly Osler, had achieved a growing national reputation, but with the exception of Welch the laboratory teachers were unheard of outside a limited circle of investigators here and abroad.

Welch was delighted when the school began with seventeen entrants, fourteen men and three women. "In view of our extremely lofty and severe requirements for admission this is considered a good beginning," he wrote his stepmother. "In addition there are forty to fifty physicians doing graduate work. Everything seems most prosperous and successful here this winter." We can discern an apparent breath of relief. In his capacity of dean, Welch even interviewed the entering class with enthusiasm. "I must meet the medical students presently . . . and examine their qualifications. Tomorrow I have to talk to them like their grandfather and then I hand them over to their regular professors for the first year." With pride he added: "We shall have four Yale men . . . apparently about the best trained of the lot."

In other words, the country was reacting well. The curricular developments followed essentially the course charted in Welch's

1886 commencement address. Laboratories took the place of the lectures traditional in American medical schools—the hospital patient was nature's laboratory—and experiments the place of precepts. Textbooks were subordinated to consultation of original sources which the possession of a reading knowledge of French and German made possible. There were struggles, of course, but diligence and example and enthusiasm engendered by the fresh, pungent air about soon overcame any inadequacies in preparation and in foreign languages. Almost immediately the young men and women began to taste the joys of self-training, because so much of their time was placed at their own disposal and they were so closely in contact with their professors.

Research was, of course, carried on at the same time as teaching, and the abler students, without intent, found themselves enmeshed in the intellectual atmosphere it created. The feature of the school which became most distinctive was that undergraduates sometimes conducted investigations of their own. As a result, some discoveries were made and many independent men turned out.

When the school's second-year enrolment reached forty, of whom eight were women, Welch was delighted. To his sister, faced with the choice of a medical school for her younger son, Welch wrote: "Our degree will mean so much more than that of any other medical school on account of our higher requirements that its prestige will count for much, even in New York."

Brilliant undergraduates at other medical schools began clamouring to transfer to the Hopkins, although the faculty, convinced that no other schools could supply them with adequately prepared students, had resolved to admit no one to advanced standing. The first to apply was Eugene L. Opie, who was at the University of Maryland; his appeal was refused. When somewhat later William G. MacCallum of Toronto was accepted, Welch rushed off a note to Opie telling him to come, as well. A few years later Rufus Cole, who had almost completed his work at the University of Michigan, was admitted to the senior class. The rule had been thrown into the discard, but more significant was the perspicacity with which the faculty recognized the qualifications of three young men who were to play major parts in the development of American scientific medicine.

The new school was growing almost too fast for the physical accommodations available. At the outset two new stories had been built on the Pathological, one for anatomy and the other for pharmacology and physiological chemistry. Fortunately the Women's Fund Memorial Building was finished in time to free the Pathological for the second-year classes; its completion, however, brought with it a problem which showed that the bad feelings which had attended the laying down of conditions by the ladies had not been entirely dissipated.

Again we find Welch in the role of mediator. With typical tact he wrote Gilman: "I learn from Dr. Hurd that Miss Garrett has expressed an earnest desire to have the inscription 'Women's Fund Memorial Building' placed on the outside of the new Anatomical Building and will feel dissatisfied if it is not so placed. I understand that your preference is for a tablet inside of the building. I agree with you that it would be in better taste to place the inscribed tablet inside of the building but it appears to me that the choice is not of sufficient importance as regards the appearance of the building or any principle involved to make it worth while to act in opposition to Miss Garrett's wishes in this matter. . . . It may be that there are objections to placing the inscription outside which do not occur to me, but if there are not, do you not think it would be better not to run the risk of alienating Miss Garrett's interest in the Medical School as I do not know to whom else we are to look for additional endowment? Mr. Gwinn and Dr. Thomas, who are supposed to know something of Miss Garrett's intentions, have repeatedly said that she would probably give more money to the school some time. If she ventured to dictate concerning the instruction or policy of the medical school, I should oppose any concession, but it seems to me that as regards the position of the inscription she may properly express her preference and that it would be wise to conform to it. . . . Possibly this whole matter has been fully considered and the decision reached after knowledge of Miss Garrett's wish, but thinking that possibly it may not have been, I have taken the liberty of writing you about the way it appears to Dr. Hurd and myself."

Although Welch's counsel prevailed, Miss Garrett made no additional gift for the endowment of the medical school. Yet in 1906 she commissioned John Singer Sargent to paint the portrait of The Four Doctors, one of the most valued treasures of the Hopkins, and in her will she made the university the final legatee of the Garrett residence in Baltimore.

Welch's stand in the matter of the inscription did not indicate that his suspicions of coeducation had been entirely allayed. Indeed, his worst fears seemed to have been realized when one of the first three women students came to him during her third year to say that she thought she ought to drop out, since she had become a Christian Scientist. This change of point of view, she continued, was largely due to Osler, who, she was sure, must be a Christian Scientist at heart, for his methods of treatment were indistinguishable from those of Mrs. Eddy. Welch, Barker reports, "felt her leaving the school a narrow escape for its reputation."

When Mall became engaged to one of his students, Welch wrote him: "I fear that you have struck a death blow to coeducation in medicine. It is much better that you should be placed hors de combat for the interest of future generations of women medical students in the Hopkins. What will Miss Garrett say?" This, of course, was written jocosely, but as late as 1897 Welch advised Gilman against accepting a scholarship offered exclusively for women, since he felt it would be a mistake "thus to emphasize the coeducational feature, which at best is no help to us."

In a few more years, however, Welch was won round. "The necessity for co-education in some form," he was to write, "becomes more evident the higher the character of the education. In no form of education is this more true than in that of medicine. . . . I might say with reference to the opening of the School of Medicine at Johns Hopkins to women, that the Faculty deserve very little credit . . . for opening the doors to women. This, however, I may say—that we regard co-education as a success; those of us who were not enthusiastic at the beginning are now sympathetic and friendly. The embarrassments which one can conjure up have not materialized at all. The presence of women, as Dr. [Stephen] Smith has said, has lifted the tone not only of the students, but I may also say of the professors of the School, and our Hospital is thrown open to women graduates. One of the most successful teachers on our Faculty is a woman." [9]

He was even to become involved in the suffrage movement. Concerning a suffrage convention in Baltimore, he wrote his sister in January 1906: "I am to preside at one of the evening sessions—think of it! Miss Garrett and Miss Thomas made a special appeal to me to do so, and I consented." After the convention he added: "I have been hobnobbing with woman suffragists, Susan B. Anthony, Julia Ward Howe, and others. Last night I presided at their meeting devoted to municipal affairs, which was largely attended. They seemed pleased with what I said, although I did not commit myself on the suffrage question. I told them the administration of a city was largely housekeeping on a large scale, and that the more women's influence was felt in such matters the better for the people. . . . The suffragists are not such a queer lot of women as many suppose, and they could hardly have selected me to preside on account of their supposed preference for long-haired men. Still I am told by some Baltimore ladies, not in sympathy with the movement, that I was called in to discover the germs of the disease."

Welch's amusement at himself in the chair of a suffrage meeting must not be interpreted as opposition to "votes for women"; he probably just thought it a peculiar place for a stout old bachelor to be. His attitude toward suffrage, as other evidence shows, was not unsympathetic. He did not think a ballot in the hand of the female of the species would entirely drive evil from the world, as the militant supporters argued, but if the women wanted the vote he did not see why they should not have it. He had learned that his opposition to coeducation at the Hopkins had been a mistake.

When at the end of the second year of the medical school the students were about to enter their clinical studies at the hospital, Welch wrote Gilman: "I expect to hand in my resignation as dean at the next meeting with the expectation that Dr. Osler will be appointed to supervise the general organization of the clinical work of the third and fourth years." Actually the transfer was not made till the fall of 1898. "I have resigned every year, but this is the first time that I have succeeded," Welch told his sister. "Osler will not have time to attend to it long, but I did not want to drop the reins without his taking them if only for a short time." Osler served one year, and then the office passed into the capable hands of Howell.

The deanship, which Welch had relinquished with such pleasure, had taken a vast amount of his time, since he had carried out all its duties himself, without assistance of any sort. He conducted the voluminous correspondence in his own hand, even writing detailed letters about requirements to candidates for admission. Howell recalls that the minutes of the faculty meetings he kept "were not bare statements of attendance and actions taken, but quite elaborate accounts of topics presented and discussions which followed. . . . They were written *con amore* and Welch read them with the interest he would take in making an address. They were in the nature of essays."

Unfortunately, these minutes have disappeared. Howell tells us, however, that the meetings were open forums of discussion. "What Welch said carried the greatest weight, but Welch never seemed conscious of his own importance and never adopted an *ex cathedra* manner. When he had occasion to differ from a colleague he was careful to state the person's views very fairly and give due weight to them while expressing his own preference in a convincing way. So that his discussions were always pleasant and devoid of any emotional bent that might give rise to irritation." [10]

Welch's manner as dean was like his manner in the laboratory; he did not talk over problems with the members of the faculty, and it is doubtful whether he was often consulted by them. Since his method was to leave men in responsible positions alone, the impression he made on his colleagues was less that of facility in originating ideas than of helpfulness in passing on suggestions made by others. "His wisdom," writes Howell, "wide knowledge, and tolerance made him a wise and safe arbiter."

Year by year the entering classes had grown in numbers. Welch wrote his stepmother in the fall of 1897: "Our Medical School is prosperous so far as number of students is concerned, beyond all of our anticipations. More Yale students come here now than even to the College of Physicians and Surgeons in New York and we also have a fair representation from Harvard, which is remarkable considering the excellence of the Harvard Medical School. We expect to put up a new laboratory building this year.[11] I am of course kept very busy and I seem never to catch up with my work."

Indeed, as Welch pointed out, the high standards of admission, far from restricting enrolment, had brought students flocking, since it had been demonstrated that "far better methods of teaching and better results can be secured with highly trained students." The medical school, which less than five years before had been afraid it would have no scholars, was now faced with a serious problem of overcrowding. "It seems evident, if we can provide suitable accommodations, that our classes will continue to grow," Welch wrote Gilman in the fall of 1897. "I should say that we can reasonably look forward in a year or two to at least one hundred in the entering class, which would make a school of four hundred students."

Welch, who had remained dean until two classes had been graduated, had carried the Johns Hopkins Medical School through its critical period, and when at last he was permitted to step down, that radical experiment had been proved a success.

CHAPTER XII

The Public Arena

I

WELCH'S part in the success of the Hopkins experiment had not been limited to his activities within the university walls; already he had begun to appear on the national stage as an outstanding propagandist for the new medical science. Already he was being called on to play a role which he had never imagined for himself. When he arrived in Baltimore he had meant to spend the rest of his days quietly developing a laboratory where he could pursue his sequestered way teaching and investigating. But it seemed only natural that in 1886 he should be chosen as the spokesman for the projected medical school at the tenth anniversary exercises of the university. And on that occasion he drew so alluring a picture of modern medical education, and revealed so sympathetic a personality, that unconsciously he imperilled his dearly bought laboratory career.

A year later he was asked to give the annual address before the Medical and Chirurgical Faculty of Maryland, and he could not resist this opportunity to bring before the physicians and surgeons of that state the implications of the newer bacteriology. Again he made a great impression that brought him more invitations to speak. Even in New York he had expressed a fear of talking too much in public; now he wrote his brother-in-law: "In an evil moment I consented to deliver the address at the Yale Commencement and shall not be happy again until it is over. I am appointed to deliver the address on State Medicine* at the meeting of the American Medical Association next year. I think

---

* In those days the phrase "state medicine" connoted what we now call preventive medicine. It is indicative of his position as spokesman for the new bacteriology that Welch was twice asked to deliver the address on this subject before the American Medical Association, first in 1889 and then in 1903.

that I had better decline this or I shall have a reputation for nothing but talk."

The opportunity was too valuable to decline; both doctors and laymen must be taught the importance of the new laboratory methods of teaching and research, and these methods could not be effective until medical schools ceased being private associations of doctors, and were keyed into the university structure of the nation. Again and again the opportunity came to him to expound these truths in major centres of learning, and he could not find the heart to refuse. Educators all over the land who wished to bring their institutions up to date called on Welch to throw his persuasive personality into their local battles; and when, the fight being won, new laboratory buildings were ready to be dedicated, Welch was called on to speak at the ceremonies to drive home the significance of the reform.

Welch's persuasiveness on the platform was not based on oratory; he appealed to reason rather than to emotion. His speeches contain no hyperbole, no metaphor, no piling of phrase on phrase. Indeed, read over now when the reforms he fought for have been almost universally accepted, his talks carry with them little sense of excitement; it was his method not to make his ideas seem startling and new, but rather obvious and inevitable. Yet in those days, when the doctrines he advocated seemed visionary, his lucid expositions struck with a force much greater than the finest tricks of speech-making could have done.

Welch carried conviction through perfect command of his subject, through his ability to make the complex simple without deviation from truth. His fine head, the healthy, rosy colour which suffused his face once he got well into his discourse, the beard trimmed to a short imperial, gave him distinction on the platform. His pleasant voice carried well and filled a large auditorium without being raised. Sometimes his first few sentences were a little slow and hesitant, but once self-consciousness had disappeared his well-chosen words flowed without apparent effort. When occasion demanded, his voice would become earnest and expressed feeling without perceptible change of pitch; his tone was powerful and even, carrying his hearers on by the intrinsic interest of the subject and the lucidity of its expression.

Superb teacher that he was, Welch was not afraid of repetition. He boiled the complex of ideas he wished to put over down to a few simple, basic points, and on these he dwelt again and again, often employing in several speeches almost identical words. He would size up the local situation, however, modifying his argument for the occasion on which he was speaking; tact was among his most powerful weapons.

At first he wrote out his addresses and read them, but soon he found this unnecessary. An outline jotted down quickly on the train sufficed; when he stood on the lecture platform his mind would automatically clothe the bare skeleton with words. If he read up on a subject in advance, he would make copious notes, but he would not take them with him to the meeting; by writing the facts down he had engraved them on his memory. As the years passed, he found it increasingly arduous to resurrect for publication speeches thus delivered; getting up the material had been fun, talking it out had been easy, but the labour of putting it all on paper when the occasion was over he found almost too dull to be borne. He could, however, if persuaded to try, write out a speech almost as fluently as he had delivered it and in almost the same words.

Many stories exist of the strength of his concentration once he forced himself to composition. He did not begin the Ether Day address he delivered in 1908 until he was actually on the train to Boston. He took a handful of cigars to the smoking car which, Cushing tells us, "was full of drummers all smoking furiously. They moved up and gave Popsy a seat in the corner where like a Buddha he sat on his feet and began writing . . . with no apparent hesitation. He nevertheless was aware of what was going on and every now and then joined in the conversation." He explained to Cushing that every page of the block-size paper on which he always wrote his speeches took a minute and a half to deliver; occasionally he would count the pages to see where he stood. When Cushing finally went to bed about eleven, Welch had accounted for twenty-three minutes, but by the next morning an exact hour of talk was down and ready to be published without change.

Once he spoke about diphtheria on an occasion so formal that a written address seemed indicated; he unfolded a sheaf of papers and began to read. Having finished the introductory paragraph, he requested the permission of his audience to put aside his written speech and continue extemporaneously. Unfortunately he forgot to take his papers with him from the rostrum. Eager to preserve Popsy's words for posterity, I retrieved the sheets, only to discover that all except the one containing the first paragraph were entirely blank.

Welch's talks were by no means all directed at doctors; "the time has come," he said, "when the needs of medical education should be brought forcibly before the general public in this country." Indeed, the newer scientific teaching was so expensive that endowments which could only be supplied by laymen were a first requisite. Medicine, as Welch pointed out, was at that time the stepchild of philanthropy. He quoted from the report of the United States Bureau of Education for 1890–91 to show that there were only five endowed chairs in American medical colleges, and not a single one south or west of Philadelphia, while there were 171 endowed chairs of theology, many of them in the South and the West. In 1889 the entire productive funds for medicine in the United States amounted to $249,200, contrasted with $11,939,631 for theology. In 1892 the figures were $611,214 for medicine and $17,599,979 for theology. Yet there were twice as many students of medicine as of theology, and medical instruction was much more expensive than theological. "If the public desires good physicians it must help to make them," Welch argued so effectively that the speeches he delivered all over the nation played a major part in making medicine the favourite object of American philanthropy.

Welch never tired of arguing, as he had done in his addresses outlining the plans for the Johns Hopkins Medical School, that modern medical education, far from producing visionary scientists, made better practitioners, since their therapy was based not on tradition but on knowledge. He also referred again and again to the fact that the best teachers were research workers; "the teaching of him who has questioned nature and received her answers has often, and I think commonly, in spite it may be of defects of delivery, a rarer and more inspiring quality."

Provisions for research, Welch insisted, should not be confined to a few medical schools. "The field must be a wide one in order to attract many to a scientific career, for of the many only a few will be found endowed with the power of discovery. There is no possible way of recognizing the possessor of this power before he has demonstrated it." No error could be greater than to suppose that the duplication of research is a waste of time and money, for it is out of the efforts of many men working in different environments and each led on by his individual light, that discoveries are made.

In his advocacy of laboratory teaching Welch was not unaware of its shortcomings. The methods are "extremely timetaking, and are not adapted to present the entire contents of any subject. Their great service is in developing the scientific spirit and in imparting a living, abiding knowledge, which cannot be gained by merely reading or being told about things." Some important subjects, of course, "either for lack of time or from the nature of the subject-matter, cannot readily be taught in the laboratory. The attention of the student in the laboratory is likely to be concentrated upon isolated facts . . . while other groups of facts and particularly broad general principles are in danger of being lost to view. There is, therefore, risk of loss of perspective in relying solely upon instruction in the laboratory." For these reasons Welch would supplement laboratory work by didactic and demonstrative lectures.

"It is important that the student should carry away from the medical school a certain mass of positive knowledge. It is still more important that he should acquire some measure of medical wisdom and of the scientific spirit, and that he should have that methodic training in observing and in drawing logical conclusions, and that familiarity with instruments and methods of examination which will enable him to continue independently his education, to follow and incorporate new discoveries in medicine, and critically to judge and to make the most of his own observations. Medical education is not completed at the medical school; it is there only begun. Of the various subjects in a medical course, the fundamental medical sciences are especially those which afford to the student this methodic training, and are calculated to develop habits of accurate observation and to stimulate interest in the practical side of his profession. The medical art is becoming more and more the application to practice of medical science."

Welch's conception of medical education was, as we should expect from his temperament, a carefully balanced one. Thus, although he would have pure science freed, as far as possible, from philosophical theory, he advocated "the study of languages, history and philosophy, which give a culture not to be derived solely from the study of the natural sciences and which should add greatly to the intellectual pleasure, satisfaction, breadth of vision and even efficiency of the man of science."

While expounding the importance of pathology for the understanding of disease, he insisted that it must be studied not merely from a narrow practical point of view. Speaking at the dedication of the Hull Biological Laboratories at the University of Chicago, he said: "The relations of pathology to practical medicine are so intimate that the broader conception of this science as a part of biology is not always appreciated." Pathology, "the pure science of medicine as distinguished from the art of healing," should be studied in the same spirit as biology is studied, since the two are closely allied, one dealing with the norm of nature, the other with nature's abnormal functions. "Experience has shown that the most important discoveries in science come not from those who make utility their guiding principle, but from the investigators of truth for its own sake, wherever and however they can attain it. It is shortsighted to fail to see that the surest way to advance pathology, even in its relations to practical medicine, is to cultivate it as a science from all points of view."

Welch's favourite among his addresses was the one on "Adaptation in Pathological Processes," which he delivered in 1897 as president of the American Congress of Physicians and Surgeons.[1] He defined adaptive processes as "the entire group of pathological processes whose results tend to the restoration or compensation of damaged structure or function or the direct neutralization of the injurious agents. Processes which may be described variously as compensatory, regenerative, self-regulatory, protective, healing, are thus included under adaptive pathological processes."

Welch began by rejecting the debated proposition "that the conception of adaptation has no place in scientific inquiry; that we are justified in asking only by what means a natural phenomenon is brought about, and not what is its meaning or purpose; in other words, that the only question open to scientific investigation is How? and never Why?"

The human mind, he said, is so constituted as to desire to seek an explanation of the adaptations which it finds everywhere in organic nature. "From the days of Empedocles and of Aristotle up to the present time there have been two leading theories to explain the apparent purposefulness of organic nature—the one, the teleological, and the other, the mechanical theory." The first implies something in the nature of an intelligence working for a predetermined end. The other is the only one open to scientific investigation and is the one which forms the working hypothesis of most biologists; it seeks an explanation for adaptations in organic evolution. Now Welch disclosed his purpose, which was to bring pathology into conformity with physiology, by showing that the doctrine of evolution helps explain both.

From ancient times to the present, he pointed out, disease has been viewed as a combative process in the presence of harmful influences. "Whole systems of medicine have been founded upon this conception, clothed in varying garb," and such theories have "profoundly influenced medical practice and were the origin of such well-known expressions as *vis medicatrix naturæ* and *medicus est minister naturæ*."

Modern investigation carries all the various physiological adaptations, the reactions of the body to normal stimuli, back to the cells, which "are especially fitted by innate properties, determined . . . in large part by evolutionary factors," to respond to changed conditions. Do the cells similarly possess peculiar fitness to meet the changes in the body created by disease? "Can we," Welch asked, "recognize in adaptive pathological processes any manifestations of cellular properties which we may not suppose the cells to possess for physiological uses?" His answer was that "most pathological adaptations have their foundation in physiological processes or mechanisms. . . . Evolutionary factors have not in general intervened with any direct reference to their adaptation" to the emergencies of illness.

Since the cells, which are fitted to respond to normal stimuli, have no separate and distinct powers of reaction to stimuli created by disease, the reaction of the cells to a morbid condition need not necessarily have curative value; indeed, many pathological reactions are harmful rather than beneficial to the individual. This led Welch to point out that "we see here, as everywhere, that 'Nature is neither kind nor cruel, but simply obedient to law, and, therefore, consistent.' " Did Welch, as he repeated this quotation, remember that twenty-seven years before, in his commencement oration at his graduation from Yale, he had exclaimed about an almost identical expression of the scientific point of view: "Oh is there not bitterness in such a thought? Does it not make life hopeless and not worth living?" Now, however, there was no trace of emotion in his voice; he proceeded to his conclusion with the irrevocable logic of a scientist.

The body's adjustments to morbid processes, he said, "present all degrees of fitness. Some are admirably complete; more are adequate, but far from perfect; many are associated with such disorder and failures that it becomes difficult to detect the element of adaptation. The teleological conception of a useful purpose in no case affords an explanation of the mechanism of an adaptive process. . . . For the most part, the agencies employed are such as exist primarily for physiological uses, and while these may be all that are required to secure a good pathological adjustment, often they have no special fitness for this purpose.

"The healing power of nature is, under the circumstances present in disease, frequently incomplete and imperfect, and systems of treatment based exclusively upon the idea that nature is doing the best thing possible to bring about recovery or some suitable adjustment, and should not be interfered with, rest often upon an insecure foundation. The agencies employed by nature may be all that can be desired; they may, however, be inadequate, even helpless, and their operation may add to existing disorder. There is ample scope for the beneficent work of the physician and surgeon."

II

Welch had created a laboratory and was encouraging the creation of others; but once investigators had completed their work, they could find no place of publication in the United States. All the existing medical magazines were clinical journals, designed to serve practitioners, not laboratory workers, and unadapted to scientific papers. This was not remarkable, since a scientific journal had of necessity to wait until there were many productive laboratories to supply it with a steady stream of suitable articles and an audience capable of understanding them. Furthermore, a subsidy would be needed. A journal could not be started until the nation was ready, but in the meantime its absence hindered the contact between laboratory and laboratory so essential to the investigators who were trying to prepare the nation.

The lack of organs of publication was not a new problem for the Johns Hopkins University. Gilman had already established under university auspices, but "open freely to contributions from every part of the country," special journals in subjects far enough developed to support a magazine; and in subjects where the university departments were working almost alone, he had encouraged them to publish occasional volumes made up entirely of their own work. Welch's pathological laboratory fell into the latter category; during 1888 he expressed the desire to publish a special volume. When a year later the opening of the hospital made money available for the *Johns Hopkins Hospital Reports*, which were to be similar to those brought out by several English hospitals, Welch was authorized to devote the first volume to reports of the work in his laboratory.[2]

Blithely Welch began editing the papers it was planned to publish, but he soon found himself struggling with a mass of impeding detail. The illustrations, since such plates had rarely been wanted in the United States, could be best made in Germany; Mall, who happened to be abroad, negotiated with the lithographer. Furthermore, the articles themselves required constant revision as a result of new researches the workers had undertaken.

Osler, who had started on a volume of clinical reports some time after Welch had started on the pathological volume, brought his out in 1890, long before Welch's was ready. "Our volume is Vol. I," Welch complained, "notwithstanding its appearance subsequent to Vol. II. I do not like this arrangement but it can not be changed now." He added hopefully that he was sure his volume could be published in less than a year. That summer he went abroad, partly to attend to the printing of plates for the volume, but delay followed on delay: the customs house was slow when the invaluable sheets arrived, the articles required correcting at the most inopportune moments, and it was not till 1897, seven years after Volume II had appeared, that Volume I saw the light of day.

Meanwhile the problem of publication had become more and more serious as Welch's laboratory expanded. Every expedient had to be grasped, including use of the *Johns Hopkins Hospital Bulletin,* a monthly intended primarily for the clinical department, which was the first regular periodical brought out by an American hospital as a repository for its work. In October 1893 Welch asked Gilman to meet with several members of the faculty, including Osler and himself, who were interested in founding a new medical journal to appear the following January.[3]

Two years later the matter was still in abeyance. "Abel is stirring things up for a new journal of high character for laboratory workers in this country in pathology, pharmacology, and physiology," Welch wrote Mall. "I think it may go through if we can secure Bowditch and the principal laboratory workers."

Go through it did, to Welch's delight, the Hopkins agreeing to contribute $1000 annually. But then a disturbing thing happened: "all seemed to think it necessary," as he wrote his sister, that he assume the editorship. Reluctantly he accepted, since he was convinced of the importance of the new venture. "The Journal of which I am editor will be the biggest thing ever undertaken in this country in the way of a scientific medical periodical. It has nothing to do with practical medicine, any more than I have. There are to be no editorials, advertisements, or vulgar features of ordinary medical journals, but the subscribers will doubtless be as rarified as the pure atmosphere in which the journal will float."

Indeed, the *Journal of Experimental Medicine,* as the new venture was called, was itself a radical experiment; it was generally believed that America did not produce enough scientific work to fill its pages. Eager to spread their net as widely as possible, the founders kept secret the fact that the Hopkins was contributing financial support; "every effort was made," Welch told Florence R. Sabin, "to make the journal national and not appear as a Johns Hopkins enterprise exclusively." A distinguished board of associate editors, appointed from different universities, were to pass on doubtful manuscripts if the editor called on them, which he probably never did, and, more important, they and their pupils were to contribute papers, as were the fifty-six scientists who were designated "collaborators." As soon as he was made editor, Welch began a diligent search for material. "Keep the Journal in mind as the best place to publish a scientific research," he urged Abbott in a typical letter. "Have you anything for us?" [4]

Even before the first issue appeared, Welch's editorial responsibilities added so much to his already heavy burden of work that he found increasing difficulty getting to his classes, as frequent notes to his subordinates show. "It will help me out in getting this malarial article off my hands," he wrote typically, "if you will look after the class this afternoon, although I hate to impose on you so much." He was even forced to give up a projected visit to his sister for the Christmas holidays. In addition to all his other tasks, he complained to her, "I must also see through the press and write an article for the new edition of one of Dr. Flint's books." Welch had not entirely given up preparing the lucid and encyclopædic scientific articles for books on the practice of medicine which he had embarked on during his New York period and which were his earliest activity for the education of the medical profession at large.

Welch's greatest difficulty as an editor arose less from outside engagements than from his own temperament, which demanded scrupulous attention to detail, but would not allow him to accept assistance in this time-consuming work. He rarely consulted the associate editors, and, shunning secretaries, wrote all the voluminous correspondence in his own hand.

His meticulousness began with the receipt of a paper. He read it closely, and if he found it unacceptable returned it with a kind note of rejection. If it required revision, he would often rewrite it himself. Should the author have overlooked important items in the earlier literature, Welch would point them out in a detailed letter. After telling Herter, for instance, that there were "one or two points which have occurred to me . . . which may, perhaps, lead you to make some additions or changes," he filled several pages with comments of a highly expert character. Welch introduced the system of checking every bibliographic reference, for which his excellent personal library sufficed, and of giving references in a uniform style much like that used in the *Surgeon General's Catalogue* and the *Index Medicus.* Then after the papers were in form, Welch prepared the manuscript for the printer, read proofs, arranged for illustrations, laid out with his own hand the make-up of the successive issues.

Always he found time to encourage a young investigator in his difficult path. Thus he wrote Cullen: "You are to be congratulated upon the excellent way in which you have written up and discussed these interesting cases. The drawings are works of art and make everything clear. You are taking the right way to build up a scientific reputation."

But sometimes a note of weariness is apparent. "Immune 'from' is the only correct construction," he explained to Abbott. "I was in despair when I had gone all over your manuscript and made it correct for you to change it all back with an interrogating hand in the proof. You and many others are confused because the Germans say 'immun gegen," but that is not English." And to me: "I notice you usually write it the Bacillus Dysenteriae. It should be Bacillus dysenteriae, leaving out the 'the,' and having the generic name always begin with a capital, and the specific one with a small letter." Welch was a purist concerning nomenclature. He consulted Migula in this case and noted that he had given the name I used to Ogata's bacillus, and if he had done so before Shiga wrote, his name would be the one to stand, but Migula wrote in 1900 and Shiga in 1898, so that the form Welch suggested was correct. He frequently consulted Stiles, an authority on nomenclature, in doubtful cases. This was just one more time-consuming effort toward perfection. Yet the educational value of the example set is not to be depreciated in this new country.

The *Journal* succeeded beyond all expectations, since American laboratories proved able to produce far more articles worthy of its pages than anyone had foreseen. Welch must have been greatly relieved, but success brought with it a penalty. At the end of the first six months, we find him writing Mall: "It will probably take me all summer to answer letters. The third number of the Journal will be a fat one, and will be out this month." And within a year he admonished Abbott: "I hope that the article will be made as short as may be. My editorial cry is 'Condensation.' Everybody writes too long papers." In apologizing to Herter for having to postpone the inclusion of a paper, Welch wrote in April 1897: "I have now waiting for publication enough articles to fill the next number, which have been in my hands for from six months to a year. The writers are justly becoming impatient." Welch assured Herter that he would not complain if the paper were published elsewhere.

To Nuttall in Cambridge, England, Welch wrote: "I am glad that you are pleased with the new journal. There can be no doubt of its scientific success. More material of good quality is coming in for publication than we can easily handle. We need all the subscriptions which we can get and hope that the journal will appeal to foreign scientific workers. I think that they will have to

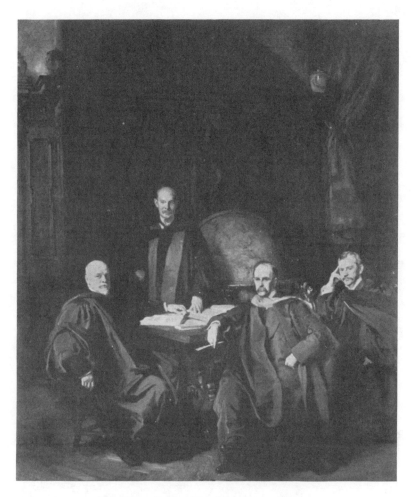

"The Four Doctors" by John Singer Sargent

WELCH, HALSTED, OSLER, KELLY

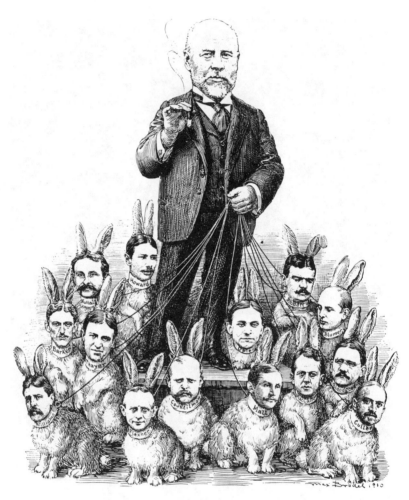

"Some Welch Rabbits"
Drawing by Max Brödel

take it if they wish to follow scientific investigations in medicine on this side of the water."

The new ferment in scientific medicine was at work, and Welch was being pressed on many sides. In 1897 the *Journal* of six hundred pages a year, at first published irregularly, was definitely established on a bi-monthly basis, and those who were afraid there would be a lack of papers for even one modest periodical were searching the horizon for signs of another magazine to help carry the growing load. As was to be expected, the relief came from the special subject that had been developed earliest in this country: the *American Journal of Physiology*, sponsored by the American Society of Physiology under Bowditch's nominal and Porter's actual editorship, began publication in January 1898. In sending Porter his subscription, Welch wrote: "As you know, I entirely approve of starting the new Journal. The pressure upon the pages of the Journal of Experimental Medicine has become excessive and your journal will afford considerable relief. When we started the Journal it was anticipated that separate departments, and first Physiology, would branch off." [5]

In 1901 Welch heard that Dr. Harold Ernst of the Harvard Medical School was planning to start another periodical in the same field as the *Journal of Experimental Medicine*. Ernst had founded the Boston Society of Medical Sciences in 1896, the year Welch's journal had first appeared, and had begun publishing its proceedings in a small pamphlet, which he now wished to convert into a national publication as the official organ of the newly organized American Association of Pathologists and Bacteriologists. Aside from this planned change of status of a local publication, the fact that the time had come for the organization of a special society for pathologists and bacteriologists in this country was significant, especially when we remember that this was also the date of the founding of the Rockefeller Institute for Medical Research.

Without troubling to consult the Johns Hopkins, which was helping to support the *Journal of Experimental Medicine*, Welch, who was finding the labours of editing increasingly onerous, offered to give the periodical to Ernst. In May he wrote me: "I am determined to give up the responsible editorship of the Journal. It is too great a burden, and some one else can do the work more easily than I, and just as well." Saying that the Hopkins "in its present financial straits" should be relieved of supporting the *Journal,* he concluded: "If Ernst is unable to take charge, then I must see what else can be done."

Ernst and President Eliot of Harvard were delighted with the idea of taking over the publication, but when Welch admitted at a meeting of the Hopkins faculty that he was giving it away, there was general surprise and consternation. "Mr. Gilman," Howell remembers, "called his attention to the fact that such a transfer was not permissible without the consent of the University which was financing the Journal in part. The situation was a bit tense and might have been awkward, but Welch at once acquiesced in Mr. Gilman's point of view and let the matter drop without argument, accepting pleasantly a resolution to appoint an assistant editor to take the burden off his shoulders." But Welch knew that he could not work with an assistant; none was ever appointed.

The first issue of Ernst's periodical, the *Journal of Medical Research,* appeared as a separate entity in July 1901; Welch was forced to return to the unwelcome grind of editing his own magazine. He got out several issues, but after March 1902 the *Journal of Experimental Medicine* suddenly ceased to appear. No explanation was given; manuscripts continued to stream in, but none was passed on to the printer. Now Welch was confining his activity as editor to attempts to give the journal away to someone acceptable to the university. In September he wrote Herter: "I should be simply delighted if the Rockefeller Institute would take over the Journal of Experimental Medicine. . . . The editorial burden weighs on me and I should be only too glad to part with it entirely, or, if that is not possible, to share it with you or Flexner or anyone suitable." He had reached the point where he would even attempt to collaborate with an associate.

Welch's final breakdown as an editor is not to be wondered at, considering the way in which he executed his office. So long as the journal appeared, he never relaxed his severe measures of editorial policy. Furthermore, his habit of leaving things to the last minute and then working under heavy pressure did not accord well with bringing out successive numbers of a regular periodical. All these labours no longer seemed worth while. It was typical of Welch that during the early days of an important enterprise he was very active in it and even willing to do chores; but once the venture was well launched, he felt it was time for others to take over. The wonder is that he published the journal for five long years with adequate punctuality.

Now he refused to budge despite innumerable proddings. Gilman's successor, President Remsen, wrote him on June 27, 1903: "Will it be possible for you to take up the work on the Journal of Experimental Medicine and complete the volume that is now hanging in mid-air? This is a matter in which the honor of the University is involved and it is necessary that the volume should be completed in the immediate future, or else the money in our hands will have to be returned to the subscribers. I sincerely hope that you will be able to take this matter up and carry it to the conclusion. If there is anything we can do here to help you we shall be glad to do so."

When all such appeals were unavailing, the Hopkins agreed to let Welch turn the journal over to the Rockefeller Institute, where Opie and I undertook the editorship. Welch's habit of procrastination prevented him from completing the necessary formalities. On December 24, 1903, Dr. L. Emmett Holt, the secretary of the institute, wrote somewhat frantically: "The Executive Committee . . . have received repeated inquiries and appeals from men who have sent articles to be published in the Journal of Experimental Medicine, under the impression that the Journal was already in the hands of the Institute. . . . As yet we have nothing to do with the conduct of the Journal and we would like to know what response shall be made to such letters."

Even after the institute secured legal possession of the journal in October 1904, Welch failed to turn over the manuscripts he had accumulated; I mentioned them to him several times, always receiving some such reply as, "Oh, yes. I'll get them out and send them to you." They never came. Finally I made a special journey to Baltimore. Welch received me with his usual graciousness, sat me down, and discoursed charmingly. When I mentioned the object of my visit, he said he would send the manuscripts to me in a day or two, and then attempted to turn to other things. "Why not get them out now?" I interposed. He answered that they would make too large a package to carry. I assured him that I had an empty suitcase in the hall which would certainly suffice. Then, with a smile of resignation, Welch began a search for the papers. He seemed to have stored them in no particular place; some were in desk drawers, some on shelves, some even piled on chairs. As I carried them away, I could almost hear him sighing with relief.[6]

III

During the arduous years when the responsibilities of editorship were added to his other back-breaking burdens, Welch needed more than ever a haven to which he could escape; trips to Atlantic City became a habit that lasted for his lifetime. He loved sea bathing, and the carnival aspects of the resort amused him. "Doubtless this is a vulgar place," he told his sister, "but I am contented and you can be as quiet as you like. There is the most terrifying, miraculous, blood-curdling affair called the 'Flip-flap railroad.' . . . After being pulled by trolley to the top, you go down from a height of about 75 feet by the momentum and then swing around the inside of the perpendicular circle, of course a part of the time with the head down and feet up, so that you would drop out of the car, if it was not for the tremendous speed. After waiting in vain to see someone killed, I tried it. They put Roman candles on the back of my car, so that the effect was a continuous circle of flame. As you go around the circle, the effect is indescribable, but it is so short in time that you really do not know what is happening to you. You are in a sort of suspended animation. Crowds stand around and say they would not try it for a thousand dollars. If you are looking for a new and thrilling sensation, this will fill the bill. It beats anything that I ever saw or dreamed of, and is said to be unique, having only just been built out on a long pier over the ocean. I should not think that Stuart or Fred would rest content until they have come and tried it. I must go now and watch it. I shall probably be here a week or so, unless destroyed on the centrifugal road."

Welch had no use for the quiet resorts to which the scholarly are supposed to want to retire. "Do you like Mohonk better than Narragansett?" he asked Emma. "It is a Quakerish sort of place, I believe, but conducive to love making. . . . I have not much idea of where it is, but picture it as a kind of twin-lakes-resort with Miss Dares' sitting in rockers on the broad piazza—very restful to shattered nerves—where it seems as if nine o'clock would never come so that one could decently go to bed. I have been told that Mr. Smiley and the whole establishment were once shaken to their foundations by discovery of a game of cards in one of the rooms. Stuart doubtless knows that colored neckties are not allowed."

Joseph S. Ames, a later president of the Hopkins, tells us: "Every now and then Dr. Welch would retire from Baltimore to Atlantic City with the avowed purpose of not having people see him eat, and down there he would order five and six desserts and nothing else." I myself remember that when I had Sunday dinner with him in Atlantic City and ordered one dessert, he told me gravely that no one orders less than two. He would never take more than his guest; it may be that he would have liked three or four desserts, but did not dare suggest that I eat so many.

In Baltimore, he always kept a box of bonbons in his desk, and it irritated him to see people eat sparingly. When I visited there during the 1900's, he was disgusted by the simple breakfasts he discovered I ate, and on one occasion he insisted that I breakfast with him at his club. I tried to escape by saying that I had to get started too soon for him—his late risings were notorious—but he opened his eyes wonderingly. "What do you mean?" he said. "I often eat as soon as the dining room opens;

sometimes I wish it would open earlier." The lesson he was going to teach me was, he felt, worth rising for at what was to him pale dawn. Sure enough, he was on hand at eight. I found the meal had been ordered—showers of eggs, griddle-cakes, sausages—and he kept a stern eye on me, making sure that I put them all down.

There is some disagreement as to whether Welch could be correctly termed an epicure. His visible girth showed that he loved food, but did he discriminate between the delicious and the merely delightful? Freeman says yes; Halsted says no. The truth seems to be that Welch's philosophy enabled him to be contented in any situation. If perfectly cooked diamond-backed terrapin came his way, he ate it with appreciative delight, but if there was no terrapin to be had, why, he would enjoy a plate of ice cream at a wayside stand.

Concerning tobacco, Welch was not particular; it was generally agreed that he would smoke anything that would burn. The cigar that was perpetually in his mouth, protruding straight forward when he walked, rising and falling during conversations, screwed to one side as he looked through his microscope, the cigar that was almost part of his apparel, cost five or at most ten cents. His favourite brand was "Robert Burns," both light and cheap. If one of his more particular friends—Dr. Buttrick, for instance—offered him a fine cigar, he accepted it, but he was too much of a realist to offer one of his own cigars in return. At the day-long meetings of some of the boards on which he sat, there would be a box of excellent cigars on the table. These Welch would smoke with relish for a while, lighting one from the other, but in an hour or two the rich and heavy tobacco would begin to cloy; then Welch would reach into his own pocket and light a Robert Burns from Havana's best. Not till after lunch would he return to the good cigars.

For years the continually enlarging figure in its wreath of smoke was a familiar sight on the streets of Baltimore; Welch was an inveterate walker. At any hour of the day or night in any part of town he was to be seen, striding sometimes in deep thought with a rapidity that belied his bulk, but just as often peering into shop windows or listening to the conversations of street urchins with a twinkling curiosity. The whole world was his province, and certainly the best way to see the world is to walk through it.

When visiting his family in Norfolk, he loved to wander about the countryside where he had spent his childhood. We can see him in our minds' eye rambling where the beauty of the hills and lanes, the variegated foliage, the profusion of wild flowers, and the outcroppings exposing the geological formation of the region offered so much to stir his interest and enchant his eye. He never owned walking shoes but walked in his everyday shoes without any thought of their suitability. Moving ahead with a quick, elastic step, he was alone except for his ceaselessly smoking cigar.

During his forty-sixth year, a faster method of locomotion caught his fancy; he wrote his sister: "I had a road bicycle lesson in New York and learned the art of mounting at the Madison Sq. Garden. The instructor there . . . said that I was sufficiently proficient to go on the road so that we went up to Central Park and I rode ten miles through the park and down the boulevard without any accident. He seemed to think I did remarkably well and could travel now on my own hook. The hills exhausted me and I was pretty well pumped out when we finished, but none the worse for it."

He carried his new skill back with him to Baltimore. "I have a Columbia bicycle and enjoy riding," he added eight months later, "but have not much time except at night in the park which is thronged with thousands of bicycles. I have punctured my tire already."

Welch was by no means averse to light-hearted amusements. He enjoyed playing whist with his friends, and exchanged all kinds of anagrams, charades, and verbal puzzles with them. He sent, for instance, to his sister the following jumble of letters, RTHDXXFRDDNSKNWGDLDPRTFRMLGWD, assuring her that by inserting a certain vowel in the proper places she would "obtain a sentence indicating the knowledge obtained at one of our oldest universities." [7] Enjoying chess, he always kept a board in his rooms so that he could work out the weekly problems in the *Times,* and upon occasion he even bested Major Venable, the club champion. When visiting players such as Lasker took on a dozen or more Baltimore experts at once, Welch sat behind one of the boards and tried to trip up the prodigy.

Those were the almost fabulous years, still discussed wistfully by Baltimoreans, when their baseball team, the Orioles, won the pennant three years running. "We are the champions," Welch wrote Emma, "and everybody here is fully aware of the fact. I have attended most of the games and have become an enthusiast, even a crank, on the subject."

His stoutish figure became familiar to the rooters in the grandstand. Between innings he would correct the proof of the *Journal of Experimental Medicine,* but once the play had resumed, he was all attention, continually scribbling on a complicated diagram he held on his knees. Welch had invented a system for keeping a record of every play which he considered far in advance of any then in existence, and he could not have been more proud of a major scientific discovery. A mine of baseball lore, he knew everyone's batting average, and the most personal facts about the players. Daily he compared form with performance, and he was delighted when Baltimore won.

It amused Welch to make out that he went to the games reluctantly. "Councilman," he wrote me, "returned Saturday, wildly enthusiastic about baseball all of the time and dragging me out daily to see the game." However, one afternoon while I was demonstrating at the microscope, Welch appeared at my shoulder. "The ball game starts in about an hour," he whispered. "We can make it; come on."

"But, Dr. Welch," I objected, "I have a class."

"I know, but can't you finish a little early?"

IV

Late in the 1890's Welch was suddenly faced with the necessity of defending scientific medicine in the United States from virtual destruction. So many triumphs were being achieved through animal experimentation that the method was being increasingly employed all over the nation as laboratories multiplied. This development stirred the antivivisectionists to greater and greater frenzy. As Welch tells us, "charges of wanton cruelty [were] brought against physiologists and physicians . . . unmatched for recklessness of statement, slanderous misrepresentations and deceit, unbounded credulity, and ignorance, not through any personal knowledge of the object of their attack or of its relations to the interests of science and humanity." And he adds that "the agitation for the prohibition of experiments on animals, conducted under the guise of an humane purpose, is fundamentally inhuman, for if it were to succeed the best hopes of humanity for further escape from physical suffering and disease would be destroyed."

Gathering from all parts of the country, publicly carrying a banner of guileless love for all animal creation, the antivivisectionists, who, although growing in power for thirty years, had been consistently defeated in their attempts to get various state legislatures to curb animal experimentation, descended on the United States Senate in 1896 to obtain in the District of Columbia what had so far been denied them in the states. The move was both astute and hazardous; a more powerful proponent of antivivisection measures might be secured, but the central government would be threatened, since the Bureau of Animal Industry of the Department of Agriculture was conducting in Washington experiments aimed at preventing disease in livestock.

An important advocate of antivivisection was found in Senator Jacob H. Gallinger of New Hampshire. Although a homeopath of the old school, the Senator was himself a doctor of medicine, a fact that carried weight with his colleagues. He presented to the Committee on the District of Columbia, of which he was a member, a bill giving the commissioners of that territory the right to license or refuse to license at will all medical research involving animal experimentation conducted therein, providing, however, that many types of research were altogether prohibited, since licences could only be given for work likely to produce altogether new discoveries in physiology or the cure of disease; the commissioners might demand a report of progress at any time, and stop any experiment when it suited them. Furthermore, the experimental procedures which might be undertaken were defined with no consideration of what the effect might be on research. Appointed official inspectors, the agents of the antivivisectionists, were to have the right of coming and going in the laboratories as they pleased, and to demand that the commissioners revoke the licence of any experimenter whose purpose or procedures seemed objectionable to their prejudiced lay minds. In other words, such scientific medicine as was not legislated out of existence was to be placed at the mercy of officials without scientific training and advised by the enemies of science. That such a bill could be passed and when passed would be a serious deterrent to research had been demonstrated by the experience of England, where Parliament had enacted an antivivisection law in 1876.

The innocuous title given the bill, which mentioned only cruelty to animals and contained no reference to medicine or research, kept the medical profession from recognizing what was happening until the morning when the committee hearing was held. The Surgeon General hurried down from the War Department to object, but he had no time to prepare his opposition or to gather evidence; accepting Senator Gallinger's assurance that there was nothing in the bill to which a reasonable doctor would take exception, the committee unanimously recommended it to the main body of the Senate.

Welch wrote Gilman: "The movement on the part of the antivivisectionists is a thoroughly organized and powerful one throughout the country. Their main effort just now is to secure national legislation and with this as a lever to agitate in the different states. . . . A petition signed by judges of the Supreme Court, bishops, distinguished clergymen and lawyers, numerous homeopathic physicians and other citizens urging the adoption of this bill by Congress must be met by vigorous action. Justice Brewer is one of the signers of this petition. He told Dr. Theobald Smith that he understood this bill was a compromise measure satisfactory to scientific men and physicians. Doubtless others signed under this misapprehension due to the deceptive appeals of antivivisectionists."

Welch drew up overnight a resolution opposing the bill which was adopted by the Association of American Physicians and, armed with this as well as such letters from distinguished people as he could collect at short notice, posted to Washington. The bill, he wrote many years later, "would have passed undoubtedly if we had not bestirred ourselves. It was then that Osler and I spent an entire evening with Senator Gorman in his house in Washington." Assisted by Welch's Yale classmate, Senator Wolcott of Colorado, Gorman succeeded in keeping the bill from reaching the floor of the Senate.

This somewhat easy victory seems to have made the champions of experimental medicine over-sanguine, for when Senator Gallinger presented virtually the same bill in the next session, they again did not get moving until it had been reported out by the unanimous vote of the Committee on the District of Columbia. Then the crisis with which they found themselves faced was so grave that Welch dropped all other activities and during the winter of 1897–98 changed himself into a political lobbyist.

As president of the American Congress of Physicians and Surgeons he organized a national committee. Securing through his friends the names of three or four principal doctors in each of the forty-eight states, he sent them form letters asking them to cooperate in heading state groups that would urge physicians and patients to deluge the Senate with protests. Particular care was taken to reach the family doctors and personal friends of individual Senators. Never did hostesses who were entertaining important guests have such ease in getting Welch to dinners as during that winter; he was sure to come early and stay late, and if the conversation turned to antivivisection, that was not surprising. Although he believed that personal letters were more effective than formal resolutions of associations, Welch used all the resolutions he could secure, often writing them out with his own hand. Medical societies of every description hurried to his assistance, as did the National Live Stock Association, which wished experimentation on animal diseases to continue.

Welch shone as the pamphleteer of the movement; his brilliant and unanswerable attack on the bill was published in the *Journal of the American Medical Association* and reprinted from there; it was read into the *Congressional Record,* reprinted again, and circulated all over the nation. In order to back up his words, Welch obtained statements from famous personalities—scientific and lay—both in the United States and abroad. "The experience in England," he wrote, "has shown the folly of the belief of some men of science and physicians that any compromise in this matter with antivivisectionists will check in the least their agitation of the subject." Later he was to receive letters from Lord Lister and Sir Michael Foster testifying that the English bill had been very hampering to science.

After giving his propaganda time to work, Welch went to Washington and talked to individual Senators; at the end of their conversation, he would pull from his pocket a statement that the Senator would oppose the bill, and usually the Senator signed. Welch would then promise to send him material for a speech opposing antivivisection. He even found his way into the White House and persuaded President Cleveland to promise to veto the bill should it pass.

As Welch's steamroller proceeded down Capitol Hill, poor Senator Gallinger seems not to have known what had struck him. Attacked by one of his colleagues, he said that "while he had his doubts as to the propriety of the bill, yet so many people were after him that he felt obliged to call it up and make a speech on it." But when he learned that Welch had got more than half the members of the Senate to sign his little papers, he promised that the measure "will not be called up for consideration at the present session of Congress."

By the next December Gallinger had found the courage to present his bill again. This time the doctors were not caught napping; when a hearing was held before the Committee on the District of Columbia on February 21, 1900, Welch appeared heading a phalanx of distinguished men. After the antivivisectionists had presented a lawyer, and an interested layman, and the late president of the Brooklyn Polytechnic Institute, and their lone physician, Dr. Matthew Woods, who boasted that he had practised for twenty-five years in Philadelphia, Welch called on Dr. William W. Keen, president of the American Medical Association, Bishop Lawrence of Massachusetts, Professor H. A. Hare of Jefferson Medical College, Professor Henry P. Bowditch of Harvard, Dr. Mary Putnam Jacobi to represent the women, Surgeon General George M. Sternberg, Dr. D. E. Salmon, chief of the Bureau of Animal Husbandry, and Drs. Osler and Kelly of the Hopkins. When all these had spoken—some of their speeches had been written for them by Welch—Welch himself arose and summed up in a devastating argument.

He welcomed the opportunity to make it clear that there was no truth in the antivivisectionists' assertion that there was "any material division of opinion in the medical profession on the subject." Pointing to the great advances in medical science achieved through the experimental method, Welch concluded: "Strange as it may seem at the turning point of the century, we are here, not as we should be, to ask you to foster and encourage scientific progress, but to beg you simply not to put legislative checks in its way. Our own contributions to this progress may now be small, but America is destined to take a place in this forward movement commensurate with her size and importance. We today should be recreant to a great trust, did we not do all in our power to protect our successors from the imposition of these trammels on freedom of research. Our appeal to you is not only in the name of science, but in the truest and widest sense in the name of humanity."

Gallinger's committee fled from him like autumn leaves during a hurricane; he withdrew his bill. Although he presented it again in various forms for several years, the antivivisectionists had been so effectively routed that Welch relinquished his lead in the matter, allowing the defence of medical science to be conducted by less busy men. He never underestimated, however, the seriousness of the danger now past; he wrote: "That was the hottest fight, I think, there has been."

The antivivisectionists continued to agitate, introducing bills whenever they could in the legislatures of the states, holding

meetings, publishing inflammatory pamphlets, occasionally se-
ducing the editors of important publications to support their
cause. Although Welch never again stepped into the forefront of
the fight, he often wrote letters and gave testimony. I remember
a later hearing before the Senate Committee on the District of
Columbia with Senator Norris in the chair. When a presentable
homeopathic physician testified that in his practice, which he had
reason to believe was ordinarily successful, he never resorted to
anything having to do with experimentation on animals, Senator
Norris asked me for a comment. Not wishing to speak before
Welch, I turned the question over to him, and he asked the physician if he ever took blood pressures. When the physician answered that he did, Welch inquired if he knew how the method
had been developed. The embarrassed doctor had to admit he
did not know, and Senator Norris interpolated: "I am interested
in the matter of blood pressure because my physician tells me
that mine is too high." Then Welch explained lucidly how the
method had been developed in Ludwig's laboratory through experimentation on dogs. The result of this simple incident was
decisive; the hearing proceeded with only listless interest on the
part of the committee, which voted the bill down.

But even more important than Welch's appearances before
legislative bodies was his role as an adviser behind the scenes in
determining the policy of the medical profession in its battle for
science. Always his counsel was the same: agitate just as little as
you can in order to achieve your ends; anything more would
serve to make the antivivisection movement seem greater than
it is. When an exhibit dramatizing alleged cruelties to animals
was moved around the country in 1910, medical leaders of each
city in turn wrote to Welch for advice; in every case Welch urged
that unless the exhibit was attracting a great deal of attention,
they should say nothing about it until it was over; then, perhaps,
"a dignified letter to your most decent newspaper exposing the
nature of the show might not be amiss."

On occasion, bills were presented to the Maryland legislature.
When the state antivivisection society tried to smoke Welch out
by publicly challenging the Hopkins Medical School to a debate

with Dr. Walter R. Hadwen, they learned that it was dangerous to defy such a champion. Welch replied: "You refer to Dr. Hadwen as 'one of the most eminent physicians in England,' and he is commonly so described in antivivisectionist publications. Dr. Hadwen is known to the medical profession at large solely as an exponent of the antivivisectionist cause. He is entirely unknown as a contributor to medical knowledge and has no claim to the position in the profession which you and other antivivisectionists assign to him. He advocates opinions entirely at variance with those accepted by the great body of the medical profession and by practically all competent scientific authorities. To enter into public debate with Dr. Hadwen under the circumstances proposed is to give him an importance unmerited by his professional reputation and to imply to the public his competence to speak with medical authority on such subjects as the germ theory of disease, serums, vaccines and the utility of vivisection. Furthermore abundant information on these subjects is readily available to the public. No useful purpose would be served by such a public debate as your Society proposes. If any public comment is made by you or your Society upon my declination of your invitation, I should like to have you publish this letter explaining the reasons for my refusal."

The antivivisectionists finally succeeded in outflanking Welch's policy of silence by having their proposed statutes brought before state electorates in referenda. This Welch regarded as a "really serious matter. . . . To educate the entire voting population on such a matter is a difficult job requiring much money and effort." Referenda were on the California ballot in 1920, and the Colorado ballot in 1922. In both instances the medical profession, having appealed to Welch for advice, succeeded in educating the public so well that the provisions were badly defeated. Yet the very existence of such a menace forced Welch to revise his attitude toward the organization of distinguished laymen to help the medical profession in its battle; formerly he had opposed this as likely to attract attention to the antivivisectionists; now he gave the movement his blessing and in 1923 the American Association for Medical Progress was inaugurated. Welch wrote: "It has essayed a difficult and a gigantic task. When we stop to consider the ignorance, the superstition, and prejudice reflected in the attitude of masses of people toward medical and health problems—people who are highly susceptible to the propaganda and misrepresentations of organized militant groups seeking to undermine the very foundations of medical progress—we get some idea of the size and the importance of the Association's program."

The antivivisection movement, however, was unable to stand up against the steady advance of medical science and the growing awareness on the part of the general public of the value of the experimental method. In 1926 Welch was able to report that antivivisection is "a lost cause and the position of the adherents is pathetic."

V

The crucial fight against antivivisection which Welch led between 1896 and 1900 was merely one of the many extra-mural duties, too important to be laid aside, which were taking Welch away from his laboratory. As he became more and more clearly the outstanding spokesman for modern scientific medicine, as institutions like the Rockefeller Institute and the Carnegie Institution of Washington made increasing demands on his energies, he found it harder and harder to secure time for his teaching at the Pathological. Welch gradually ceased to be a personal instructor of young men. Out of each week he eventually could spare only Monday for his courses: "I am there all day from eleven in the morning until ten at night. I have a recitation, a lecture, a demonstration, a conference and a medical meeting on that day. It is about the only day when I can be counted upon, and I try to make up for much remissness on that one day." When a class petitioned him to hold extra recitations on Wednesdays, he tried to do it, but his correspondence with his assistant, Whipple, reveals that he was able to keep the engagement only rarely.[8]

That Welch was not entirely reconciled to his new regimen is shown by a letter he wrote in 1907 to his nephew Fred: "I am very tired of giving these general addresses and talks at dinners and clubs, and after each one I swear off that that will be the last. They interfere very much with my teaching and laboratory work, which are my real interests."

The six days in the week when Welch was not at the Hopkins were taken up with such a vast number of seemingly unrelated activities that merely to list them for a month would be arduous. He was, as he himself realized, oppressed with an inability to say "no." When someone came to see him with an asking look in his eye, he would launch into a discussion of some unrelated topic, trying with erudition to charm his tormentor into forgetting his mission. And when, despite his best efforts, the request was made at last, Welch's face would fall; he would demur, but if his tormentor began to argue he knew the cause was lost.

"President Harper," he wrote Mall in a typical outburst, "has asked me to give the dedication address at the formal opening of the Biological Laboratories at the University of Chicago on July 2. I sat down to write a declination but I found after completing the letter that my pen had involuntarily made it an acceptance. This seems to me an interesting illustration of psychological automatism from the development of habit collaterals to ganglion cell processes in the lower regions of the central nervous system. I want you to tell me what to say. Some of your Sunday School addresses and papers in the Youth's Companion will help me. If you have got any literature, papers, addresses, etc., of a general character on biology, do pick them out for me."

Many of the chores Welch agreed to do were very important. As we have seen, his speeches went far toward changing the course of American medicine; he supplemented them by innumerable consultations, in person and by letter, with university presidents who wished advice on raising the standards of their medical schools. Dr. Ray Lyman Wilbur, president of Stanford University, wrote him in 1911: "Not to turn to you for information in regard to the best men to fill vacancies in our Medical School would be to violate all the best precedents of American Medical Education, so I am taking the liberty of enclosing a couple of slips of paper describing some vacancies that we wish to fill here."

Problems of public health administration were brought to Welch by officials, and individual scientists brought him their personal professional problems, on which he was ever ready to advise.

Welch was so skilful a presiding officer, so equitable a moderator, that he was in great demand as chairman of meetings and president of congresses. Under his direction affairs usually went smoothly, but upon one occasion he was in the chair at an evening meeting of the Congress of Hygiene and Demography when a French delegate was lecturing. After getting half-way through his speech in the most atrocious broken English, the Frenchman stopped and told his hearers who filled the auditorium of the National Museum that he felt he was not doing himself justice; he hoped that they would not mind if he started his speech over again in French. Sonorous Gallic periods flowed from his mouth for a long time; then the lights were turned out for lantern slides. While the speaker pointed with enthusiasm to the pictures on the screen, a faint rustling rose from the audience. Suddenly the lights went on, revealing empty seats; the entire audience, some fifteen hundred people, had tiptoed from the hall. On the platform, Welch sat in lonely majesty by the horrified speaker's side. "Dr. Welch," I asked him, "what did you say?" And he replied: "Flexner, what would you have said?"

Welch was trapped by his overpowering good nature into agreeing to do many unimportant favours for many people, but once he had agreed there was no certainty that he would do them. He would put the matter out of his mind. Letters sent him would be unanswered and, as far as the sender knew, unopened; even telegrams would not break Welch's silence. And when the injured party finally cornered Welch in person, with a smile childlike and bland Welch would blame his absent-mindedness. If only he were not so absent-minded!

There can be no doubt that Welch encouraged people to believe him inefficient and even lazy. It is much more doubtful that he was either of these things. There is no record of his having failed to open a letter which he considered important; never did carelessness come between him and something he really wanted to do. These things were a pretence, a shield behind which he was able to go his own way without giving the real explanation of what he was doing. And he was so generally beloved that the foibles he pretended to were regarded as an endearing part of his character, although they sometimes worked great inconvenience on the people whose projects he conveniently forgot.

VI

Before Welch was finally drawn from his laboratory to move on a wider stage, his friends and pupils found an opportunity to dramatize his importance as a teacher. In 1900, Welch, now fifty years old, had been out of medical school twenty-five years; Mall sent out a circular letter which read in part: "It is customary in Germany for the pupils of a great teacher to express their appreciation and gratitude by dedicating to him a volume of their contributions to learning. The pupils of Dr. Wm. H. Welch of Baltimore have decided to give expression to their regard for him in a similar way and the publication of a volume to mark his twenty-fifth year as a teacher and investigator is now in progress. . . . The book will contain contributions to pathology and to correlated sciences agreeing in scope with that of the leading scientific medical journals."

Asked to suggest the names of pupils who might have researches to contribute, Welch found he was not sure who had worked in his New York laboratory. "I cannot remember positively whether Starr, Gilman Thompson, Holt and Tuttle studied with me, but I think some may have done so, and you might write to inquire, not, however, mentioning my name, as I should not care to have them know whether I remembered so important a matter." Mall was finally able to state that "some seventy-five persons have undertaken investigation under Dr. Welch's leadership." Thirty-eight, two of whom had worked with him in New York and the rest at the Johns Hopkins, contributed to the volume.[9]

Welch wrote to every contributor, thanking him personally and graciously praising his contribution. Thus to Herter: "Your paper is a most valuable one and embodies the results of an immense amount of accurate research upon subjects of great importance. It is an ornament to the Festschrift and makes me proud that I may count you among my pupils, as indeed I have ever been. I had no idea of the greatness of the honor which my pupils and associates were preparing for me. I do not believe that a more valuable collection of scientific papers in medicine was ever dedicated to a teacher."

These letters were the result of unhurried examination of the volume, which was presented to Welch by Councilman at a dinner held in the Maryland Club. While Councilman showered praises ("Tone down Councilman's eulogy," Welch wrote me; "I really shrink from seeing it printed in its unadulterated form"), Welch's mind ran over the amazing changes in which he had taken part. Twenty years before in New York he had been regarded as a ridiculous visionary for desiring medical laboratories; it had been only fifteen years since he had been called to Baltimore and seven since the Johns Hopkins Medical School had opened, and now he sat at a high table looking down into the faces of some seventy-five productive investigators whom he had trained.

Rising to his feet, he spoke: "To me the most significant feature of this occasion is that the time has come in America when a group of investigators, more or less closely connected through common teachers, can bring together so large a number of important, original contributions to medical science. Twenty-five years ago this would not have been possible. That I should have been permitted to participate with others in bringing about this advance is to me a source of much gratification. . . .

"Today, pathology is everywhere recognized as a subject of fundamental importance in medical education, and is represented in our best medical schools by a full professorship. At least a dozen good pathological laboratories, equipped not only for teaching, but also for research, have been founded; many of our best hospitals have established clinical and pathological laboratories; fellowships and assistantships afford opportunity for the thorough training and advancement of those who wish to follow pathology as their career; special workers with suitable preliminary education are attracted to undertake original studies in our pathological laboratories; students are beginning to realize the benefits of a year or more spent in pathological work after their graduation; and as a result of all these activities the contributions to pathology from our American laboratories take rank with those from the best European ones. While we realize that we are only at the beginning of better things, and that far more remains to be accomplished than has yet been attained, nevertheless the progress of pathology in America during these twenty-five years has surely been most encouraging."

Among Welch's pupils were men such as Bolton, Councilman, Halsted, Mall, and Nuttall, who had been already trained in scientific medicine before they became attached to the Pathological, but who none the less acknowledged their indebtedness to Welch for their subsequent development. As time went on, some of these men and other professors at the Hopkins had assistants who, although each worked in the special field of his immediate superior, came under Welch's influence and also looked upon themselves as his pupils. We may mention Cushing and Bloodgood, who worked with Halsted, and Cullen, who worked with Kelly.

Virtually contemporaneous with this group were the young men who came to Welch, before the Hopkins Medical School opened, from other medical schools that had failed to give them the scientific opportunities they desired; Alexander C. Abbott, L. F. Barker, Henry J. Berkley, W. D. Booker, William T. Howard, junior, J. Whitridge Williams, and Simon Flexner all made careers in scientific medicine, with pathology or bacteriology as the foundation of their work. The most unusual case is that of Berkley, who studied the histology of the nervous system by the methods of Golgi and Cajal, finding under Welch a favourable environment for this work which might seem so far afield.

With the opening of the Medical School the scene changed. In successive years, young men and women stimulated by Welch's laboratory spent extra hours there and after graduation returned to specialize in pathology. This group included such brilliant men as MacCallum, Opie, G. H. Whipple, and M. C. Winternitz. These men, and many others who also made important contributions, carried Welch's influence all over the nation, until American pathology came to equal and even perhaps exceed the European schools on which it was modelled.[10]

CHAPTER XIII

The Rockefeller Institute for Medical Research

I

IT WAS an important event in the history of American medicine when the pastor of the Central Baptist Church of Minneapolis became acquainted with a boy in his congregation. Years passed and the boy, Elon W. Huntington, came to New York to study to be a doctor; a lonely student in a strange city, he often went to near-by Montclair, New Jersey, to visit his former pastor, the Rev. Frederick T. Gates, who was now one of John D. Rockefeller's philanthropic advisers.

"We used to take long walks together," Gates remembered, "and the subject of our conversation was quite naturally medicine." Fascinated, Gates asked his companion to recommend a text for him to read, and Huntington suggested Osler's *Principles and Practice of Medicine*. "I bought my precious volume in June, 1897. . . . My sole purpose was to become reasonably intelligent as a layman on the subject of medicine. Perhaps I ought to delay long enough to say that . . . my father, before he became a minister, had studied medicine. . . .

"I read the whole book without skipping any of it. I speak of this not to commemorate my industry, but to celebrate Osler's charm. . . . There was a fascination about the style itself that led me on, and having once started, I found a hook in my nose that pulled me from page to page. . . . But there were other things besides its style that attracted me and constantly . . . intensified my interest. I had been a skeptic before. . . . This book not only confirmed my skepticism, but its revelation absolutely astounded and appalled me. . . . Let me name some of the things which, commonplace as they are to intelligent physicians, were absolutely appalling to me. . . . I found, for illustration, that the best medical practice did not, and did not pretend to, cure more than four or five diseases. That is, medicine had at that time specifics for about as many diseases as there are fingers on one hand. It was nature, and not the doctor . . . that performed the cures. . . . Osler's own attitude toward drugs was interesting, and I came at length to approach his curative suggestions with a smile. . . . He would suggest that such and such had found that this or that treatment was efficacious, but such had not been his own experience. . . .

"To the layman student like me, demanding cures and specifics, he had no word of comfort whatever. In fact, I saw clearly from the work of this able and honest man that medicine had, with the few exceptions above mentioned, no cures, and that about all that medicine up to 1897 could do was to nurse the patients and alleviate in some degree the suffering. . . . I found further that a large number of the most common diseases, especially of the young and middle-aged, were simply infectious and contagious. . . . I learned that of these germs [causing disease] only a very few had been identified and isolated. I made a list, and it was a very long one at that time . . . of the germs which we might reasonably hope to discover but which as yet had never been with certainty identified, and I made a very much longer list of the infectious or contagious diseases for which there had been as yet no specific found.

"When I laid down this book I had begun to realize how woefully neglected in all civilized countries, and perhaps most of all in this country, had been the scientific study of medicine. . . . Moreover, while other departments of science, astronomy, chemistry, physics, etc., had been endowed very generously in colleges and universities throughout the whole civilized world, medicine, owing to the peculiar commercial organization of medical colleges, had rarely, if ever, been anywhere endowed, and research and instruction alike had been left to shift for themselves. . . . It became clear to me that medicine could hardly hope to become a science until medicine should be endowed and qualified men could give themselves for uninterrupted study and investigation

. . . entirely independent of practice. To this end it seemed to me an Institute of medical research ought to be established in the United States.

"Here was an opportunity, to me the greatest which the world could afford, for Mr. Rockefeller to become a pioneer. This idea took possession of me. The more I thought of it the more enthusiastic I became. I knew nothing of the cost of research; I did not realize its enormous difficulties; the only thing I saw was the overwhelming need and the infinite promise, world-wide, universal, eternal.

"Filled with these thoughts and enthusiasms, I returned from my vacation . . . I brought my Osler into the office . . . and there dictated . . . for Mr. Rockefeller's eye a memorandum in which I tried to show him the, to me, amazing discoveries that I had made of the actual conditions of medicine in the United States and the world. . . . I pointed to the Koch Institute in Berlin and at greater length to the Pasteur Institute in Paris. It was either in this connection or a little later . . . that I pointed out . . . that the results in dollars or francs of Pasteur's discoveries . . . had saved for the French nation a sum far in excess of the entire cost of the Franco-German War. I remember insisting in this or some subsequent memorandum that even if the proposed institute should fail to discover anything, the mere fact that he, Mr. Rockefeller, had established such an institute of research, if he were to consent to do so, would result in other institutes of a similar kind, or at least other funds for research being established, until research in this country would be conducted on a great scale, and that out of the multitudes of workers, we might be sure in the end of abundant rewards, even though those rewards did not come directly from the Institute which he might found. . . .

"I never saw my memorandum again. But that Mr. Rockefeller was impressed by the force of these considerations I have documentary evidence. . . .[1] The matter . . . continued to be referred to and conferred upon for a year or two, particularly with Mr. Rockefeller, Jr., who shared all my interest in it. Any active steps toward founding the institution would involve extensive conference with the leading men of research in this country, a study of similar institutions in Europe, and an amount of thought, correspondence, and travel that might well engage a large part of the time of a competent man. I therefore suggested . . . to Mr. John D. Rockefeller, Jr., that we employ a man for this exclusive service and suggested a man entirely qualified whom I thought we could command . . . my friend . . . Mr. Starr J. Murphy."

Murphy began by making a survey of the outstanding medical schools of this country, and after a delay of some two years, during which the idea was considered and matured, Rockefeller, junior, consulted his family physician Dr. Holt, who soon brought Herter into the discussions. Early in the spring of 1901 Rockefeller asked these men to propose a group of doctors to help in the establishment of an independent organization for medical research. "The first name which occurred to us to suggest was of course that of Dr. Welch," Holt remembered. "The others were Drs. Prudden, Theobald Smith, and [Hermann M.] Biggs."

Herter wrote Welch that the laboratory was to be established "in a small way at first without an endowment and hence without a board of trustees," but implied that should the plan be a success, further support would be forthcoming. A group of scientific men would be asked to act in an advisory capacity and to help in the selection of a director. Herter did not need to point out to Welch that the beginnings were conceived in so modest a manner because it was by no means certain that the United States was ready for an institution devoted wholly to medical research; the success of the *Journal of Experimental Medicine* was a hopeful sign, but laboratory instruction in this country was still a recent innovation limited to a few medical schools; the Hopkins, for instance, had graduated only five classes by 1901.

Caution, Herter's letter shows, was being exercised at every step. "It has been suggested," he wrote, "that the [New York City] Health Board be asked to give shelter to the laboratory during its first years." Sufficient time was to be taken to find a director who should combine the necessary scientific qualifications with the ability to get on with his colleagues, and with a certain amount of common sense. "It seems to me that you are in a peculiarly favorable position to help in reference to the selection of such a man," Herter continued. "Mr. Rockefeller has expressed a strong wish that you serve on the Advisory Board and would be much gratified if you could see your way clear to acting as its Chairman. . . . While Mr. Rockefeller's interest in the establishment of a research laboratory is primarily humanitarian rather than scientific, I am confident that he would never allow his desire for practical results to hamper the laboratory in its direct or indirect efforts to obtain such results."

Welch, who had known for some time that such a plan was brewing, replied that he considered Rockefeller's offer a very important and generous one which should be of great benefit to humanity. The success or failure of the undertaking, he felt, would depend entirely on who was appointed director; and he expressed his willingness to serve on the advisory board that would make the selection, "although not as chairman, for it is impossible for me to give the time and attention which I should consider necessary, and then it is better to select a New York man as chairman. . . . My preference for chairman would be either Prudden or Biggs." Then Welch sent a characteristic message of appreciation to Rockefeller, junior, expressing willingness "to co-operate in every way in my power."

The Association of American Physicians used always to convene at the old Arlington Hotel in Washington early in May, bringing together the élite of the medical profession. At the meeting in 1901 Welch, Holt, Herter, Prudden, and Biggs conferred further about the new research institution, and Welch was empowered to write an all-important letter to Theobald Smith; although neither Rockefeller nor Gates had met Welch, the group of New York physicians instinctively turned to him to guide the new enterprise.

In his letter to Smith, Welch said: "The proposition now made by Mr. Rockefeller is to give twenty thousand dollars annually for at least ten years, and place in the hands of a committee the arrangements for its expenditure." Welch admitted that he felt the institute should be connected with a university, "but it seems that Mr. Rockefeller is more favorable to the proposition of making use of the new laboratory . . . [of] the New York City Board of Health . . . with the understanding that we shall be entirely independent. . . . I do not think that it is worth while to discuss any other place for the laboratory except in New York, and indeed that is probably the most suitable location."

Having asked Smith to join the advisory board, Welch added: "but what is more important is that we were unanimous in the opinion that you were the best man—indeed it seemed to us the only man in this country available—to take charge as director of the new laboratory, and I was especially charged to write you of our decision and to learn whether you could be tempted to consider such a proposition. . . . There will of course be assistants and such arrangements as the director desires with the resources available. . . .

"I have said perhaps enough to enable you to think the matter over in the meantime, although not enough to enable you to come to any decision. Think over under what conditions you might be tempted to take the directorship of such an undertaking. While of course twenty thousand dollars a year should do much good in promoting scientific research, it is the greater possibilities for the future which have the main interest for me." [2]

On May 9 Welch gaily wrote his brother-in-law that Rockefeller, junior, was pressing him to be chairman of the advisory board "on account of my well known business talent. It is all confidential at present, so do not spread the news outside the family, I mean this conspicuous recognition of my business capacity is to be kept secret for the present." He added in a more serious mood that Rockefeller "is prepared to give a large sum of money. I am not yet clear as to the plans, but it is believed that something very great, like the Pasteur Institute in Paris, will come of it."

When Welch finally accepted the presidency of the board, his sister was not enthusiastic. "Your remarks on my participation in the organization of the Rockefeller Institute are quite to the point," he wrote her. "I really ought not to assume any new obligations, but those interested were so insistent that I was the one to start the undertaking as president, and the movement means so much for the future of medical science in this country, that I felt it my duty to accept. . . . Ultimately it is thought the work will be centralized in an institute in New York, but how soon this will be is uncertain. I should not consider any proposition to come to New York to take charge of the Institute. I prefer my present position. . . . I shall not retain the presidency of the Institute any longer than seems necessary, but shall be willing to continue as a member of the Board. I have to attend to a good deal of correspondence, and of course have received many letters from all over the country about it."

At a dinner given in New York by Rockefeller, junior, it had been decided to postpone the establishment of the laboratory, since it was felt that for the time being better results would be achieved by granting money for research to already existing laboratories; therefore no further efforts were then made to secure Smith as director. Welch wrote me, in a letter asking that I join the advisory board, that "Mr. Rockefeller wishes to begin in a rather modest and tentative way, and to let the scheme gradually evolve, as experience may indicate. . . . We suggested the name 'Rockefeller Institute for Medical Research,' but we have yet to learn whether Mr. Rockefeller will consent to this use of his name; if not, perhaps 'American' will be substituted. The Board of Directors now is composed of Prudden (vice-president), Holt (secretary), Herter (treasurer), Biggs, Theobald Smith, you and myself (president). . . .

"We meet again on Saturday evening, May 25 . . . the special object of which is to consider proposals for distribution of the funds for the coming year. Only such part of them will be used as we feel can be judiciously expended. In the meantime we are to try to learn by inquiry what various laboratories are prepared to undertake. It is not proposed to appropriate any specified sums to individual laboratories, but rather such amounts as are required for special investigations along appropriate lines and are approved by the Committee. The employment of competent persons to devote themselves to these investigations, purchase of necessary apparatus, material, etc., would be proper use of the funds."

Since I was then a professor at the University of Pennsylvania, Welch added: "Will you think over what can be done in Philadelphia, conferring with Abbott, and if you think best with others? . . . The main things to consider are first the problem to investigate, and second the men to undertake the investigations. Something relating to infectious diseases, to immunity and the like would be best."

Welch was soon busy writing the laboratory heads in a selected group of medical schools informing them of the plans under way, and inviting applications for funds. This important correspondence was almost spontaneously left to him, since his natural desire to keep informed and his key position as editor of the *Journal of Experimental Medicine* had made him more familiar than anyone else with the work being done in laboratories all over the nation.

During 1901 approximately $12,000 and during 1902, $14,450, was appropriated in individual grants ranging from $300 to, in a few cases, $1200. While aid was given only to Americans, they were allowed to work in Europe as well as at home, and in those days of rapidly advancing immunology and chemotherapy * Ehrlich's Institute in Frankfurt was a great attraction. The "research students, research scholars, and fellows of the Institute," as they were called, who received the larger sums were expected to devote themselves entirely to the work in question. Such scientific apparatus as they purchased under the grants was to remain the property of the Rockefeller Institute.

It is indicative of the resources then available for scientific research that the sums of money granted, which will seem tiny to contemporary readers, were sought with enthusiasm by such men as Victor C. Vaughan of the University of Michigan, Harold C. Ernst of Harvard, Ludvig Hektoen of the University of Chicago, H. W. Conn of Wesleyan, and J. G. Adami of Montreal. Although a few hinted that they could use larger amounts, Adami was worried for fear that even such assistance as was offered might prove harmful by over-encouraging medical scientists. He

---

* Treatment of diseases with chemicals which act specifically, as quinine in malaria, salvarsan (606) in syphilis, etc.

wrote Welch: "Since you outlined your views about the matter . . . I have thought much over the different possible methods of utilising that gift, and I see more and more clearly that your plan is that promising the best results. The objection I urged, namely the danger of encouraging a number of good men to accept simultaneously the Fellowships or Studentships because at the end of the time they would find themselves thrown upon the medical world with not a sufficiency of satisfactory openings ready for them—that in short they would glut the market—is not, after all, I think, so very serious. If the plan is, as it should surely be, successful and the results satisfy Mr. Rockefeller, the Fellows or Students, or the best of them, will form the nucleus of the staff of the forthcoming Institute: that Institute will absorb a fair proportion of them: it will in itself solve the difficulty."

It is significant that no grants were made to clinicians. This reflected no prearranged policy; clinical laboratories for studying disease in living patients were still in their infancy, far behind the laboratories of the pre-clinical sciences.[3]

The grants made by the institute involved a vast amount of detail, and all of it fell on Welch. "I am collecting the batch of reports on the work done by Rockefeller fellows, etc., to be presented at the meeting of the Board in New York on Saturday next," he wrote Abbott in a typical letter. "I do not find any detailed report from you. My impression is that you have presented the results in a paper before the Association of Physicians, which I was not fortunate enough to hear, but I should have some statement from you to show the Board. . . . If the paper is ready for publication, it will suffice if you make a brief report to that effect, perhaps giving a short outline of the general character and results of the work. Your applications for next year will be considered."

Although papers had to be approved by Welch and the board and due acknowledgment given to the institute, they could be published anywhere, provided that in each case five hundred reprints in the page size of the *Journal of Experimental Medicine* were prepared at the expense of the foundation, so that the studies could be bound together and distributed gratis to selected persons and libraries.[4]

The only part of the management of the institute which did not fall on Welch was paying the stipends, the duty of Herter, who was treasurer, but even in this matter Welch was consulted when there were any difficulties. Thus he wrote Herter in 1903: "The Rockefeller grants . . . are all straightened out without any serious inconvenience and you must not give yourself any anxiety in the matter." He then listed the appropriations outstanding, amounts he had received, and what he had paid to various fellows of the institute, summing up receipts and disbursements in business-like manner. "I hope the foregoing, which I dare say might be presented in a simpler way, will make the situation clear to you."

It is curious how history, with Welch, repeated itself. When the Hopkins Medical School was launched, he took charge of the negotiations with most of the first professorial group, the correspondence with prospective students, the functions of the deanship, the official responsibility for graduation, while also carrying on his teaching in pathology and bacteriology. In the early years of the *Journal of Experimental Medicine,* he was editor, proofreader, make-up man, etc. Just so, when the Rockefeller Institute came along in 1901, he assumed almost all the duties in getting that institution started. As always, he accepted no assistance, not even clerical; every detail was attended to with his own hand, every letter handwritten. It must have been a great joy to him when Barker, then at the University of Chicago, wrote him in 1903 that Mr. Gates "told me what you must already know, that Mr. Rockefeller was more pleased with the way the Institute for Medical Research had been and is being handled than with any other benefaction he has ever made. He says that there is practically a 'blank check' for you to be filled in as desired. He praised the 'very, very wise' gradual method of development."

II

The policy of grants-in-aid, which had encouraged investigations all over America, had been conceived partly as a method of determining the country's readiness for an institution devoted purely to research. Welch was so greatly pleased with the result that on January 13, 1902, he wrote Rockefeller, junior, with whom he had dined a few days before: "My own feeling after the conversation with you on Saturday is that we should consider the establishment of a laboratory, provided we can secure a good working staff. I do not think the time has come to start out with a large plant with the permanent location and connections fixed, or to abandon our present plan of aiding investigations elsewhere, provided these are important, in the right field, and really need our help. It seems best, when we are ready, to start a laboratory in a comparatively modest way, and let time and experience indicate the best lines of organization and development. The most important matter is to secure a man of first-rate scientific and administrative ability to direct the work of a laboratory. At our meeting we asked Dr. Theobald Smith to let us know on what terms he would consider an offer of such a position, and he agreed to take the matter into consideration. I believe that we should be fortunate, if we could secure him. He has, however, an exceptionally attractive position at Harvard. Still I believe the head of our laboratory would have opportunities for investigation and a field of usefulness unsurpassed in this country.

"I do not consider that there is any such urgency in making a change in our present plans as to prevent us from waiting until we are sure that we have the right men to recommend for the staff of the laboratory."

To this Rockefeller replied: "As I said to you the other night, I am prepared to take up with my Father any recommendations that your Board shall present. As soon as you have come to some decision regarding the advisability of establishing a laboratory in, for the present, a rented building, and have a director in mind for the same, or any other plan for enlargement which seems to the Board wise, do not hesitate to communicate the same to me." *

---

* The plan, which had been considered at first, of placing the institute at least temporarily in the laboratory of the New York City Board of Health had long since been abandoned. A member of the Board of Directors of the institute since May 1901, I did not know, until I examined the correspondence on which this chapter is based, that such a suggestion had ever been made.

Smith had from the first been regarded as the natural choice for the director of a laboratory when it should be established, since he had been proved America's leading investigator by his brilliant investigations of Texas fever of cattle, which demonstrated conclusively the principle of insect transmission of disease, thus opening a new chapter in the study of parasitology. Smith, however, declined the directorship, giving as a main reason his fear that "my interest for years in animal pathology and my firm belief in its great usefulness in the study of problems in human pathology might give an impress to the work of the laboratory which might eventually arouse adverse criticism."

The new laboratory, Smith continued, should in his opinion concentrate on "the study of infectious diseases from all points of view. They are the great threatening dangers of our present social system." He suggested three "mutually contributing" laboratories: for the study of the morphology (forms and structure) of disease; for pathological physiology, including the study of infection, immunity, etc.; and for physiological and pathological chemistry. These he regarded as the minimum requirements, remarking that "there need be no fear that the laboratory would not grow steadily in other directions."

On receipt of Smith's letter Welch wrote to Prudden: "It seems desirable to continue our efforts to secure a Director and working staff of a laboratory. I think that Flexner is inclined to consider an offer such as we made to Smith, and if he could be secured I believe that we could not find a better man. Still I do not feel very hopeful that he would accept. I have sounded him in this matter, and he seems to be more tempted than I thought he would be. . . . I write this especially to learn how you feel about making the offer to Flexner and perhaps you may have opportunity to sound some of the other New York members of the Board on the subject."

At the board meeting of March 8 at which Smith's declination was presented, Welch turned to me and said: "Now, Flexner, we hope that you will accept the directorship." And I was thereupon officially asked to prepare a statement of my views on the future establishment of a research institute. I was, of course, not entirely unprepared for the invitation. Indeed, I had given anxious thought to the possibility and had made special journeys to Baltimore to talk it over with Welch. I had misgivings: I was happy at the University of Pennsylvania, where pathology was developing satisfactorily and a new laboratory would soon remove the discomforts and disadvantages of inadequate quarters for teaching and research in the old medical building. I was very doubtful of my competence to conduct a purely research laboratory. So far I had been both teacher and investigator; I had often found the balance strenuous, but the combination had worked well enough. What would happen if the prop of teaching were wholly removed? I was concerned also by the indefinite tenure of office, for although a permanent endowment of the almost unimaginable sum of $5,000,000 was hoped for, its receipt was not certain, depending in no small measure on the success of the initial venture into pure research. It was only sure that the institute would be supported for ten years. Ten years would go around quickly; what then? I hesitated, but Welch seemed free from doubts and tribulations. He said to me one day: "Flexner, they will never desert you." Then I was shy about the great commercial city of New York. Welch had once said to me in Baltimore that New York was cold to scientific medicine. The prospect seemed to me full of terrors.

While I was still in the throes of indecision, Prudden with Welch's assistance drew up a statement adopted by the board of the institute which read in part: "Existing institutions in this country . . . do not afford adequate facilities for many phases of investigation. . . . This is in part due to lack of sufficient endowment, in part to the large demands made upon the time and energy of the workers by their duties as teachers." As to the grants-in-aid, "the highest aims of the Institute cannot be secured in this way alone." What was needed was an organization fitted to "secure the unity of aim and the coordination and mutual stimulus which are essential to the highest achievements in research. These are to be secured . . . by the centralization . . . of the work of the Institute under a competent head in a fixed place, with adequate equipment and permanent endowment . . . large enough to provide full compensation for the directors of the departments and the associates, as well as a liberal allowance for the equipment and running expenses. . . .

"There is in this country no institution in which the elements of high scientific achievement in medical research are now brought together in the most effective way. In this regard America is less fortunate than France, Germany, Russia, or England, which possess well-endowed and productive institutions for medical research. . . .[5]

"The scope of the Institute should be broad enough, when fully organized, to cover the entire field of medical research in respect both to man and animals. . . . The problems of human disease should always be close to the Institute. While the study of the diseases of the lower animals is highly important both from an economic point of view and from their bearing upon the understanding of many forms of human disease, and while the work of the Institute will of necessity be largely experimental, yet intimate relation with the problems of human disease should not . . . be lost sight of. In order that the causes and treatment of human disease may be studied to the best advantage, there should be attached to the Institute a hospital for the investigation of special groups of cases of disease."

Prudden continued that the major aim should at first be the investigation of infectious diseases. Although he did not specify in detail what this involved, the directors, as I remember, hoped to establish, in addition to the hospital, laboratories devoted to the pathology, bacteriology, and immunology of the diseases of man and the lower animals. Only one line of major research was omitted in the original formulation, namely, the diseases of plants. Later a laboratory for this important subject was added, making the scope of the institute complete.

After conferring with Welch, Holt, and Herter, Rockefeller, junior, telegraphed his father on June 13, 1902, that the directors were now ready to purchase land and erect buildings, which with provision for endowment would probably require as much as $5,000,000. However, $1,000,000 to be used over a period of ten years would suffice to get the institute started; he strongly recommended such a gift, expressing his confidence that it would be "conservative and wise." The following day Rockefeller, senior, telegraphed his pledge of $1,000,000 to be spent over a decade, but deferred consideration of the proposed $5,000,000.

On June 20, the younger Rockefeller wrote Welch confirming the gift. The understanding was, he said, that between $300,000 and $400,000 would be needed to purchase land in New York and construct "the building now required," and that the work outlined in Prudden's memorandum would "require for its support annually from forty to sixty thousand dollars." He added that the $1,000,000, which was to be paid out as it was needed over the ten-year period, was to be an addition to the original grant made in 1901, "the unpaid balance of which shall continue to be used by the Board either for the carrying on of research in other laboratories than its own or in connection with the new work as above outlined, at the discretion of the Board." [6]

III

The year 1903 was for the Rockefeller Institute a period of transition. Grants-in-aid were given for the last time, since from then on the money would be needed for a laboratory. In February the present site of the institute on the East River was bought, and plans for the building were under consideration. Many of the details still fell on Welch, since I was abroad preparing myself in the rapidly enlarging science of physiological chemistry whose importance for physiology and pathology was being increasingly recognized. I studied in Berlin with Salkowski and, more important, with Emil Fischer, who was doing his basic work in the chemistry of animal tissues and organs.

In the fall of 1904 I returned and laboratories were opened in New York. Now the institution was well started and Welch, as was his habit when enterprises needed his active direction no longer, stepped back into the advisory position from which he continued all his life to make important contributions to the welfare of the Rockefeller Institute.

Since the buildings on the East River were far from completion, the laboratory opened in a three-story residence on the corner of Fiftieth Street and Lexington Avenue which had been altered at small expense. Welch was, of course, consulted about the original staff appointments, which were necessarily opportunist in character; until the institute should prove itself and receive an endowment, successful investigators could not be expected to leave university positions to take part in what might easily prove a temporary venture. Pathology and bacteriology were represented by myself, Hideyo Noguchi (whom I had brought with me from the University of Pennsylvania), and Opie, a member of the first class at the Hopkins Medical School and since then an assistant at the Pathological under Welch. The physiologist was Meltzer, the man who had co-operated with Welch in the only piece of research done in his Bellevue laboratory. Since Meltzer was now a highly successful New York practitioner and consultant, it was with trepidation that I offered him a half-time job at the meagre salary of $1500, which I knew would involve a financial sacrifice. He replied: "Heretofore I have always paid laboratories to be permitted to work in them; now you propose to pay me to work. Of course I will come." The original staff was completed a few months later with the addition of P. A. Levene in chemistry; a Russian who had worked in Fischer's laboratory, he brought something of the problems and atmosphere of that exciting place to the infant institute.

There had been no thought of any exercises to mark the beginnings of the institute in New York, but when the new laboratory building, with its attached animal and power houses, was ready for occupation, it seemed appropriate to make the public aware of the new enterprise. On May 11, 1906, the building was opened with a formal ceremony at which Welch delivered an address on "The Benefits of the Endowment of Medical Research." He pointed out that the ferment of medical science was beginning to move so effectively in American life that since the Rockefeller Institute had been founded in 1901, Harold McCormick, a son-in-law of the elder Rockefeller, had in 1902 endowed the Memorial Institute for Infectious Diseases in Chicago; and a year later Henry Phipps had, with a gift of more than $1,000,000, established in Philadelphia the Phipps Institute for the Study, Treatment, and Prevention of Tuberculosis. Also in 1902 Andrew Carnegie had founded with $10,000,000 the Carnegie Institution of Washington, which, Welch said, "includes within its scope the support of biological and chemical investigations of great importance to medical science, so that our country now stands in line with Germany, France and Great Britain in the opportunities afforded for research in medical and other sciences."

The new laboratory provided the institute with adequate facilities for the pursuit of medical science, but the future remained uncertain until in November 1907 Rockefeller gave $2,620,610 for a permanent endowment. Formerly, when the institute had needed some of the money granted it, a requisition had been sent to the Rockefeller office; now it was necessary to set up machinery so the institute could administer its own funds. Two boards were established, the trustees made up of three financiers and two directors, and the old board of directors, renamed "scientific directors." At Prudden's revolutionary suggestion, Rockefeller and his advisers agreed to a delegation of power such as may never before have existed in an American philanthropic institution. The trustees agreed merely to take care of the funds, leaving the decision of how they were to be spent to a joint committee containing a majority of scientists.[7]

This unprecedented step had been made possible by the past history of the institute. During the years when there had been no endowment, the directors themselves had determined the use of funds, often in the presence of the three financiers who were to be the original trustees. Rockefeller, junior, precise and penetrating in his thinking; Gates, always urbane and imaginative; Murphy, the agreeable, sound legal adviser: these men attended the directors' meetings, taking a deep interest in the scientific matters discussed and sharing in the formulation of general principles. An intimacy and sense of common purpose quickly sprang up, very pleasant and permanently enduring. Furthermore, the business men were impressed by the cautious and efficient way in which the directors, under Welch's presidency, handled their financial affairs. As we have seen, Gates had said that the directors, and Welch in particular, could have a "blank check" to develop as they pleased; now the blank check was signed.

Indeed, the success of the institute encouraged the Rockefeller office to consider further support for scientific research; the developments following a fire that destroyed two buildings of McGill University in 1907 showed that Gates hoped to utilize the scientific directors as an advisory body in this connexion. Osler and others having appealed to Rockefeller for assistance in rebuilding McGill, Gates referred the request to the institute directors. "The only question which interests us here," he wrote, "is this: Is the Medical School at McGill University a center of investigation so highly adapted and so important as to justify Mr. Rockefeller or to justify the Rockefeller Institute, if it had the funds available for the purpose, in placing several hundred thousand dollars at the disposal of McGill to be exclusively devoted to investigation? . . . You would confer a great favor upon us if you and your co-laborers could answer this question."

Entrusted by the directors with preparing their reply, Welch widened the specific question of a gift to McGill into a consideration of "a broad policy of advancing in the most effective manner possible the advancement of medical knowledge." Since this was "the main function of the Institute and the controlling purpose of the founder in its establishment," the institute "should not be indifferent to the conditions of education in our better medical schools and should not rest upon the assumption that the educational side can be safely left to take care of itself." The institute had been made possible, he pointed out, by the improvement in medical education which had preceded it; its staff would have to continue to be drawn from men trained in the universities.

"What character of medical school is it desirable to aid in

the expectation of advancing medical knowledge? We believe that such aid should be granted only to certain medical schools which possess the following characteristics:—The school should be upon a university basis, an integral part of an important university, completely controlled by the trustees of the university, the teachers being supported by salaries paid by the universities and not by a division of fees of students. The school must already be in possession of laboratories which have been productive in research. It must be clear that the heads of these laboratories and the teaching staff in general are selected primarily for their demonstrated capacity to advance and stimulate research and to train young men to become independent investigators. . . . The school should furthermore have advanced requirements for the matriculation of students, either a college degree or collegiate training in sciences fundamental to medicine, such as physics, chemistry and biology, being required for admission."

It is indicative of the great progress since the Hopkins Medical School was founded that Welch was able to list as satisfying these requirements "Harvard, Columbia, Johns Hopkins, the Western Reserve of Cleveland, the University of Chicago, and in part McGill, leaving out of consideration the medical departments of State universities."

The best way to further scientific research in such medical schools was by furnishing "permanent gifts of money, under certain well defined conditions, to be used for construction or equipment of laboratories or endowment of laboratories or of chairs connected with them or the provision of opportunities for hospital clinics associated with laboratories." Such clinics he considered to be, together with "laboratories of hygiene," of the first importance. "In every instance very careful investigation would be required to ensure the proper bestowal of such gifts and their utilization with the ultimate aim of improving the conditions for the promotion of medical science. It is believed that occasional grants for specific purposes could not be made to serve the same useful purpose as permanent endowment, for it is only upon assurance for the future that the proper organization and work of laboratories can be securely effected."

Dwelling at length on the great advantages to humanity which might come from such gifts as he described, Welch said that the directors of the institute would be willing to advise the Rockefeller office on the most useful way of disposing funds to advance medical science. They would, he promised, "endeavor to exercise the same care and thought which they have hitherto given to the interests of the Institute." But he added: "It is desired by the Directors before expressing a definite opinion upon the application of the McGill Medical School to learn how far the general policy of granting aid to medical schools along the lines suggested in this statement meets the approval of the founder of the Institute and his advisers."

Welch was obviously trying to influence the Rockefellers into taking up on a large scale the support of American medical education and science. No one can tell how much effect this letter had on later developments that were to bring the Rockefeller-endowed boards most effectively into the very activities Welch described, but the time was not yet ripe. Nothing was given to McGill, and the board of scientific directors of the institute was not called on again for advice concerning gifts to outside institutions.

Probably it was fortunate that the great responsibility of distributing funds on a continental scale was avoided, for the scientific future of the institute might easily have suffered from the resulting division of energies, and the directors could not have escaped a certain amount of criticism and even jealousy, which would have worked to the detriment of the research institution they represented.

As it was, the institute was permitted to develop unhampered along its own lines. It had departed at the outset from the two European models on which, more than any others, it had been based, for the Pasteur and Koch Institutes, as a few years later the Ehrlich Institute, had been built around a single remarkable man, while the Rockefeller Institute relied more on the co-operation of a group of talented division heads. Thus it was not confined in its growth by the interests, however great, of a commanding personality; it could look forward to a broader foundation of science, one limited in compass only by its material resources and the speed with which its own staff developed in scope and power. Furthermore, its usefulness could not be so seriously impaired by the death or retirement of one man.

Between 1888 when the Pasteur Institute was founded and 1904 when the first laboratory of the Rockefeller Institute was opened, the outlook on medical research had undergone rapid changes. Bacteriology as such, without losing its pre-eminent position, had become more closely linked with pathology and with immunology, this last a new science dating virtually from the 1890's. Biology as a whole, including physiology and pathology in the broadest aspects, was fast taking on a chemical guise and was therefore being more and more affected by the swift developments occurring in organic and physical chemistry and in physics. The Rockefeller Institute took part in this growth by providing in its original organization for the new biological chemistry, now called biochemistry, in its organic and physical forms. Biophysics, the corresponding new discipline, was added later.

The primary purpose of the institute may be defined as the attempt to add to knowledge by discovery, and to apply that knowledge to the prevention and alleviation of disease. When findings were made, they were at once rendered generally available; the time soon came when practical applications could be carried out in a hospital added to the laboratories. Thus both pure and applied science were cultivated side by side. It was recognized that the atmosphere which the pursuit of pure science creates is highly favourable to the promotion of applied science, a fact of special importance in respect to medicine, which has so long been moving along empiric lines, urged forward by the insistent need of alleviating suffering and of saving human life. How many centuries, indeed, had the practice endured of putting drugs of which the doctor knew little into human bodies of which he knew less! The way, therefore, to make the art of medicine more effective was to make it more accurate, that is scientific, and thus to purify it by replacing empiricism with knowledge.

Only an exceptional person, of course, is gifted with the power to extend knowledge, but a much larger number of persons can, under direction, add to the sum total; both kinds of ability were utilized by the growing institution. The power of the more gifted was enlarged through the use of the less, and the incidental training secured by the latter became a valuable asset in the educational expansion of the country. For research institutes are places for the instruction of all their staffs; no real distinction exists between them and a university, except that in laboratories dedicated purely to investigation the more elementary forms of training are not given but taken for granted on the part of its incoming appointees.

To recognize and then to secure men of the highest talent is always a difficult and often a dubious and baffling undertaking, requiring an endeavour to look some distance into the future. There is no royal road to discovery, and a discovery made is not an unfailing guide for the years to come. The ablest men are often the most diffident and self-depreciatory; they require in many cases to be reassured and made to believe in themselves. On the other hand, the self-assured are not infrequently the most self-deluded.

I remember well a question put to me by Professor Anton Dohrn when I was in Naples the year before the laboratories opened. We were sailing together toward Ischia in the collecting boat of the zoological station which he directed. "Will you permit workers in the medical institute to make fools of themselves?" he asked me suddenly. This was quite a startling query, but before I could attempt an answer Dohrn added: "Unless you permit the investigators to make fools of themselves you will make no great discoveries." The profound meaning of the question now became apparent: the greatest discoveries often seem fantastic. "It's a poor institution," Dohrn remarked, "that cannot afford to make an occasional mistake."

In the years to come, the sail to Ischia and that searching question were not forgotten.

It would have been possible, of course, to get the institute under way with much more rapidity had trained scientists been imported from Europe; some foreigner of great reputation could perhaps have been secured as director, who would have brought with him an aura of distinction and acclaim. Such expedients, however, were never even discussed; from the first, the institute undertook to develop American medicine through the training of American scientists. This meant, in practice, choosing promising young men, affording them suitable opportunities for work under little or no direction, and retaining over a term of years those who showed the greatest aptitudes in finding themselves and dealing successfully with the problems on which they were engaged.

Moreover, it was sound tradition to explore American capabilities by developing latent talent. The home of science has never remained fixed; from Italy it passed to England, France, Holland, and Germany in the course of three centuries. Now in a sense it was America's turn. Ludwig had recognized the potentialities of America when he said to Welch: "What becomes of the young men from your country who work in our medical laboratories? While here they do good work and show an aptitude and capacity for scientific investigation, certainly not less than our native students. But after their return to America, we hear no more of them." It is interesting to recall in this connexion that when the Kaiser Wilhelm Institute was founded at Berlin in 1911, it was avowedly based on the Rockefeller Institute and the Carnegie Institution of Washington.

Welch's judgment and wisdom were utilized as far as possible—more, in fact, than those of any other scientific director —in the finding of young men of promise and then in the elevation of the most talented to permanent positions. Sometimes his suggestions of subjects for researches were very fruitful, as when he wrote me in 1905, calling my attention to Schaudinn's discovery of the germ of syphilis: "Can you not get at the syphilis spirochete? It seems to me the most exciting thing just now." This hint started Noguchi on the investigation which yielded such important results.

Welch's great usefulness as an adviser, exemplified not only in the board meetings of the Rockefeller Institute but in innumerable other council chambers, was becoming increasingly recognized on a national scale. In 1906 he was made a trustee of the Carnegie Institution of Washington, which is for the physical sciences what the Rockefeller Institute is for the medical. Two years later he wrote me: "They have made me chairman of the Executive Committee of the Carnegie Institution in spite of as vigorous protest as I could make. I think that perhaps Mr. Carnegie desired it. This position involves a good deal of responsibility, as the Executive Committee meets once a month, and directs all the expenditures and determines the policy of the Institution. This policy is still in flux on fundamental matters, and I shall have to give my thought carefully to it for a time. There are some points regarding it about which I shall want your advice. This position will not divert my interest from the Rockefeller Institute, which is my first love of the two great foundations. It is rather remarkable that I should have so much responsibility in connection with these two institutions."

At this time as at many others, Welch tried to resign from the presidency of the scientific directors; year after year he urged that Prudden, vice-president from the beginning, should be promoted. "It is not so much that the presidency is any burden to me," he wrote in this letter, "as that I feel that I have held the office long enough, and that Prudden should enjoy the honor. I thought that notwithstanding his reluctance, he would appreciate such a mark of esteem and confidence coming at the time of his retirement from the professorship [at the College of Physicians and Surgeons]." But Prudden would not consent.

Welch remained president of the scientific directors for thirty-two years. He conducted the meetings with easy deliberation, listening with unwearied patience and showing no eagerness to express his own point of view. After a long and perhaps intricate discussion, he would sum up the subject so clearly that no vote had to be taken; either the proposal was accepted or simply dropped. As in all free discussions, there would be minutes of repetition or dullness; Welch would then draw odd or geometrical figures on the pad of paper before him. But he never lost touch with the opinions expressed, for at the right moment he would either close the discussion with his own remarks or merely pass on to the next item in the agenda.

Each year the scientific directors were presented with detailed reports on the work of the institute, reports often difficult to understand, since they were highly technical and extremely complicated. The scope of the work was so wide that at times the subject presented seemed remote from medicine, although this apparent remoteness grew smaller year by year until it disappeared altogether. Organic and physical chemistry, physics, mathematics even, all were drawn into the medical orbit; all required specially trained and gifted workers, and all touched borders with medicine as represented by pathology, physiology, and pharmacology and as practised in the hospital wards and even in the homes of patients.

The two men who studied the scientific reports most assiduously were Welch and Gates. In spite of his want of real scientific education, the latter made a good deal out of them, for his vigorous intellect so far bridged the gap that he could feel, if not wholly understand, that the institute was working fundamentally in medical science and thus building for the future as well as traversing established paths in laboratories or hospital. He had no itch for rapid practical conquests; his faith in the eventual triumph of the scientific method was invulnerable.

Welch was of course better informed. As a technical specialist, it is true, he was limited to pathology and bacteriology, but he was widely read and upon occasion he sought information from his Baltimore colleagues. His understanding of the theory on which the institute was being developed proved invaluable; he saw that for maximum effectiveness such an institution should be made up of highly trained specialists at the head of individual laboratories and that, as far as the resources of the organization allowed, these men must be encouraged to carry out their research in their own way. Now that scientific medicine in this country had got the start which he had done so much to bring about, no one knew better than Welch that the time had definitely gone by when a committee of medically trained men might hope to determine the problems to be studied. And yet of all the members of the board he was the one most competent to deal with a wide variety of fields.

As the years passed, the institute earned so completely the confidence of the Rockefellers and their advisers that it was in less danger of being starved for funds than of being encouraged to proceed too rapidly. By 1928, gifts from the Rockefellers personally and from the Rockefeller Foundation for endowment, buildings, and land reached in round numbers $65,-000,000.

Thus supported and encouraged, the institute gradually expanded along the lines planned until it became complete in its organization, which included the study of all living things. Its hospital opened in October 1910, under the directorship of Rufus Cole, a Hopkins graduate recommended by Welch. Herter was associated with Cole until ill health forced him to retire after a few months of active service. Since hospitals devoted exclusively to research hardly existed anywhere in the world, the institute had to work out a new method of organization. The hospital staff was appointed on precisely the same terms as the staff of the laboratory; not permitted to engage in outside practice, the physicians were required to give their full time to their scientific work. Patients were admitted only if they were suffering from diseases which were being studied at the time, and in order to make sure that the choice should never be determined by financial considerations, at Gates's suggestion it was agreed that no payment should be accepted.

The establishment of a department of animal pathology had been under consideration since the beginning of the institute, but in accordance with the principle of gradual development the directors had left the matter in abeyance until in 1913 a chance occurrence brought it forward again in a concrete and compelling fashion. A devastating outbreak of hog cholera in the West had alarmed J. J. Hill, president of the Great Northern Railway, since the resulting impoverishment of the farmers had affected the business of his road. He consulted Biggs, his physician, who brought me into a conference which resulted in his offering the institute $50,000 with which to investigate the disease. Although as a result of Hill's death his offer lapsed, the subject, thus reopened, received the approval of Rockefeller and his advisers. It was decided to establish at Princeton, New Jersey, a clinic for sick animals and laboratories for investigation.

Welch, who had studied comparative anatomy with Leuckart and had himself worked on hog cholera, was a firm believer in the importance of investigating the diseases of animals. Certain illnesses are transmissible from animals to man, and the reverse transmission, from man to animals, is of the first importance to research, since once an illness is given to a member of a lower species, the experimental method can be applied much more successfully. Results must then be interpreted through a knowledge of both human and animal pathology.

The directorship of the new department was, of course, offered to Theobald Smith, but Welch feared he would decline; "no one gives up a Harvard professorship," Welch said. There was great rejoicing when, on April 16, 1914, Smith accepted. The ideal director had been secured, and in 1917 the department of animal pathology was opened.

One link in the chain of subjects remained to be forged, namely, plant pathology.[8] The urge to develop this subject was increased by the growing awareness that the so-called "virus diseases" were as great a source of danger to human beings as diseases caused by bacteria, if not even greater. The first virus disease was discovered through the study of plants, which seemed to offer valuable opportunities for further discoveries. Plans for the establishment of a division of plant pathology were begun in 1926 and culminated in 1931 with the appointment of Dr. Louis O. Kunkel, of the Boyce Thompson Institute for Plant Research, as director, and the erection of laboratories and greenhouses adjoining the buildings for animal pathology, the two divisions being merged under the general directorship of Dr. Carl TenBroeck, Smith's successor.[9]

Just thirty years after the tentative beginnings of the Rockefeller Institute, its several departments were thus completed and unified. Welch's presidency of the board of scientific directors extended even beyond this time, and his influence is discernible in all the major developments that made the institute an outstanding contributor to medical science.

CHAPTER XIV

Science at the Bedside

I

IN 1901, the year that the Rockefeller Institute was founded, Welch, in his address as president of the Association of American Physicians, made a statement which, although perhaps not especially noticed by his hearers, contained the germs of the next great revolution in American medical education. His speech presaged a reform in clinical teaching that was achieved only through a controversy that raged for more than a decade and is not altogether silent today.

As a young man Welch had organized the first pathological laboratory in all America; now, twenty-three years later, he was able to say: "In astonishingly few years the laboratory side of our teaching has advanced in several of our institutions from the weakest to the strongest feature of the medical curriculum." The United States, he pointed out, possessed "far from enough, but still a fair number," of anatomical, physiological, and pathological laboratories, which offered students training that "compares favorably with that provided anywhere in the world." Furthermore, an able laboratory worker in these fields "can look forward with reasonable assurance to securing a desirable position as a teacher and a director of a laboratory of his special branch of science." However, "young physicians who wish to fit themselves for corresponding careers in clinical medicine and surgery" found that with one or two exceptions American hospitals offered them no such opportunities for training, and that when they were trained they had little chance of obtaining positions in which they could carry on their work.[1]

Welch, who never publicly advocated a reform until he believed it possible of completion, made at this time no suggestion as to how research and instruction at the bedside of the sick could be raised to the standard of the basic medical sciences. But by examining the movement in which he was now cautiously taking part, we may see what he had in mind.

Except at the Hopkins, the professors who expounded actual methods of treating patients were still, as all American medical teachers had once been, selected from among the leading local practitioners; the Harvard Medical School, for instance, failed to call a clinical professor from the outside until 1912.[2] Even the minor clinical posts were held by local doctors who often retained their appointments for most of their lives, in sharp contrast to the assistants or assistant professors in laboratory departments, who were young men appointed for a short term and expected to improve scientifically so that they could be advanced or called elsewhere. Thus, as Welch pointed out, ambitious scientists could obtain clinical positions only if death or resignation happened to create a vacancy in some medical school in the city where they practised. And, of course, they had to be successful practitioners before they could expect any appointment at all. There was no way for a young man to get a clinical position through the whole-hearted pursuit of the scientific side of medicine.

Furthermore, the pay was so small in the clinical departments that the staff had to support themselves primarily by private practice, giving only a limited part of their time to medical school and hospital duties. Laboratories in the clinic were still very few and, with an occasional exception, of the simplest nature. Research in the clinic languished. The contrast could scarcely have been greater between the active scientific atmosphere of the pre-clinical laboratories and the atmosphere of the hospital clinics where patients were actually treated. Indeed, the clinical situation was very similar to the situation Welch had faced when he returned from Germany as a young pathologist.

In the meantime, the steady progress of medical research coming more from the laboratories than from the clinics was widening the gap long existing between the discovery of new useful knowledge and its applications to the prevention and alleviation of disease. It became almost impossible for clinical teachers, engaged as they were in the onerous duties of private practice, to keep up with the rising tide of literature on scientific medicine. So much that was new was being found out not in physiology only, but in physiological chemistry and pharmacology as well, while Koch's epochal discoveries were revolutionizing medicine in respect to the infectious and epidemic diseases. All this new wine could no longer be safely poured into old bottles; the clinics, it became clear to advanced thinkers, would have to be reconstructed.

For a long time, an occasional worker had revolted against the *status quo*. Louis, the great French physician who attracted many American pupils in the first half of the nineteenth century, had withdrawn from practice to devote several concentrated years to the study of tuberculosis in the hospital, and he advised his brilliant young American pupil, James Jackson, junior, to do likewise.[3] In Germany also some professors of clinical medicine voluntarily gave up consultative practice to devote their whole time to teaching and studying in the clinics.

The first man, however, really to start an alternate system was Hugo von Ziemssen, who became so dissatisfied with the organization of medical clinics that in 1873 he set up at Erlangen in Bavaria a small laboratory of a half-dozen rooms. The next year he was called to Munich, where a new hospital was built for him into which he introduced an "Institute for Clinical Research." In 1884 this innovation led to the establishment of the first hospital laboratory in which investigators and students worked side by side. It was subdivided into departments of physiology, pathology, and chemistry, and Welch, who saw it in operation during its first year, was to regard it as the first modern medical clinic.[4]

The physiologist Ludwig in Leipzig followed von Ziemssen's innovations with close interest. Seeing more clearly than others that part-way measures would not suffice to meet the ever-growing demands of scientific discovery and invention applicable to the treatment of disease, he began to argue that clinical instruction should be raised to full university status. Paid on a scale that would enable them to give all their time to their teaching and scientific work, the professors should be expected to do so. Private practice would then no longer encroach on the energies that should be spent in the pursuit and application of knowledge. This was not the point of view of a narrow academic physiologist, for Ludwig had long pondered the relation of that branch of biology to all of medicine, itself a complex biological science. "Every disease," he said, "is a physiological experiment, which is the more important for us, since we can rarely reproduce it experimentally."

General discussions were in the spirit of Ludwig's laboratory, which besides being the busiest workshop in Germany was also the most genial anywhere. The professor himself emanated good will and the talk that went on around him was stimulating in high degree. Everyone was encouraged to take part, just as everyone profited from the diversity of researches going on in the laboratory. Thus Ludwig often expounded his ideas on clinical reform to his American pupil Mall, who worked with him in the winter of 1885–86. That Ludwig admired Mall's intellectual qualities is clear from the letters that were to pass between them, which show a rare devotion between teacher and pupil, an old man and a young. Indeed, they had many temperamental traits in common which tended to bring them into sympathy with each other. They stood together on the anatomical basis of their investigations into the physiology of the organs, and each possessed a certain elegance in the manner in which his scientific work was completed and presented for publication. The order and meticulousness of Ludwig's laboratory in the eighties were repeated in Mall's much simpler one of the nineties, a similarity in organization and conduct which probably grew as much out of Mall's temperament as out of the example set him by his adored teacher.[5]

Fired with a belief in the importance of clinical reform, Mall returned to America, but he bided his time before expressing such revolutionary ideas until he was in a position sufficiently important to make people listen with respect. The moment came in 1892, when, as professor of anatomy at the University of Chicago, he found himself one of a brilliant group of young men who worshipped scientific medicine with a visionary zeal. The American history of modern clinical reform begins with heated talks between Mall, George E. Vincent, the sociologist who was to become president of the Rockefeller Foundation, and Jacques Loeb, a medically trained biologist whose subsequent scientific work was to be of first importance. Chicago medical circles began to resound with discussions of "full-time," as the movement came to be called, since a basic tenet was that clinical professors should devote their entire time to teaching and research.

In 1893, Mall returned to the Hopkins, where he continued to argue for full-time, and again he found willing ears. The young laboratory group in Baltimore were all potential reformers. The hospital was flourishing under Osler, Halsted, and Kelly as the Pathological had done a decade earlier under Welch. The pervading enthusiasm kept everyone at fever heat.

Mall's method of work, acquired in Germany, was different from that of the pathologists. One experiment a day was his rule, after which, if other duties permitted, he was free. The pathologist's lot is more commonplace. There is always the pressure of routine: autopsies to be made and written up, bacteriology to be worked out, besides teaching and research in a catch-as-catch-can manner. The day has not hours enough for him.

I would hear Mall's footsteps on the stair as, around noon, his experiment finished, he would yield to a passion to be moving—around the building, into the adjacent part of the city. He would look into my room, and not infrequently we would roam the streets of East Baltimore together. During these chats he often talked his best, discoursing on problems of research, on advanced educational and other reforms. Brilliant arguments for full-time flowed from his lips.

Mall's method of propagandizing was personal, limited to discussions between man and man; he left public arguments to others. After Lewellys F. Barker, who had been Mall's associate in Baltimore for five years, was called to the chair of anatomy at the University of Chicago, he became Mall's mouthpiece. In an inspiring address delivered before the western alumni of the Hopkins on February 28, 1902, he changed full-time from a local aspiration to almost a national issue.

Having defined the university hospital clinic as a place which should train students to carry on research in the wards and the laboratories, Barker said it should be staffed by men possessed of the same talents, attainments, and personality as other professors in the university, men who had already made important contributions to knowledge. They should, "like other university professors, give their whole time and energy to the work of the university, to teaching and to investigating in the hospitals. . . . They should be well paid by the university. They should not engage in private practice." Consultations should be permitted in exceptional cases, and the fees received from them "might be contributed to the budget of the hospitals themselves." Although the services of part-time men might also be used, Barker considered that the greatest need then was for full-time "physicians and surgeons trained in physiology and pathology" who, after careful observation in the wards and over the operating table, would submit the ideas there gleaned to experimental test "in laboratories adjacent to the wards." [6]

The *Journal of the American Medical Association* took notice of Barker's talk, although only to criticize the plan as impracticable. It would be prohibitively expensive, the editors insisted, and furthermore professors needed the experience gained from daily private practice. Other champions, however, entered the lists on Barker's side. Also in 1902, John M. Dodson, professor of pediatrics at Rush Medical College, contributed an article to the *Journal of the American Medical Association,* and a year later Frank Billings, the dean, argued in his address as president of the association that professors of medicine, surgery, and obstetrics "should give their whole time to the work of teaching and to original research in the hospital." He went on to say that, in addition to such men, professors who engaged in private practice would also be needed, for they would "impart to the student a better idea of medicine as a whole" and "coordinate and arrange the isolated facts of clinical and laboratory investigation."

Although the movement was attacked by Arthur Dean Bevan, head of the department of surgery at the University of Chicago, Abraham Flexner remembers that "Dr. Frank Billings once stated in a speech that a resolution was adopted by the Faculty of Rush Medical College after it became affiliated with the University of Chicago [in 1898], pledging the school to the establishment of full-time clinical teaching whenever funds could be procured."

The first Hopkins professor publicly to endorse full-time was, the record indicates, Howell, who in an address at Yale in 1909 asserted that "the university school which shall first establish departments on this basis may . . . secure both reputation and students as compared with schools organized on the present system. . . . Our country is in a peculiarly favorable position to make such an experiment. Our system of medical education has heretofore simply developed along lines laid down by the experience of foreign countries; perhaps in the direction suggested . . . we may have the opportunity to take the lead instead of trailing along in the rear." [7]

In the meantime, what of Welch? In 1901, as we have seen, he had pointed out the inferiority of clinical instruction to the pre-clinical; he returned to the same subject in 1906 at Harvard: "The most urgent need in medical education at the present time in this country I believe to be the organization of our clinics both for teaching and for research in the spirit of this modern movement and with provision for as intimate, prolonged, personal contact of the student with the subject of study as he finds in the laboratory." * But of full-time itself he said not a word.

---

* In 1925 Welch said: "Unfortunately in the minds of many the term 'clinic' means no more than . . . a clinical demonstrative lecture. A clinic as here understood signifies something very different from this—it includes an elaborate plant consisting of hospital wards, rooms, laboratories and equipment, an adequate supply of patients, a well-trained professional staff of higher grade than the ordinary hospital interns devoting their time to the care of patients, the training of

Welch had a canny perception of the right moment for active intervention in any cause, an essential element of his statesmanship. It has been said of Queen Elizabeth that the essence of her foreign policy was her successful use of procrastination, which gave "a breathing space . . . for the English people to discover a middle way and to grow contented, prosperous, and respected throughout the world." The new Hopkins Medical School also needed a breathing space in order to establish itself. It was part of its strength that the pre-clinical chairs should first overtake and then outdistance the clinical.

Furthermore, Welch knew that full-time would be so expensive that its discussion was useless as long as medical endowments lagged far behind other endowments, when there was no possibility of securing the necessary funds. So he kept himself aloof from the excited talk of Mall and his colleagues, awaiting a suitable occasion with the patience that was fundamental to his character.

In 1907, in an address at the University of Chicago, he took a very cautious step forward. "The heads of the principal clinical departments, particularly the medical and the surgical, should devote their main energies and time to their hospital work and to teaching and investigating without the necessity of seeking their livelihood in a busy outside practice and without allowing such practice to become their chief professional occupation."

A year later the hospital of the Rockefeller Institute, in the organization of which Welch had taken a prominent part, got under way on a full-time plan. It is important to recall the part taken by Rockefeller's adviser Gates in establishing the clinical services on the same basis as those of the laboratory, and in promoting the scientific study of the sick by providing that patients accepted for investigation be treated without charge. A significant, practical blow had been struck without excitement

---

students, and the investigation of disease. . . . Such a clinic . . . is comparable to the scientific laboratories; its problems are those presented by living patients; the investigation of these problems is conducted by the methods and in the spirit of scientific research with every regard for the best interests and treatment of patients."

or fanfare. Now Welch quietly awaited the opportunity to strike another blow.

It came in 1910, when the distinguished Viennese children's specialist Clement von Pirquet, who had spent one year in Baltimore as professor of pediatrics, accepted a professorship at Breslau, but expressed willingness to return to the Hopkins if his appointment were placed on a university basis. On November 22 Welch wrote me: "I believe that if we could secure an endowment of say $200,000, for the chair and department of pediatrics, we could at last establish a clinical department of pediatrics on the ideal basis of a laboratory department. Von Pirquet would fall into such an arrangement perfectly. The idea is to have at the head of such a clinical department a productive investigator, who would make his hospital work, his teaching and the conduct of research the main things. He could build up a great school of pediatrics and would be a great stimulus and inspiration to the country. . . . Do you suppose that we could present this matter to Mr. Rockefeller through Mr. Gates, Mr. Murphy, and his advisers with a prospect of interesting them?"

There is no evidence that Welch presented the von Pirquet matter to the Rockefeller office at this time, but if he did, as seems probable, it failed to appeal to Gates as an isolated undertaking. The next relevant document that has come down to us is a letter from Gates to Welch dated January 6, 1911. "I have not forgotten the main subject of conversation on the occasion of your visit to my home, so delightful to me and to us all. Nor has my interest in medical education in the United States decreased, nor my belief that the Johns Hopkins Medical School should occupy in the future a position even more important than in the past. I am looking, therefore, with deep interest, I might almost say solicitude, for the estimate you are preparing of the needs of the institution. I should like to have the estimate cover two things: First, the necessary expense of furnishing an entrance class of one hundred each year as good facilities throughout their course as the institution can now offer to an entering class of fifty each year. Second, the expense of conducting the institution in such a way that none of its professors (I speak now of an ultimate ideal) shall be permitted to make anything beyond the merest nominal charge for consultation or other service."

Welch replied that it would be "a comparatively simple matter to supply a statement of what is needed in the way of increased laboratory facilities to meet the demands of teaching efficiently one hundred students," but that "the perplexity comes in taking up the hospital side, and mainly on account of the largeness of the proposition." He admitted that he hesitated sending Gates an estimate of what it would cost.

Gates, however, was never frightened by the size of undertakings; he wrote Welch: "It seems to me that the thing to do is to figure out now the ideal thing, whatever it may come to and however appalling the financial total. This will include the enlargement of the Hospital as well as the enlargement of other facilities. If we cannot compass so large an undertaking all at once, or if we cannot compass it at all, we can still have it before us and can build toward it so that everything that we shall do will mean progress toward a definite chosen end, and nothing that we shall do will be inconsistent with it. . . . I will agree, therefore, not to be discouraged at your figures. Your letter prepares me in advance."

In fact, the requirements, whether they exceeded his expectations or not, proved beyond Gates's powers. "The job which they offer is, I am afraid, too big a one for me to tackle at this period of my life," he wrote on January 30. But he saw some possible economies and asked Welch to give him an hour or two on his next visit to New York. "You have told me some of your troubles, and I want an opportunity to tell you some of mine and perhaps we can mutually comfort each other."

II

The contrast between the clinical and the pre-clinical departments was becoming increasingly clear all over the nation as medical school after medical school raised its standards. Although Welch, having in mind the contributions of such schools as Harvard and Michigan, claimed no monopoly on the part of the Johns Hopkins University for these advances, the changes that were being put into effect had a tendency to follow the lines laid down by the Hopkins experiment. Entrance requirements were gradually raised, the period of study lengthened, the course graded, and pre-clinical laboratories established, often under the directorship of Welch's pupils.

Welch wrote his sister during 1903: "Progress in these respects has been really very great during the last fifteen years, so that America is now contributing her fair share to the advancement of medical science, whereas a quarter of a century ago almost no scientific work in medicine was done in this country. I have had a share in this, but others have also worked successfully to the same end. Far more remains to be accomplished than has been done, but now that the public and men of wealth realize that medical education and institutions for research are worthy objects of endowment, and that advancement of medical and sanitary knowledge is of immense importance to the welfare of mankind, the outlook for the future is most hopeful."

In 1904 the movement which had been growing steadily within the walls of isolated medical schools was organized on a national scale: the American Medical Association founded its Council on Medical Education. Six years later Abraham Flexner, under the auspices of the Carnegie Foundation for the Advancement of Teaching, published his epoch-making investigation of medical schools in the United States and Canada. He showed that out of the 155 institutions in existence, 50, or a little less than a third, were integral parts of universities. Only Harvard and the Hopkins required a college degree for entrance; Cornell required three years of college; and 20 other schools required two. One hundred and thirty-two schools admitted students with a high school education or less. Laboratory instruction, Flexner reported, was given in most of the more advanced institutions.

Publishing a detailed study of every school, Flexner laid bare

conditions in many of the privately owned ones that were so un-
believably bad that a national revulsion took place. His report
touched off a great movement of reform that in a decade or so
made the new departures of the Hopkins experiment standard
all over the continent. The shoals of little schools, possessing
almost no modern facilities, were forced either to raise their
standards or to go out of existence. This movement was greatly
assisted by a stiffening of requirements in the State Licensing
Boards, which no longer automatically granted licences to practise to every graduate of every so-called medical school.

Abraham Flexner's rigorous, impartial analysis appealed to
Gates, who, as we learn from Rockefeller's *Random Reminiscences of Men and Events,* used virtually the same method in
his investigations of business affairs. After all, medical education
around 1910 was as much a business—perhaps even more so—
as a profession. Flexner spoke to Gates in a language he could
well understand on a subject which lay near his heart and to
which he had already devoted much study.[8]

Inviting Flexner to lunch, Gates asked him what he would
do with $1,000,000 to be used for medical education. "I should
give it to Dr. Welch," Flexner replied. The upshot was that
he was sent to Baltimore to make a detailed study of the situation there. Welch instantly asked him to dine at the Maryland
Club with Mall and Halsted, and after a marvellous dinner had
been served, Mall argued eloquently that every penny of any
new funds that might be obtained should be spent on putting
the heads of the clinical departments on full-time.

After examining the situation further, Flexner made a report
to Gates which presented three alternative plans. Number One
proposed that the school should be endowed and reduced to
250 students (a cut in the enrolment for that year of 97) and the
main clinical chairs placed on a university, or full-time, basis;
Number Two proposed a school of 250, the organization of a
department of bacteriology and hygiene, the erection of a new
building to house among other things a library, and additions
to the dispensary, the clinical departments being left as they
were; Number Three was based on a school of 400 students, a

department of bacteriology and hygiene, and a new building, with the clinical departments left as they were. "My judgment," Flexner concluded, "inclines strongly to alternative I."

This suggestion, involving as it did full-time, contained dynamite, as everyone saw. On May 10 Welch wrote Gates apologizing for the delay in coming to any conclusion concerning Flexner's report. "We have had numerous conferences both in the Faculty and with the Trustees and the ideas are taking concrete shape. . . . There are considerable differences of opinion on essential points. The experiment proposed cannot be undertaken without full deliberation. . . . You can hardly appreciate the keen interest which has been aroused. Something has leaked out, but nothing definite and I think nothing prejudicial to our instituting reforms, if given the opportunity. I am more than ever convinced that the next great step in advancing medical education is along improvement on the clinical side, and I expect to be able to tell you that we shall be prepared to introduce desired reforms in this direction."

On June 11, 1911, Welch finally reported to Gates that "the opinion prevails in our medical faculty and among the trustees of the University" that the proposition involving full-time, "if it can be carried out upon an adequate financial basis, is the one which meets the most urgent needs and promises the largest benefits not to the Johns Hopkins School alone but to medical education in general."

There was unanimous agreement, he said, to limiting the size of the school to 250, provided the loss in tuition was made up. "The quality of students will be improved by the necessity of more careful selection. . . . There is need of a conspicuous example that the ideal of the medical school should be not bigness but the best adjustment of the means of training to the end of making the best physicians and medical thinkers."

Full-time, however, involved "such radical changes in conditions which now exist and have always existed in medical schools both here and in Europe that entire agreement of opinion as to the wisdom of the change is not to be expected. Nor can the plan be carried out without some hardship to individuals and some disturbance of personal relations. These are among the reasons why it has been deemed necessary or expedient to allow full time for deliberation and discussion and to endeavor to bring about a situation where the changes can be effected with the least possible disturbance of the exceptionally harmonious relations which have always existed in our faculty."

Welch then listed the main objections to the proposal. The first, "the alleged difficulty or impossibility of securing and holding the best men for the positions with such salaries as could be contemplated," he regarded as most serious, although only temporarily so. "It would be hazardous in the extreme to start the new arrangement with young men in the clinical chairs without considerable experience and without established reputations, however promising they may seem to be. At present the field of choice is a very restricted one, but one of the great benefits to be expected from the suggested plan is the wide extension of this field by the training of men for the higher clinical walks." Once the new system was established, it would create its own professors, who had never become used to living on the scale of successful practitioners.

Other objections were, Welch pointed out, "the difficulty of keeping the public and the profession away from men with the reputations these clinicians should have, and the loss to the community and medical practitioners by withdrawal of such men from outside practice, and third the contention that limitation to practise within the hospital would deprive the teachers of opportunities and experience valuable to them in their own development, in their training of students destined to become practitioners." But he argued that such difficulties would be overcome by the fact that the salaried clinicians "should be permitted to have consultations at the hospital and to have patients in the private wards, but the professional fees from such patients should go to the hospital or university. . . . The number of these private patients should be limited and determined mainly by the scientific interest of the cases." Furthermore, "the new plan of course does not contemplate dispensing with the service of men engaged in practice who can give only a part of their time to teaching. . . . Among the practitioners are some who love to teach and are really excellent teachers, whose services it would be a great detriment to the school to lose."

To the objection "that the imposition of fixed rules and regulations upon the conduct and the use of the time of such men as would be entrusted with these clinical chairs would be harassing, improper and unnecessary," he answered that once the tradition had been established rigid stipulations regarding the full-time service would no longer be needed. Moreover, he foresaw that while "the principle must be safeguarded contingencies may arise which might make proper and desirable an exception to the rule that the salaried, full-time professor should not receive a fee for professional services."

Since the attraction of the new chairs would not be salary, but the opportunity for scientific work and teaching of a high order, it followed that the occupants should not be "overburdened with administration, teaching, and the care of patients," that they should have "a staff of capable young men (and it may be also young women) acting as associate professors, associates and assistants, who are themselves in training for the higher positions elsewhere, that various laboratories for clinical teaching and research shall be provided and that there shall be an adequate budget for running expenses."

All the disadvantages of the plan, Welch insisted, were small compared with its advantages. "The establishment upon the clinical side of the medical school of academic ideals like those which prevail in other departments of the university would be a forward movement of far-reaching significance. These ideals imply single-minded devotion to the work belonging to the university chair. An absorbing outside practice is not a part of this work and is incompatible with that devotion to teaching, to investigating and to the duties of a hospital physician or surgeon which should characterize a university professor and which is required to obtain the best results in the activities which properly belong to his chair.

"It is inspiring to contemplate the possibilities of a well-supported and properly organized medical or surgical clinic upon a true university basis. It would introduce new opportunities and higher standards of teaching and of productive research. It would place before students and the profession higher ideals of the mission of the physician and of his relations to the community. It would advance both the science and the art of medicine by training investigators, by making better physicians, and by contributing to useful knowledge. . . . We who advocate this change believe that it will initiate a reform in medical education so far-reaching as to constitute a new era."

On August 2, 1911, Rockefeller, junior, wrote his father that he united with Murphy and Gates in recommending a gift of $1,200,000 to the Hopkins for the establishment of full-time. Gates pointed out in an enclosed memorandum that medicine had up till then "been neglected by philanthropy." As a result, medical colleges, unlike other colleges, had been organized by private individuals and too often had become business ventures for profit, so that, with a few honourable exceptions, there had been stagnation in the science of medicine. "There have been occasional discoveries, just as there will be eddies in every stream."

The gift now recommended, Gates continued, offered "more productive results than anything in sight. I think that this sum, so invested, will probably result, in the course of some years, in a beneficent revolution of medical education, first in the United States, second in Europe, and finally in the remotest parts of the world. This revolution, when effected, will place medicine throughout the world on a scientific and a disinterested basis, like other forms of beneficent learning, and will be of unimaginable value to the human race."

On this recommendation to the elder Rockefeller no immediate action was taken. Although the reasons for the delay are not stated in the documents that have come down to us, Abraham Flexner remembers that it was due partly to the size of the sum involved. The General Education Board, which was at that time handling most of the Rockefellers' donations to institutions of learning, had made so many commitments to be paid out of accruing income that a pause was required in which to accumulate the fund for full-time. Furthermore, there continued to be controversy at the Hopkins concerning the wisdom of the change. "The trustees," Abraham Flexner writes, "endorsed the plan subject to ratification by the medical faculty. Within the medical faculty the scheme was unanimously endorsed by the laboratory men, but there was a rift among the clinicians. Dr. Welch made no endeavor whatsoever to push the idea. Every member of the medical faculty had a copy of the report [A. Flexner's], and Dr. Welch bided his time." He seems to have been working behind the scenes in his quiet way for a general agreement which would make it unnecessary to hurt feelings by the use of force; the friendly, co-operative atmosphere of the Hopkins was too valuable to be unnecessarily shattered for the sake of speed.

Barker, Osler's successor as professor of medicine, had in an address at McGill receded from the advanced position on full-time he had occupied as a young man. And Osler himself, who had been away from Baltimore for six years, was not enthusiastic, although in 1889 he had taken a long step toward the reform now contemplated by establishing clinical clerkships, extended terms of service at the hospital, and the beginnings of a clinical laboratory.[9] Osler's opinion was given great weight not only at the Hopkins but throughout America by doctors and the laity alike, because during his sixteen years in Baltimore he had made the greatest contribution to the teaching of the practice of medicine that had been made by anyone in this country. Furthermore, his charm of personality and his literary talents had captured many hearts.*

---

* On learning that Osler intended to resign, Welch wrote him: "Your letter drove me into a fit of the blues and nearly wrecked one of my lectures. Your going will be an irreparable loss to us in a multitude of ways, but of course I cannot blame you. I understand what a tremendous pressure there has been on you, and how you must welcome a quieter and more peaceful existence. It is splendid that you should have been chosen for the professorship at Oxford, but it is not surprising. Of course they were sure to want you.

"I shall miss you, we all shall, more than can be told, and I do not like to think of it. It is after all a fine thing to have had you for fifteen years, and that

On May 23, 1911, he wrote Welch that since he had not heard the proposal in detail, he found it difficult to express an opinion. He was, however, concerned lest the payment to clinicians of salaries on the academic scale "would spell ruin for the hospital. You could, perhaps, get the good men for a few years for that, but they would flit off, inevitably. On the other hand if the Trustees paid liberal salaries of 15 to 20 thousand dollars, they could always command the best men, and I would be strongly in favour of it. Careful provision should be made that the Hospital was not converted into a Sanatorium, and a large part of the time of the professors taken up with earning money for the Hospital from its private patients. I think this is the whole matter in a nutshell." To Dr. H. M. Thomas in Baltimore Osler had previously written: "Personally, I feel that to cut off the heads of departments from a practice is a Utopian scheme, admirable on paper; but the very men who would be most in favour of it would be the first to get the professors to break their rules. . . . It is an experiment I would like very much to see tried, but not at the Johns Hopkins first. It might have been different if we had started so, but I do not believe that there is any possibility of success at present."

While the issue of full-time at the Hopkins was gradually working itself out through peaceful discussion, Welch was moving quietly on another aspect of the clinical problem. If the great public hospitals could be brought into close connexion with the university medical schools, it would, he felt, be an important step toward advancing teaching and research in the clinic; even when the schools possessed hospitals of their own, the growing ward teaching called for more beds than were thus available. On January 1, 1911, Welch wrote MacCallum, then professor at the College of Physicians and Surgeons, which was now allied with Columbia University, "I am delighted at the prospect of the union between Columbia and the Presbyterian Hospital. President Butler has sent me the confidential report,

---

you have laid the foundations, established the traditions and given things medical an impetus which I hope will continue to keep them in the right track."

and I had previously had a conference with Mr. [Robert W.] de Forest at his request, so that I have been informed for some time of the developments." MacCallum called on Welch to use his influence with the trustees of both institutions, and when the time came to make the issue public, de Forest asked Welch to speak at the forty-third anniversary of the Presbyterian Hospital on "The Advantages to a Charitable Hospital of Affiliation with a University Medical School."

Welch, who had already referred to the matter in an address at the Jefferson Medical College Hospital in 1907, stated that an ideal hospital "shall serve not only in a restricted sense the philanthropic and humanitarian purposes for which all hospitals are created, but also in a more extended sense the educational and scientific needs of medicine. . . . The type of hospital contemplated by the alliance is in no sense an experiment," he continued, giving examples to show that all over the world "the hospitals that have made the most important contributions to medical science . . . have won the greatest reputation."

The three functions of the ideal hospital, he said, were the care of the sick, the adequate training of the medical men of the future, and the advancement of medical knowledge. "The care of the sick stands first and is never to be forgotten, for the welfare of the patient is the primary purpose of the hospital." Welch did not dismiss lightly the fears which "laymen are apt to conjure up in their minds [of] conditions under which the inroads of medical students into a hospital would be disturbing to the order and quiet of the wards, and where the examination of patients for purposes of teaching might be harmful to the sick." He told his hearers that "instead of weakening the humanitarian efficiency, the educational and research functions increase the value of the service which a hospital fulfills in the care of its patients." The sufferers in the wards are better served because the very best professional staff is made available, men talented and singularly devoted, "who realize that their first duty is to the allied interests of the hospital and the school. . . .

They are men who will not become absorbed in a large outside practice, be it even a consulting practice, which would interfere with this work."

Ward teaching, Welch continued, was very important from an educational point of view, since "that vital knowledge—which enters into the fibre of being and gives power and wisdom—can come only from intimate contact with the objects of study." And the resulting improvement in training would be of advantage to patients not only in the future when the medical students themselves became practitioners, but at the very moment the teaching was going on, because the staff physicians themselves would profit from the scientific and questioning attitude created.

To the advancement of knowledge, the third important function of the hospital, Welch gave special attention. Pointing out that medical research "makes the strongest possible appeal to philanthropy," he implied that the hospital which fosters it would have an advantage in obtaining funds. That the patients would reap rewards from research was clear from the progress already made which had in less than a half-century reduced the mortality rate "from thirty-five deaths per thousand inhabitants to about fifteen," adding some twelve years to the period of human life. This saving in life had resulted from the better control of infectious diseases; little had been done for the organic diseases of advancing years. "The ideal hospital," Welch said, "can be a workshop for new knowledge in that direction." [10]

In his closing words Welch showed that he had a vision of the great medical centre that was to come two decades later: "I should like to see the College of Physicians and Surgeons and the Presbyterian Hospital situated side by side, and the destiny of the two institutions brought closer together."

That Welch's speech had made an impression is shown by the fact that when the American Medical Association formed its section on hospitals the following year, it asked not a clinician but Welch, the pathologist, to make the opening address. His argument on this important occasion, when thousands of physicians and surgeons were assembled, followed closely on that of his Presbyterian Hospital speech, but he added a plea for the utilization in hospitals of the new sociological techniques.[11]

Welch was an ardent believer in publicly supported hospitals. Congratulating the citizens of Cincinnati on their new municipal institution, he said: "You have a hospital without any equal in this country in its possibilities for medical education. . . . The future of medical education is not going to lie with endowed hospitals. Their clinics can never be as large as yours. It will not be possible for them to provide for the care of hundreds of patients on account of the vast amount of money which would be required. . . . You have here a hospital equal in all essentials to the great one in Vienna."

The movement for the union of medical schools and hospitals made rapid headway. In 1914 the Peter Bent Brigham Hospital became affiliated with the Harvard Medical School; speaking at the exercises, Welch was able to point to several other examples of close association: the New York Hospital and the Cornell Medical School, the New Haven Hospital and the Yale Medical School, the Barnes Hospital in St. Louis and the Medical School of Washington University.

While contributing to these advances, Welch, of course, had not forgotten the cause of full-time at the Hopkins. Obviously trying to forge an entering wedge, in March 1912 he tried again to interest Gates in bringing von Pirquet back as professor of pediatrics. An additional annual income of $15,000, he wrote, would open the Children's Hospital and establish a pediatric clinic with von Pirquet in charge. "It is something of a surprise that he is willing to relinquish the leading chair of pediatrics in the world to come to the Hopkins, but he was most favorably impressed with the general spirit and environment here and especially with the high class of our students. . . . I am sure that you will be especially interested and gratified to note that von Pirquet makes it a condition that he shall not engage in private practice and that he shall be paid a salary sufficient to enable him to do this. His condition that any income received from private consultations shall go to the development of his own department I consider to be admirable. . . . If we could secure von Pirquet on these terms we could at least demonstrate in a conspicuous instance the merits of the much discussed plan of 'Whole-time professors,' and I know that this point will make an appeal to you, as it does to me."

Gates, however, was still uninterested in this smaller approach. On September 23 Welch wrote Osler: "We could not raise the money to put the children's department into the shape which would justify von Pirquet in leaving Vienna, and we have secured Howland, who begins in October. I think that we are fortunate and that he will fit in admirably and make a success of it, but we need more money for the children's hospital."

In January 1913, when President Remsen resigned because of illness, Welch was forced into a position of greater power. He wrote Wallace Buttrick: "In spite of my protest they have coralled me for chairman of the Faculty Committee to run the University until a new president is secured. The Trustees, the Academic Council and the Medical Faculty all met and were unanimous in their desire that I should take the position. They seem to have conspired to shut off every avenue of escape, and I have been forced to yield. I feel that they made a mistake, but I shall do the best I can under the circumstances. My interest in getting a president for the University as soon as possible is now more lively than before."

To many of his friends Welch wrote complaining letters. The *Baltimore Evening Sun* tells us how he protested: "He had never known what it was to have office hours, he said. He had never been accustomed to routine work. He had never dictated a letter in his life. He did not want an executive position." But once he had assumed the job, a frightening thing happened: his popularity "began to bring in rich returns to the university. . . . The trustees saw this and they believed they had made a find. Dr. Welch's character was counting for more than executive training might count for. The trustees asked him to resign his temporary chairmanship for the purpose of accepting the permanent presidency; this although he was older than men they had in mind."

In March Welch, who was usually so well, was hurried off to the Johns Hopkins Hospital, "railroaded," as he himself described it. Surrounded with flowers and detective stories, "as my failing is well known," he was forced to rest. "I suppose that I have been overworked, and I have quite a capacity for loafing when the opportunity offers. I am perfectly comfortable—no pain—no fever."

In July he was sent abroad by his doctors to take a cure at Carlsbad for the gout, an ailment which had first attacked him six or seven years before and from which he was to suffer periodically for the rest of his life. Although his doctors were inclined to ascribe the ailment to his eating habits, Welch always insisted that his gout was "absurd and unmerited"; he refused to change his diet except when actually suffering from an attack.

He was not pleased at being sent to Carlsbad. He did not need the treatment, which he had heard was very debilitating, he wrote his niece, "but I came over ostensibly for it and I must go through a course of the waters, or rather they must go through me." A month later his point of view had changed: "I have completed my three weeks cure at Carlsbad with great success. The waters and the place agreed with me finely. . . . I was invited a good deal to luncheons and dinners and automobile rides, but the life is or should be simple. I lost only five pounds; some take off a pound a day, but I was not very abstemious in my diet. . . . Whether the good comes from the early rising and the early to bed, or the much walking and life in the open, or the simple and abstemious diet and life or the waters, it is hard to say. . . . When one has nothing to do, one is always very busy, and so the days were very short and full, and at the end I was sorry to leave." After that, he visited Carlsbad many times, but rarely without writing that it was ridiculous for him to be taking the cure, which he obviously did not need.

That summer he went from Carlsbad to Vienna, to the Lido for the sea bathing—"it was the full moon in Venice and I spent my substance on gondolas up and down the Grand Canal"—and to Munich for the opera. "I have been foot-free, if not fancy free," he wrote; the Hopkins presidency was chasing him. "I must get back to Baltimore before the president of the Johns Hopkins board of trustees sails for Europe the latter part of this month. They have not yet selected a president for the University, and are altogether too satisfied to let things drift along with me in the President's office. I have positively declined to accept the presidency, and am extremely anxious to be relieved of my temporary duties in this capacity. It is important that I should get back to Baltimore without much delay to push matters along as fast as I can."

At first professors at Columbia, Chicago, Harvard, and Illinois were prominently under consideration. They were eliminated one by one until the leading candidate became William H. Buckler, a many-sided trustee of the university who was an attorney, an archæologist, and an economist. But when Welch met him in Europe, Buckler expressed disinclination to be considered for the post. Welch was forced to remain chairman of the administrative committee, and he complained: "The man we want seems to be as yet unborn." [12]

Push as he would, Welch could not get rid of the job until the end of that academic year. At the 1914 commencement he was able to announce the selection of Frank Johnson Goodnow. The next day he wrote to his niece: "He seems just the man for us. He is now in China advising Yuan Shi Kai, and I imagine that it is a relief to both that he is released from this duty. I sang my swan-song—as the paper says—at our Commencement yesterday —and I shall get back to my ordinary routine."

III

While he was still acting head of the university, Welch had brought the full-time negotiations to a triumphant close. On October 21, 1913, he wrote the General Education Board that "the Faculty of the Medical School are fully convinced of the wisdom and necessity of commanding the entire time and devotion of a staff of teachers in the main clinical branches," and that the trustees of the university and the hospital had authorized him to ask for funds to place the departments of medicine, surgery, and pediatrics on this basis. Should the funds be provided, he continued, in each department the professor and his staff, "consisting of Associate Professors, Associates, Assistants, etc. . . . would be free to render any service required by humanity or science, but from it they would be expected to derive no pecuniary benefit." Such fees as would upon occasion be charged would be paid to the hospital and used "to promote the objects for the attainment of which this request is made.

"The changes here discussed can be introduced immediately into the department of pediatrics, because this department has been established recently; medicine and surgery can be reorganized by the beginning of the next academic year. Certain men now holding important posts but partly engaged in practice can be utilized to advantage in the service of the school, but from the start the public hospital service would be entirely in charge of men on the full-time basis. In the dispensary, in clinical teaching, and in the teaching of special topics men engaged partly in practice can be advantageously used to some extent."

Two days later the General Education Board took action. "RE-SOLVED, that the General Education Board hereby agrees to appropriate the funds necessary [$1,500,000] to carry out the full-time scheme described in Dr. Welch's letter under date of October 21, 1913, and empowers the Finance Committee to take the necessary steps looking to the execution of this agreement.

"RESOLVED, that in view of Dr. Welch's great services to the cause of medical education in America, the fund appropriated as above be called 'The William H. Welch Endowment for Clinical Education and Research.' " [13]

Welch, who was waiting at the offices of the General Education Board when the appropriation was made, was called into the meeting room; the trustees rose, shook hands with him, and expressed their gratification. "It was one of the great moments in my life," he said many years later.

The Baltimore press took this occasion to shower personal tributes on Welch. Recalling President Eliot's words, "Dr. Welch is beyond all question the leader of the medical profession in America," the *Baltimore News* continued: "His is a familiar figure to the people of this city. He is a typical Baltimorean and would rather live here than anywhere else, although he was born in Connecticut. . . . Dr. Welch is a bachelor . . . and is in demand as a dinner guest and for other social diversions, but his taste runs not to society." And the *Sun:* "His modesty is such that even a presumptuous newspaper finds opportunity but rarely to say just how highly he is regarded in this community. He is a splendid influence in the general as well as the professional life of Baltimore. . . . His knowledge of and interest in many departments of our civic life [are] so unusual, that it is not strange his name should have been proposed for the presidency of the Johns Hopkins University, for United States Senator,* and other positions of honor and importance. . . . Having regard first for the substance of things, he is almost equally scrupulous concerning the form. But with his splendid poise goes a capacity to arouse enthusiasm in the people around. . . . He is one of those exceptionally well-informed, well-balanced beings whom it is almost impossible to appraise without seeming to exaggerate. Those who meet him and deal with him instinctively feel that here is a man with whom Huxley or Goethe or Leonardo would have delighted to converse. One such man is a mighty factor in the life of any community; two or three such would make any city great."

The reaction of the medical press was, however, mixed. The *Boston Medical and Surgical Journal* said that such gifts "of the type which medical education most needs in this country today, will be gratefully welcomed, not only by the institutions which they benefit, but by every member of the profession." But the *Medical Record* referred to "this somewhat doubtful experiment" and went on to state that full-time would make clinical professors into laboratory workers and that laboratory workers were narrower than practitioners. The powerful *Journal of the American Medical Association* started out by declaring that full-time "will not only elevate the standards of clinical instruction, but also develop a more extensive research along

---

* On July 23, 1907, Welch wrote his niece: "I am not taking my senatorial boom seriously, nor are the politicians. Of course, I should not even consider the idea, if I could get the Senatorship, but it is absurd to say that one would not consider the impossible. The movement, if it may be so dignified, started with the doctors, and I think that I have put a stop to it, as I do not care for the notoriety."

the lines of clinical medicine, leading to a wider application of new discoveries in the treatment of disease." But within a year the editors had changed their minds. During 1914 they published a series of attacks on what they termed "the Hopkins plan," contending that first-class clinicians could not be expected to make the financial sacrifice of accepting university salaries. "If a great clinician is willing to give half or two-thirds of his time to research and instruction, but wishes to reserve two or three hours a day for consulting work for which he can readily secure large fees, is there any real advantage gained in compelling him to surrender these fees to the university?"

The Council on Medical Education of the American Medical Association,[14] the body immediately concerned, took a hostile attitude toward the new departure. Full-time became a *cause célèbre* that was vehemently discussed over a period of years, the main bone of contention being the payment of consultation fees not to the consultant, but to the university. A committee of experienced clinicians, appointed to study the matter, made their report at the annual meeting of the council in Chicago in February 1915. "Is some private practice by clinical teachers essential to keep medical education in sympathetic touch with the human side of medical practice?" they asked. "Will the placing of clinical chairs on a full-time basis result in a gradual separation of medical teachers from perhaps some of the most vital problems of active medical practice? . . .

"The principle that the practice of clinical teachers should be restricted appears to have general acceptance. In determining to what extent that practice should be limited, there are two extremes somewhere between which it is possible to construct a rational scheme. On the one side is the whole-time requirement as adopted at Johns Hopkins, and on the other side is the condition in some medical schools where clinical teachers are so busy with their private practice that their teaching is badly neglected. Opinion is by no means unanimous that the whole-time requirement is ideal."

The conclusion reached was that schools must appoint a teacher "whose chief business is to instruct medical students, who chooses the work because he loves it, and who is qualified by education and by personal experience in experimental work to be a productive teacher. Given such teachers, the limitation of their practice will take care of itself." [15]

Welch, who took part in the discussion, wrote me: "You will be amused at the latest attack on the full-time scheme, which I encountered in Chicago last week from Bevan, Rodman and others. It is fee-splitting, dichotomy, unethical, immoral, wicked!!! If you cannot see it, it is because you are a laboratory man and not a clinician."

Despite an attempt by Welch to stem the tide, the Council on Medical Education went further than its committee. They violently attacked the Hopkins scheme and recommended that the full-time members of the clinical staff should not include the professors, but be young men who would hold their positions from five to ten years while they received not only the training to be clinical professors but also to be great consultants. [16]

Faced by the most bitter controversy of his long career, Welch felt that the best way to confound the critics was to make full-time work successfully. As he well knew, the scheme was only a piece of machinery; it had to be implemented with men. Welch sent identical letters to the three clinical professors involved, expressing "the earnest wish of the Board of Trustees" that they accept the new chairs. Halsted's continuance in surgery was a foregone conclusion, since he had always been more interested in scientific work than in private practice. Howland, who had been attracted to the Hopkins by the opportunity to investigate the diseases of children, could also be counted upon. Concerning Barker, however, there was considerable doubt. To him Welch wrote a second letter, expressing his personal wish that he retain the professorship of medicine. Indeed, Welch went beyond his authority by offering Barker a higher salary than had been offered the other clinical professors; Welch wished to avoid even the appearance of violent measures, and also to safeguard the university in case it should become necessary to offer a larger salary to a successor.

After Barker had declined, the chair was offered to W. S.

Thayer, then clinical professor of medicine. When Thayer proved unwilling to move into the full-time position, Welch turned to Theodore C. Janeway, professor of medicine at Columbia and son of Welch's old associate at Bellevue. Despite the heavy pressure of teaching and practice, the younger Janeway had carried on investigations on the diseases of the heart and circulation, and had published an important book on the subject. An advanced thinker and accomplished writer, he was already concerned with giving more scientific content to clinical medicine in classroom and hospital.

Janeway accepted on April 28, 1914; Welch wrote him: "Your telegram . . . brought great joy. . . . That you have decided as you have is the best warrant of the high ideals which guide you, and will go far in commending the new plan of organizing the clinical departments and in contributing to its success."

Another letter to Janeway shows that Welch had not forgotten an old wound. "It seems to me hardly fair for the Columbia people to represent that you are under any moral obligations to stay. That is an attitude of mind which institutions are only too ready to assume under similar circumstances, and with which I have no sympathy. Surely every man has a right to order his life and to seek the place where he feels the largest opportunities for his own development and service lie. . . . In a smaller way I encountered the same line of argument when I was called to the Johns Hopkins, and I hope and believe that you will have no more cause to regret your decision than I have had in all these years. It gave me my great opportunity, and I trust that it will you."

As we have seen, the full-time movement was not limited to Baltimore, but was being actively discussed in advanced medical schools all over the country. Encouraged by the success of the Hopkins in obtaining distinguished and scientific-minded professors, the General Education Board announced, in the newspaper release telling of the completion of the full-time faculty there, that "a grant of $750,000 has been made to Washington University, St. Louis, and of $500,000 to the Medical School of Yale University, upon an understanding that they also reorganize their work so as to put their clinical teaching upon a full-time basis."

Six months after full-time went into effect at the Hopkins, the three main participators wrote out their impressions. Halsted said that "a keen and wholesome rivalry has been aroused," that "the range of my clinical experience seems not to have been affected," and that he had found much more time to devote to his research. Howland felt that full-time had increased his clinical opportunities, since "it allows more time to devote to the observation of patients." With this statement Janeway agreed, adding that the students were receiving better training, and "the development of research in the wards has gone ahead with great rapidity."

In 1917, however, Janeway resigned with the intention of returning to private practice in New York, partly, as he said, because of his financial obligations to his family, and partly because he was no longer altogether in sympathy with the full-time scheme. Although he agreed that clinical teachers should give most of their energies to teaching and scientific work, he felt that "no inconsiderable part of my own knowledge of medicine upon which I now draw in my teaching has been derived from . . . outside engagements." Furthermore, it was "unnatural and repugnant to the patient's sense of justice" that a consultant "should not receive the usual fee for such service." His basic belief was that if the right men were selected for clinical chairs, the question of outside practice would take care of itself. "To me the spirit is everything, the letter nothing."

Before his resignation became effective, Janeway died, his health having broken during the early months of America's entry into the war under the strain of working both at the Hopkins and at the Surgeon General's office in Washington.

Opinions on full-time were changing both ways. Thayer, who had refused the professorship of medicine when Janeway accepted it, now accepted it after Janeway's death. And, even more encouraging to Welch, in 1919 Osler yielded to the new order. He wrote Welch asking him to use his influence to persuade the General Education Board to "help McGill start up-to-date clinics in medicine and surgery." Exactly what Osler had in mind is shown by a circular letter which he sent to prominent physicians in Montreal: "The situation is this—McGill simply cannot afford to fall behind other first-class schools in the development of modern clinics in Medicine and Surgery, and Obstetrics and Gynæcology. New conditions have arisen." And he added that each professor should be "a whole-time man, or if thought wiser, largely so." Although the General Education Board could do nothing, since its charter limited it to making grants in the United States, in 1924 the Rockefeller Foundation gave $500,000 to McGill for the establishment of a university clinic, the director to be the professor of medicine on a whole-time basis.

Despite occasional set-backs, the reform was making headway. At the Hopkins the department of obstetrics was placed on a full-time basis in 1919, that of psychiatry in 1923, and that of ophthalmology in 1925. In the meantime, the leaven was working elsewhere; several more leading schools in this country, aided by the General Education Board and the Rockefeller Foundation, placed major clinical chairs on full-time.

During 1940, the *Journal of the American Medical Association* stated: "In the United States today our medical schools vary from some which have a majority of full-time teachers in the clinical branches to one of our leading medical schools which still has none." Although disagreement on its advisability has by no means died, the experiment at the Hopkins has been influential in raising the standards of clinical teaching and research all over the country, even in those schools which have not embraced the exact plan put into effect in Baltimore. As Welch said, "Doubtless when the traditions have been established men of the character fitted for these high positions could be trusted to conform to the spirit of the understanding that they will be expected to give their whole time to their university and hospital work without rigid stipulations."

The reform was also taking place abroad. Abraham Flexner writes: "In 1915, quite independently of the American development, the British Medical Research Council established a full-time clinical chair for Thomas Lewis, now Sir Thomas Lewis, at the University Hospital, London. Since that date, full-time units, living side-by-side with part-time units, have been established at other British schools." The English movement reached its climax in 1936 with Lord Nuffield's gift of £2,000,000 to Oxford University for whole-time departments in medicine, surgery, and gynæcology.[17]

Strong support for full-time has continued in America. As this book was being prepared for the printer, during April 1941, the Rockefeller Foundation set aside $168,000, with the understanding that a similar sum will probably be appropriated in 1943, to establish fellowships in internal medicine. To be administered by the National Research Council, this gift will enable mature clinicians, men from thirty to forty years of age, to pursue the paths of science, so that when the present incumbents of full-time chairs retire, there will certainly be available to succeed them brilliant clinicians who have devoted themselves primarily to the advancement of knowledge. Remembering the contributions to full-time of "one of the Foundation's wisest advisers," that body has resolved that the gift shall be called the Welch Fellowships in Medicine.[18]

CHAPTER XV

Tragedies and Triumphs

I

THE spring of 1910, four years before full-time became an actuality, was in many ways an epitome of the life Welch now led. One aspect was the growing isolation of an ageing man. His stepmother had died in 1901; his brother-in-law in 1905; and his sister, who had been an invalid for many years, now followed them. "The death," Welch wrote, "was as nearly instantaneous as any that I ever heard of, and must, I think, have been due to plugging of a coronary artery of the heart. She was unusually well and cheerful that morning, her son, Fred, have [having?] arrived from New York to visit her about two hours before. Such a mode of death is fortunate except in the shock to the friends. My sister, as you know, was very near and dear to me, and she had practically so far recovered from the severe illness of two years ago as to enjoy life."

Indeed, of all the people Welch ever knew, his sister was his closest friend. To her he wrote his most intimate and revealing letters, to her he confided his pleasure in success. "It sounds horribly conceited to be telling these things," he added after writing of some honours he had received, "but I suppose I should not mention them except to my sister. They are subjects which should not be talked about outside of the family. Every family has some skeleton." Always he was eager to have her present at his moments of triumph; when she was too ill to attend one of the many testimonial dinners he was given,[1] Welch wrote Frederic Walcott: "Lights of the social world, men and women, have attended, and I have often thought how much your mother would have enjoyed it all, and how much pride, even if too generous, she would have had in seeing me in the seats of the mighty." His letters to the companion he had now lost contained his rare bursts of emotion, as when he spoke of "re-reading a package of your cherished letters, as I do from time to time to refresh my soul."

Honour followed quickly on the heels of tragedy. The year of his sister's death he was president of the American Medical Association, the largest and most representative body of physicians in the land. "I was not desirous of the presidency," he wrote, "but there was no ready escape without giving offense." Using his position as an excuse, a group of his friends commissioned Victor D. Brenner to make a medallion portrait of him, a gold replica of which was presented to Welch at a dinner in honour of his sixtieth birthday.[2] On paper surrounded with a black mourning band, Welch wrote his niece: "Your letters are a great comfort. You really must not believe that I am such a great man as that newspaper article represented. I do not know where the reporter got all that information. . . . They are preparing a testimonial banquet for me for next Saturday, but I am kept in profound ignorance of all the arrangements and do not know who are coming. . . . I consented with the understanding that it would be a small affair with a few friends, but I am beginning to be embarrassed, not to say frightened, by what I see in the papers. . . .

"I thank you very much for that last letter from your mother. I am glad to have it. I have thought much about you these last weeks. It seems most fitting that you should live in the old house, and I am glad that you and Fred are to do so. . . . I shall be interested some time in looking over that box of scraps and memorabilia [of Welch's own life] which your mother kept so lovingly and faithfully."

The testimonial dinner broke into Welch's mourning for his sister; since her death he had made no social engagements. It was a majestic affair, attended by five hundred of the most distinguished physicians and laymen in the nation. The tables were adorned with spring flowers, an "enlarged orchestra" played in the corridor, and the Hotel Belvedere provided its richest foods and rarest wines. Welch was led into the dining room between two long lines of his friends, who cheered and applauded. Thayer, the toastmaster, read letters and telegrams from all over the world, from Koch, Ehrlich, Osler, Calmette, Gibson, Marchiafava, Bignami, Bastianelli, Wright, Salomonsen, Madsen, Billings, Janeway, Hektoen, and others. Then Weir Mitchell read a poem he had written especially for the occasion, and Abraham Jacobi, Major General Wood, Councilman, Samuel Alexander, J. A. Witherspoon, and Henry Barton Jacobs vied with one another in praising Welch.

When Welch finally rose to his feet, he gave the credit for his achievements to his teachers and colleagues, who sat around him: Delafield, "to whom I owe my first introduction to and first interest in pathology"; Jacobi, "I rejoice indeed that my old master has honored me by coming here"; and Dennis, " my dear friend," who seemed to have forgotten their old conflict. Welch's other associates and acquaintances were there by the score. But his sister was not there, and his closest remaining companion, Major Venable, looked old, drawn, and ill. Time was passing; he himself was sixty; did the honours of age satisfy the bright ambitions of youth?

As in this moment of triumph he surveyed in his mind's eye the young man he had once been, he remembered the eagerness that had burned within him to do research in a laboratory isolated from the world in which now he so brightly shone. "I cannot but regret," some of those present must have been amazed to hear him say, "a certain amount of dissipation of energy which comes from undertaking so many things. I do think my experience ought to be a warning to younger men. I have been more or less driven into it—resisting sometimes—yet at the same time pleasures and privileges have been placed upon me. But I do think younger men should guard against undertaking so many different things as I have undertaken." Perhaps the faces of those before him showed that he had struck an unexpected note; in any case he turned quickly to humour. "It reminds me of the story of the little boy who was found crying. A kind gentleman asked him what he was crying about and he said: 'Nothing happens at our house unless I get blamed for it, and I never do nothin' neither.' I feel as though that was in some sort my fate."

Then he spoke of the bright side of his career. "Now, ladies and gentlemen, there have been in these thirty-five years great advances in American medicine. . . . Many have been concerned in this development. I have had only a share with many others, but it has been an immense gratification to see such progress in the opportunities for the cultivation of medical science. I believe that the recognition that has been won for American medicine on the other side of the water has been one of the most important developments of the last half century."

When Welch had finished speaking, everyone rose and sang "Auld Lang Syne." The toastmaster said: "The hour is late or rather early; the patient has been on the table for nearly three hours, and although his condition seems excellent . . . we must reluctantly send him to his bed, and bid him a loving goodnight."

Welch wrote his niece: "Your presence with that of the two Freds at the celebration on Saturday really more than doubled my pleasure. What is the use of such a demonstration if you cannot share it with those you love?"

By the middle of April, Major Venable had been rushed to a hospital, seriously ill. Welch left him there when he went to St. Louis for the convention of the American Medical Association over which he was to preside. He had hoped that his sister would help him with the social duties of his office; after her death he had tried in vain to secure his niece. As all by himself he received the plaudits of his profession, he must have felt lonely. When it was all over he wrote: "While it would have been pleasant to have Bessie at my side at the reception, I am glad that I did not insist, for I had not a moment of leisure, and she would not have cared for that kind of a reception. . . . I was exhausted, and my side-partner, Mrs. Mudd, nearly succumbed at over two hours of continuous handshaking and calling out the names to the next in line. I managed to get through my address successfully and should not have minded the presence of my relatives on that occasion.

"I am leaving to-morrow for the Princeton Commencement where they contemplate decorating me with another LL.D. I already have six which ought to satisfy the most voracious appetite for such empty honors."

Late in June he attended a wedding at which he saw his childhood sweetheart, Alice Eldridge, now an old lady "who is suffering from a severe attack of neuritis." That this contrast with the past did not depress him is shown by his gay letter to his niece. "The church was beautifully decorated—largely with laurel from Norfolk. All the aunts and other relatives were present, and the bride was beaming with joy, to all appearances genuine. Dr. Moffat was as unobtrusive as is becoming to a bridegroom. He made a good impression. . . . Mr. Swift, the father, is rather overcome, but Mrs. Swift seems cheerful. The wedding breakfast was gay, and indeed the wedding seems to be a great success."

On his return to Baltimore, Welch learned that Major Venable's condition had become serious. "I am with him a good deal of the time. It seems hardly possible that he can recover, but he is holding on remarkably." The *Baltimore Sun* tells us that on the morning of July 10 Welch was awakened by a request to come immediately to his friend's house. He found him in a coma, the pulse scarcely detectable. "There was no struggle and, seemingly, no pain, and but for the fitful breathing, the Major might have been asleep. Only the last gasping breath or two told that death had come. . . .

"Dr. Welch was at the house the greater part of the day. Major Venable and the Doctor were almost inseparable companions, and the death of the former has proved one of the greatest shocks in the lifetime of the eminent physician. Indeed," the paper continues, repeating a story that would be very agreeable to Baltimore, "the last words uttered by the Major were ones of esteem and appreciation of the friend who had assisted him so valiantly in his hopeless battle for life. While the attendants at his bedside Friday, in answer to a motion from the Major, bent down to catch his trembling words, he said to them, 'I want to express my great admiration for Dr. Welch.' This commendation from such a source touched Dr. Welch deeply, and when the incident was told him he plainly showed his grief."

As the years passed, Welch's circle continued to shrink. In 1917 Mall died, in 1919 Osler, and in 1922 Halsted. His letters mentioning the passing of these friends were almost entirely given over to the medical details of their illnesses; he was unable to express deeply felt emotion.

Walter C. Burket had been editing Halsted's surgical papers, and Halsted, before his death, had collected autobiographical material for Welch to use in preparing the introduction. Although he had agreed to attempt this task, Welch could no more characterize his departed friend on paper than he had been able to write a memoir of his own father many years before. In 1923 and again in 1924 he took the material abroad with him, carrying the special suitcase everywhere, "as it is too frail to check," yet he failed to write a word. By 1926 the Halsted volumes, printed but unbound, had been lying on the shelves of the Lord Baltimore Press for nearly a year, waiting for Welch's introduction and running up a financial loss that the university had to assume. Both Burket and President Goodnow begged Welch either to finish the sketch or to turn it over to someone else, but received no answer.

In 1927 the handbag again crossed the ocean with Welch. He wrote his friends from Italy and Sicily that he was working on Halsted's biography as well as on that of Dr. Biggs: [3] "it is a slave's existence to have to put in my time in this way"; actually, he had left the material in Paris and his diaries indicate that he never put pen to paper. When in May 1928 he received a letter congratulating the "Johns Hopkins and all concerned" on the fine volumes of Halsted's surgical papers, he noted: "First I have heard of the appearance of these." The volumes carried in place of Welch's introduction a memorial address on Halsted delivered by Dr. Rudolph Matas of New Orleans.

Welch's relief was shortlived, for MacCallum now asked him to write the introduction to his life of Halsted; again Welch docilely agreed and again he procrastinated. During the summer of 1930, when he was in California, he received urgent letters and telegrams from MacCallum, which he answered with his usual promises. Toward the end of the summer, MacCallum spoke of publishing the book without an introduction, and Welch firmly announced in his diary that he intended to seclude himself in his hotel room until he had written it. He really did absent himself from the Huntington Library for ten days, but he spent all but the last two on sightseeing trips, social engagements, and motion pictures. On the ninth day he finally sat down at his desk, only to find that he had forgotten to bring the necessary material with him from Baltimore; he did, however, write several pages extolling Halsted's great contribution in general terms: "Halsted combined, in a degree rarely matched, the interests of the practical surgeon with those of the experimental biologist in his fundamental studies of the processes of wound-healing and of the handling of wounds, as well as of surgical injuries and diseases in general." One sentence gives the key to his eight years of delay; he said that when he tried to write a biographical sketch for the collection of Halsted's papers, he "became aware that our relations had been so intimate that . . . an adequate portrayal of Halsted's life and work required a more detached point of view than it was possible for me to occupy."

Among the younger men who surrounded Welch after most of his contemporaries had died, he was most friendly with Alfred Jenkins Shriver, a prominent lawyer who wrote books on the law and who, like Venable, enjoyed a practical joke and remained a bachelor. Welch was president of the University Club; Shriver was vice-president; and the two men spent many evenings there together. Like Welch, Shriver was a careful host who made a hobby of giving perfect dinners, and they were both active in the affairs of the Johns Hopkins. Shriver, however, never became as close to Welch as Venable had been.

Welch's most intimate letters were now written to his niece, Mrs. Kellogg, and to Frederic Walcott, his nephew; the letters, however, were not so frequent or so revealing as the letters he had written to their mother. Mrs. Kellogg shared with him a taste for serious books, and much of their correspondence deals with the exchange of volumes that took place at Christmas. Every year he gave her a list of works he would like to receive from which she could choose his gift, and often his gifts to her were munificent; in 1911 he sent her the entire *Dictionary of National Biography*. He liked to visit his family in the holidays and was irritated when, as often happened, he was prevented from doing so. "I have got entangled in these various scientific societies which meet at this season, but it is simply impossible for me to give myself to them every year at this season, and I am determined to escape." On another occasion he wrote: "I hope that I shall not have another interrupted Christmas. There are no more societies left for me to preside over, so far as I can foresee." But there were always more societies. When he was able to get away, he was very pleased. "I am looking forward with the greatest delight to seeing you all at Christmas at Englewood [Frederic Walcott's home]. It will be a joyful occasion to be all together again, and I am so glad that the Kellogg family is migrating to Englewood."

Welch enjoyed playing jokes on his relatives. Thus he revealed at the Kellogg dinner table the most amazing erudition on the most out-of-the-way subjects, and he was delighted when it was discovered that he had been reading them up in the *Encyclopædia Britannica* directly before each meal. The game continued despite this exposure, the point now being to catch Popsy as he subtly led the conversation to the topic which he had prepared.

He possessed an airplane pilot's licence, he told the Kelloggs with such wealth of detail that his relations, although they knew he had never learned to drive a car, believed his story. He had been taught to fly in Atlantic City by one of the Wright brothers during the first years of aviation; he made a successful solo flight, although when he finally brought the seaplane down it was one of the "wettest landings" in history. Since that was before the days of federal licences, the Wright brothers themselves gave him a certificate showing he was a pilot. Welch also repeated versions of this story to his friends, writing Dr. T. S. Cullen, for instance, that Selskar M. Gunn "is the one who arranged for my lessons in aviation and is responsible for my pilot's license to run an air-plane."

When Welch's matter-of-fact biographers questioned Gunn,

they were told that Gunn introduced Welch to Earle L. Ovington, who had some seaplanes in Atlantic City and took passengers up for a fee; Welch flew with him several times. Gunn was
sure that Welch had never taken a flying lesson or obtained a
licence. And alas for so fine a legend, among Popsy's papers the
following document came to light: "No. 1695. Certificate of
Flight. This is to certify that Wm. H. Welch of Baltimore flew
in Atlantic City in a Curtiss Aeroplane piloted by Earle L.
Ovington, licensed aviator. Date August 25, 1919."

Welch gave his grandnieces and nephews Christmas presents
every year, but he usually asked Mrs. Kellogg to buy the gifts
for him, since, as he admitted, it was difficult for him to conceive
what a child would like; his natural tendency was to give them
serious books suitable for adults. As he wrote one of his name-
sakes, then aged five: "I am afraid that you will have to grow
up to those books which I sent you, and perhaps by that time
you will rather read them in the original Latin and Greek."
Presents suitable to the very young seemed to him trivial, and
he resented their being quickly outgrown. "As to the children,"
he wrote Mrs. Kellogg, "if you think phonograph records the
best, I shall be content, but I really want to give them something to remember me by. I intend to grow up with them."

His grandnieces remember that whenever he was present at
Christmas he dressed up as Santa Claus, a part for which nature
seems to have designed him. He succeeded in fooling the smaller
children so completely that they were furious with Uncle William for being still asleep when they tiptoed downstairs to catch
the rotund, jolly sprite in the very act of filling their stock-
ings. Except for his role in this traditional masquerade, Welch
never took part in their games. Sometimes, his grandnieces recall, he accompanied them on walks, and they imagine that they
must have chattered to him as children will, but they do not
remember that he ever made any effort to answer in kind or
discuss their childish concerns.

Once he took Mrs. Kellogg's three children for a stroll through
the barnyard. Finding some newly laid eggs, he gathered them
in his derby hat, and then he lifted little Stuart up to a corn-

crib; the boy stepped into a hornets' nest. Hastening to snatch Stuart down, the great pathologist clapped the derby hat on his head, and his grandnieces saw a yellow flood, which they were certain was bees' blood, spread over their uncle's features. This scene comes back to them even today not as amusing, but tinged with horror.

Welch was greatly concerned with the physical health of his young relations, refusing their kisses while he lectured their parents on the hygienic dangers of allowing children to be kissed. Whenever there was illness in the house, he was consulted; he listened gravely to all the symptoms and asked questions, but he never prescribed himself; he referred the sufferer to a specialist in the field where he thought the malady lay.

Such medical consultations were his greatest contribution to the well-being of the young; he seemed unable to enter far enough into their affairs to understand their personalities. It is remarkable then that the children looked forward to his visits with great eagerness, and would sit quietly by the hour listening to him talk about adult concerns. His grandnieces cannot explain this fact. Undoubtedly they learned from their parents that he was a great man whose presence was an honour, but this in itself does not inspire love. Furthermore, he never interfered with their pleasures, for their highest crescendos of noise never bothered him and, although he failed to take part in their games, he never objected to their playing around him. If a toy train collided with his foot, he would lift the foot imperturbably and go on with his talk. The real explanation of their affection must have lain in the same intangible quality that enabled him to convince hundreds of adults that he was their close friend, while he never encouraged familiarity.

His grandnieces remember that Welch's interest in their characters increased the closer they came to adulthood. Among his letters is one that showed great sympathy with a boy of fifteen. When his namesake, William Welch Flexner, was forced by ill health to go to a school in Arizona he dreaded, Popsy sent him cards of introduction to Western celebrities. "I know," he wrote, "that you must regret leaving the Lincoln School, but I am sure that you will find there are compensations in what is before you, and I consider that you will get a very important kind of education by living in the Southwest and that you will always look back upon this experience as a delightful one. Perhaps you will be a bit homesick at first; this is natural, but you are to see your father about Christmas and with will and determination you will settle down to a very interesting life. I fear that I never thanked you for sending me a copy of your play 'Cooks is Cooks.' I thought it very clever and amusing, and have allowed several persons to read it. One tells me that it would make a hit on the stage, to be sure she said vaudeville stage. I wonder what family experience you have had to elicit such a funny plot. I cannot help thinking your father is the overconscientious householder. With all best wishes for your year in Arizona and much love . . ."

Probably the young person he saw most of was Frederica, the pretty daughter of his landlady, Mrs. W. Edward Heimendahl. When she returned from parties late at night the door of Welch's study would sometimes open, and he would ask her in. Sitting in his swivel chair with his back to the desk, he would listen to the young girl chatter about gay young things, but suddenly, in the middle of a story sometimes, he would turn his chair back to the papers that awaited him. Then Frederica would know the visit was over; she tiptoed out into the hall and closed the door noiselessly behind her.

Welch's correspondence with this young lady at the time of her marriage to Henry May Gittings in 1924 shows that their friendship never outgrew a formal note. "Thank you," he wrote the recent bride, "for remembering me with that charming letter, so full of happiness as to rejoice my heart. I am delighted that all is going so well and the future is so full of promise. Both you and Henry have taken over a large responsibility, each for the other, and I am counting on neither falling down on it. I am sorry that I cannot drop in on you or accept your invitation before I sail."

After a matter-of-fact description of what he intends to do in Europe, Welch adds: "I am greatly envied to have been the sole guest outside of your families at the wedding. Someone asked me at the Club what we three old bachelors—George Cator, [Henry M.] Warfield and I—are going to do now that Henry Gittings has appropriated you! . . . Love and goodbye to you and Henry."

There is no evidence that Welch was ever really lonely; he had long taught himself to live without intimates and get his human satisfaction from a horde of acquaintances who admired him. When he wanted to meet some of these, he had merely to go to the medical school, or to his club, or for that matter out on the streets of Baltimore. His lodgings supplied him the type of home that suited his temperament: a place where he could be entirely free and where his every need was looked after. His succession of landladies adored him. "I am so glad that Dr. Welch is safely home," one wrote. "I always *feel* so *safe* when he is in the house. Do you think there is any great man in this world quite so good and kind as he is? I don't."

CHAPTER XVI

The Health of the Nation

I

WELCH had played a major part in revolutionizing American medicine, but there were still some ideas of his young manhood which had not been carried to fruition. He had, for instance, written Gilman from Germany in 1884: "I have been particularly impressed with the hygienic institute which is the pride of the Medical School in Munich. I hope that we may have a similar institute in Baltimore, and if possible in connection with the institute someone who has been trained in the Pettenkofer school of hygiene. Pettenkofer and his institute have accomplished wonders in improving sanitary conditions of Munich which from one of the most unhealthy has become one of the most healthful cities in Germany. Hardly another department would attract in greater degree the favor of the general public than such a hygienic institute as that of Munich to which are referred such problems as those pertaining to ventilation, heating, sewage, school-lunches, etc. Important discoveries pertaining to the causation of epidemic diseases have also been made here."

Thus in his early days Welch testified to his interest in hygiene. Called also sanitary science, public health, and preventive medicine, this subject involves the application of a group of sciences, not all primarily medical, toward the common end of alleviating sickness through the wise organization of community life.

The first teacher of hygiene at the Hopkins was Billings, who began in 1883 to commute from Washington to deliver courses of lectures; he was in Garrison's words "a philosophical hygienist," who expounded accepted principles. Eager to organize instruction on a basis more in accord with modern laboratory science, in 1886 Welch sent Abbott to study the subject with both von Pettenkofer and Koch, and, after his return in 1889, organized a miniature hygienic laboratory copied after the Munich institute.* It lasted for only two years, however; before the department was well started Abbott was called to the new hygienic laboratory established under Billings's direction at the University of Pennsylvania.[1]

Forced to begin all over again, Welch used special lectures by Billings as a stop-gap, and persuaded Nuttall, then assistant in bacteriology, to return to Germany in 1893 for the study of hygiene. Welch hoped that this brilliant young man, who had already done important work on the power of normal blood serum to kill bacteria, would provide the link uniting bacteriology, hygiene, and pathology into a comprehensive subject dealing with the causes, the effects, and the means of preventing epidemic diseases. Nuttall's subsequent career showed that Welch had chosen the right man, but there was one contingency on which he had not counted; becoming engaged to be married in Germany, Nuttall required a larger salary than the Hopkins was able to offer him. To a letter admitting that he could not, under the circumstances, urge Nuttall to return, Welch added with perfect good humour: "Councilman is in the seventh heaven. He has recently become engaged to Miss Coolidge of Boston, whom he represents as the flower of her sex, and he is evidently over head and ears in love. You and he should get together." [2]

Welch, thus frustrated in his plans for a department of hygiene, invited Abbott year after year to give a series of weekly lectures. Following somewhat in the tradition of von Pettenkofer's laboratory, Abbott spoke of vital statistics and the part they play in public sanitation, especially as used at that time in

---

* A few months before, in January 1889, the first special laboratory in America devoted to teaching and research in hygiene had been opened at the University of Michigan. Described in the university catalogue as containing "all of the improved apparatus employed by Koch," it offered a three months' course in bacteriology apart from the regular medical curriculum and available only to students who wished to do original work under the director, Victor C. Vaughan, professor of both hygiene and physiological chemistry. A year later laboratory courses in hygiene for the second and third years of the medical course were instituted.

England; he dealt with habitations, water supply, sewage disposal, influence of occupation, ventilation, etc. These occasional lectures were continued until 1907, when W. W. Ford took over the subject in the medical school, lecturing and later offering laboratory instruction to a small number of students.

In the meantime Welch was propagandizing all over the nation for the study of hygiene. Again and again he pointed out in addresses delivered at many places that bacteriology was destined to be very valuable "in the prevention of disease, especially of epidemic diseases." Arguing that public health workers should be trained to take advantage of the new knowledge, he deplored that in America "opportunities are not afforded for the study of hygiene in a manner at all commensurate with its modern development and importance." He did not despair, but foresaw that, "with increased facilities for higher medical education, hygienic laboratories will be established which shall meet the demands of the times."

In 1892 the role of modern hygiene was brought dramatically to the attention of the American people; a severe epidemic of cholera broke out in Hamburg and seven ships brought almost a hundred cases to New York. The foremost bacteriologists of the country sprang into action; Biggs, Prudden, and Welch conferred; and the first municipal bacteriological laboratory in this country was hastily fitted up by the New York City Board of Health. Dr. Edward K. Dunham, working under Biggs's direction, obtained cultures of cholera bacilli which were confirmed by Prudden, Welch, and Ernst, as well as by the Imperial Board of Health in Berlin. The disease was arrested in the port of New York.[3]

Welch, of course, did not miss this opportunity to point out the importance of the bacteriological control method. In a popular article entitled "Asiatic Cholera in Relation to Sanitary Reforms" he argued for permanent public health laboratories. "The same measures which are needed to protect a city against occasional epidemics of cholera are needed at all times to protect it against other infectious diseases, such as typhoid fever, which are spread in a similar manner, and which, although they do not come with the terrible impetuosity of cholera, steadily do their deadly work, and in the course of time destroy among us far more lives than cholera."

The lesson thus brought home by Welch and others was so quickly learned by the American people that in 1899 Welch was able to say: "The development of laboratories connected with boards of health is one which is peculiarly American." Their greatest usefulness, he continued, had been their assistance to physicians in making diagnoses of such diseases as tuberculosis, typhoid fever, malaria, and diphtheria; the work they had done in furthering the treatment of diphtheria by antitoxin had been particularly valuable.[4] Welch went on to argue that university laboratories of hygiene served a function equal in importance to that of the state-operated laboratories, since they were needed to train scientific hygienic workers and to make new discoveries for the state laboratories to apply. He regretted that "one could count upon the fingers of one hand the laboratories connected with medical colleges and universities in this country which are appropriately called hygienic laboratories."

With other members of the Hopkins group, Welch had taken advantage of the cholera scare to propagandize for specific public health reforms in Maryland. There was much to be done. Although two generations of citizens' committees and public health officials had urged cleansing the soil and providing a safe water supply for Baltimore, sewage contamination in Lake Roland, the source of drinking water for a large part of the city, was known to exist, and in other public health matters Baltimore was equally backward. Welch believed that "under our existing political conditions, experience seems to show that more can be accomplished by the quiet, intelligent and well-directed efforts of individuals and of such organizations as societies for city improvement, which do not directly antagonize those who wield political power, and which receive the approval of the general public, than by spasmodic political movements for reform."

Welch welcomed the opportunity of doing what he could, but he was unable to resist complaining to his stepmother: "I have become without any effort of my own involved in work relating to public sanitary matters in the city here, and I rather begrudge the time given to this. . . . The public is stirred up and perhaps some good will be accomplished, but the political conditions are adverse to much reform. . . . The anticipation of cholera next summer is the main thing in arousing public interest."

Delivering public addresses before Maryland audiences, Welch shrewdly followed other public health propagandizers in arguing that "merely from a mercenary and commercial point of view it is for the interest of the community to take care of the health of the poor. Philanthropy assumes a totally different aspect in the eyes of the world when it is able to demonstrate that it pays to keep the people healthy. . . . It is estimated, and of course such an estimate can be only a rough one, that nearly 100,000 deaths occur annually in this country from preventable causes. For each death there are of course several cases of illness not fatal, due to preventable causes. One can form from such a statement some idea of the enormous loss in money and productive labor which we suffer from preventable causes of illness and death."

It is of present-day interest that Welch went with careful detail into the matter of housing as a sanitary problem. He also argued for a public disinfection station, and the hospital for infectious diseases that as a result of continuous agitation was finally opened in 1909.[5]

In urging an improved sewerage system, Welch fastened attention on typhoid fever as the index of existing sanitary conditions. Starting with the examples of Munich and Vienna, where by the gradual elimination of soil pollution the death rate from typhoid fever had fallen from 24.2 per 10,000 inhabitants to 1.4 and even 1 during the decade of the eighties, he turned to Danzig, Stockholm, Breslau, Frankfurt, Berlin, Brussels, London, New York, Boston, and Brooklyn, to show the progressive lowering of the death rate from that disease to a quarter, a sixth, an eighth, a twelfth, and even a twentieth of the former rate through the introduction of a sewerage system and of pure drinking water. The same results, he said, could be achieved by Baltimore and other cities.[6]

Harry S. Sherwood, of the *Baltimore Sun*, tells us that Welch played an important part in changing the city "from a cesspool of outhouses and wells in the back yard of every dwelling to a modern sanitary city. Interviews which he gave to the public press of Baltimore furnished the first impulse toward the construction of the excellent plant for the filtration of the city water supply. He was the chief influence in that community in making an end of the ancient order of milkmen who sixteen or twenty years ago drove their wagons up to the front door, thrust a long-handled dipper into a milk-can, and sloppily poured milk into the upheld pitcher. . . . This old institution was replaced by the modern bottle of Pasteurized milk. . . . Doctor Welch and his associates have introduced a system of guarding the public schools against contagious disease. The politicians of Baltimore have been taught that the Health Department must not be interfered with by them."

Welch's influence extended beyond the city of Baltimore. Appointed to the Maryland State Board of Health in 1898, he was elected its president two years later, an office from which typically he at once tried to escape. "My main use on the Board is to prevent interference with Fulton [the secretary] and to keep politics out," he wrote after serving one year. "If I am convinced that my presence is not needed for either of these purposes, I shall prefer to let someone take the place who can give more attention to it than I can." Yet he remained president until the office was abolished in 1922, and he did not resign from the board until 1929.

Ford tells us that during this period of thirty-one years, "not a single important project was carried out which he had not considered carefully and hardly a single one which he had not approved. . . . His particular contribution may be said to have been his broad outlook for the health needs of the State, his intuition as to which should and could be met first, his grasp of the ways and means of initiating and carrying out new projects. Finally, his strong personality, his popularity, his ability to inspire confidence, and the clarity and ease with which he could present his views to the various Governors and the members of the Maryland Legislature were practically always guarantees that any undertaking to which he gave support would be carried out successfully."

According to Sherwood, during Welch's presidency of the Maryland Board of Health, "the old politically minded county health officers who gave a part (and a small part) of their time to such duties, and who made no pretense of being scientific, have been replaced by men who have real zeal for science and who give their whole time to their work. A corps of sanitary engineers, supervising the construction of sewerage systems in the rural districts and doing other sanitary work, has been created. In rural Maryland the farmer whose house is not equipped with a bathroom and a sanitary toilet is ashamed of that fact. In Maryland people no longer go to the country for their summer vacations and return in the fall to die of typhoid fever with which they were infected while seeking health close to nature. What has been done in Maryland is typical of what has been done by men trained by Doctor Welch, or by others who taught what he brought to America as the new bacteriology, throughout the country."

In addition, Welch took an important part in the passage of a pure food and drug bill, and in the organization of bureaux of child hygiene and tuberculosis prevention. When in 1909 work was begun on a new home-rule charter for Baltimore, he was placed on the commission. "It is responsible and important work," he wrote his sister, "and as I have the subjects of health, charities, corrections, playgrounds, baths, and schools assigned to the Committee of which I am chairman, I am kept pretty busy."

As the value of preventive medicine became increasingly clear to American minds, more and more national organizations sprang up to promote different aspects of an intelligent public health program. Usually Welch was importuned to serve on the boards of such bodies, and he usually accepted. His contributions to these groups varied greatly: to some he merely lent the prestige of his name; in others he played a determining role as strategist and adviser. An annotated list of the organizations to which he belonged will be found in Appendix B; we shall content ourselves here with discussing two of the most important.

During 1904 Welch helped organize the National Association for the Study and Prevention of Tuberculosis (now the National Tuberculosis Association), and in 1911 he was its president. He was an active propagandist for the better control of "the disease of the people" which was responsible for one-third of the deaths suffered during the prime of life. Adequate sanitariums, though important, were not enough, he argued; the disease could be prevented by giving all the people fresh air, proper and sufficient food, and opportunities for exercise and play. To achieve these ends, he advocated the building of well-ventilated and sanitary homes and workshops, the establishment of shorter working hours and a living wage.

Welch would not admit that his programme was visionary; he said in 1908: "At least one-half of the existing sickness and mortality from tuberculosis could be prevented within the next two decades by the application of rational and entirely practicable measures." And the passing years proved this wild-sounding statement not wild at all; in 1933, after twenty-five years, the mortality from tuberculosis had dropped 62.5 per cent.

Welch's contribution to this great advance was evaluated as follows by Livingston Farrand, the first executive secretary of the national association: "Those who were concerned in the first organization of the great fight against tuberculosis remember very clearly the counsel and the encouragement that Dr. Welch gave and the wise lines of action which he laid out and indicated, lines which have been followed throughout this country and throughout the world."

In 1908 Clifford Beers's extraordinary autobiography, *A Mind That Found Itself*, which told the story of his experiences during a period of temporary insanity, shocked the American people with its picture of the inadequacy and the stupidity of the treatment of even well-to-do mental cases. Instantly a clamour for action arose; within eleven months of the book's publication, we find Welch attending the meeting at which the National

Committee for Mental Hygiene was formed. From the first a member of the board of directors, he was successively vice-president (1909–23), president (1923), and honorary president (1924–34). On the organization of the American Foundation for Mental Hygiene in 1928, he was again made honorary president.

Beers tells us: "He attended many of the meetings and was kept informed of details of the work through talks with Dr. Salmon [the medical director] and me and other officers of the National Committee. Few important questions of policies and plans were ever adopted without prior consultation with Dr. Welch. He gave many hours of his time to the consideration of our plans and policies and actively intervened on many occasions in important negotiations that led to the securing of financial support for our National Committee."

Welch regarded the mental hygiene movement as "one of the great movements of all time," and was eager to help create a sound, scientific basis for the care of the mentally sick.[7] Two months after Beers's book was published, he received a letter from Henry Phipps saying: "When I had the pleasure of lunching with you in Baltimore you dropped a remark that set me to thinking in regard to the treatment of the insane in cottages as is practised in Holland and Belgium." Phipps offered to pay the expenses of two doctors selected by Welch for a trip to those countries "to make a full report, and [determine] the approximate cost of carrying out the idea in Baltimore on a small scale of say twenty-five to fifty patients. We could then decide whether it would be advisable to go on with the project or not. . . . It seems to me a very good work, and under the management of the Johns Hopkins its success would be assured." Welch's reply must have contained a tactful disclaimer of his intention of obtaining any money from Phipps, since that gentleman wrote four days later: "I know that your remark was just a chance one, and not made with any intent to encourage me to aid in the care of the insane, but I am very much pleased at the prospect of doing so."

Taking Barker with him, Welch called on Phipps and persuaded the philanthropist not to wait to send investigators abroad. In June 1908, less than a month after his first letter,

Phipps sent Welch a formal offer of gift, "nearly identical with the terms of the letter you kindly prepared for me yesterday." He promised the Johns Hopkins Hospital "the funds necessary for the erection and equipment of a psychiatric hospital on its grounds . . . to provide for about sixty patients, and to contain the necessary laboratory and other facilities"; he promised the university "additional funds for the establishment of a professorship of psychiatry, and the assistantships thereto, the professor to be also the director of the psychiatric hospital." Welch secured Adolf Meyer, who had helped Beers with his epoch-making book, as the first director of the Henry Phipps Psychiatric Clinic.[8]

Welch's activities in the hygiene movement as a whole sometimes went far afield; his influence, for instance, was important in the successful building of the Panama Canal. Yellow fever and malaria had defeated previous efforts, and they seemed likely to defeat those of President Theodore Roosevelt, since the sanitary aspect of the problem was neglected by the engineers, who thought that the eradication of mosquitoes was nonsense; it was obvious, said the engineers, that mosquitoes could have nothing to do with fatal disease. Welch intervened, and in February 1904 received a letter from Roosevelt: "I sincerely wish that more people of your standing would write me in reference to possible candidates exactly such letters as you have written. I enclose you a copy of the letter which I have sent Admiral Walker in regard to it."

The President's letter to Walker read: "I enclose you a letter from Dr. Welch. It gives exactly what he thinks of Dr. Wright, and I wish to Heaven we could get from other people, whose opinions we desire, such exact and straightforward information as this letter contains. As you know, I feel that the sanitary and hygienic problems in connection with the work on the Isthmus are those which are literally of the first importance. . . . I wish the Commission to get the very best medical man in the country to have the headship and supervision over this work, and I desire the Commission to consult Dr. Welch, Dr. Osler, Dr. Polk of New York and others of their standing in securing this man."

Welch headed a delegation to Roosevelt that secured the appointment of William C. Gorgas, who had already eliminated yellow fever from Cuba, as Chief Sanitary Officer to the Commission to Panama. Gorgas had his troubles with incredulous and obstructive superiors, but in the end he eradicated yellow fever on the Isthmus, enabling the canal to be built.[9]

II

The public health movement was advancing on many fronts. A most important development took place in the fall of 1908 at a conference in connexion with the work of President Theodore Roosevelt's Commission on Country Life, the purpose of which was to report on the economic, social, and sanitary condition of American farms. Since at that time the General Education Board was supporting agricultural improvements in the South, its secretary, Wallace Buttrick, attended the conference, and there he was introduced to Charles Wardell Stiles, a zoologist and public health official who was profoundly concerned with the hookworm problem.[10] During most of a long night, the two men sat up together while Stiles explained the devastating effect hookworm had on life in the coastal plain east of the Mississippi. Entering the body through the bare feet and legs, the worm travels to the small intestine, where it clings with a little hook and lays such a multitude of eggs that as many as 4500 worms have been expelled from one person. The parasites feed on blood corpuscles, producing anæmia, and further disturb the nutrition of the victim by interfering with proper absorption through the intestinal wall. Communities afflicted with this scourge sink into a collective torpor that makes any cultural, social, or economic improvement almost impossible.

On his return to New York, Buttrick told the hookworm story to Gates, and after Gates himself had conferred with Stiles, he is reported to have said: "This is the biggest proposition ever put up to the Rockefeller office." For a year Rockefeller representatives investigated the disease, verifying its extent and the fact that it could be cured and prevented. Then on October 26, 1909, Rockefeller, junior, called a meeting at his office attended by Welch, Gates, Murphy, Stiles, E. A. Alderman, H. B. Frissell, David F. Houston, Walter H. Page, and myself. Rockefeller gave the group a letter stating that he hoped the conference might "lead to the adoption of well-considered plans for a cooperative movement of the Schools, the Press, and other agencies, for the cure and prevention of this disease [hookworm]. If you deem it wise to undertake this commission I shall be glad to be permitted to work with you to that end and you may call upon me from time to time for such sums as may be needed during the next five years for carrying on an aggressive campaign up to a total of one million dollars."

The Rockefeller Sanitary Commission was thereupon organized, and in 1910 Wickliffe Rose, who as agent of the Peabody Fund and trustee of the John F. Slater Fund was already concerned with the furtherance of education in the South, was chosen administrative secretary. Thus began his amazing career for the betterment of health and the upbuilding of science, a career which was to assume world-wide dimensions.[11]

Concerning the Sanitary Commission Welch was to write: "Both the purpose of the gift and the opportunity thereby created were unique in the annals of preventive medicine. . . . This was the first entrance of private philanthropy into the field of public health—a field now recognized as one of the most rewarding for such support in benefits to mankind."

When in October 1914 the five-year term of the Rockefeller Sanitary Commission came to an end, public health administrative methods in a number of Southern states had been greatly improved; the fight on hookworm had reduced not only its incidence, but also that of other diseases spread through soil contamination, notably typhoid fever and dysentery. The work, too important to be discarded, was carried on by the Rockefeller Foundation under the leadership of the International Health Commission, whose name was later changed to the International Health Board and finally to the International Health Division of the Rockefeller Foundation. Rose was appointed director general.[12]

By 1916 hookworm was being fought in eight Southern states

with the co-operation of the federal government, and in fifteen foreign countries of the tropical and subtropical belt, the native habitat of the disease. Moreover, the work had been extended to include experiments in malaria control, and two yellow fever commissions led by General Gorgas had been sent to South America "to ascertain what measures were necessary and feasible to eradicate the disease from the localities responsible for its dissemination."

A major problem which had confronted the Sanitary Commission and which continued to confront its successors was the lack of competent, trained personnel. So much of the success of their campaigns depended upon the nature of the field staff itself that training stations for recruits were found necessary. Such stations were established on the islands of Trinidad and Ceylon, and later transferred, for greater efficiency, to North Carolina. But as the projects undertaken by the board multiplied, these provisional arrangements proved inadequate.[13]

In December 1913, shortly after the General Education Board had made its grant to the Hopkins for full-time, the Rockefeller Foundation asked its sister board to inquire into the best way to increase the number and the competence of practical health officers. Inquiries were addressed to those universities which included some form of hygiene in their medical curricula, and a year and a half later a committee of the General Education Board undertook visits of inspection. No institution in America was found to possess adequate facilities for teaching public health.[14]

These preliminary studies led to an important conference, presided over by Gates, on October 16, 1914. In the light of future developments the remarks of Biggs, Welch, and Rose are of special interest. Having just taken part in the formulation of the modern public health law enacted by New York State in 1913, and having become State Commissioner of Health early in 1914, Biggs saw the problem in the light of his own difficult task. He reminded the conference that at that time there were 1200 health officers in New York State and for them he thought elementary courses, even correspondence courses, the greatest present need. The current rewards of public health, he added, were so small that only an elementary course was practicable. For a higher type of work a one- or two-year course would be requisite, while the outlet for men so trained was very limited.

Welch took a broader view. "It is very clear in my mind," he said, ". . . that the great need in improving the health conditions of this country is to provide the great lack in our medical schools, the striking deficiency, the absence of a department of hygiene at least equal to those in foreign universities. I should regard as necessary for a center for the training of health officers the establishment of a first-rate department of hygiene, and all that that embraces. . . . I should emphasize the training in the science of sanitation. The rest is application, and everybody knows the risk of starting men too soon in technical training without a good knowledge of general principles. The rest requires specialized training, which takes care of itself and is easily supplied. The department of hygiene should include chemistry, bacteriology, physical science—Pettenkofer's conception brought up to modern times."

Welch argued against establishing a school of hygiene as an independent institution, since connexion with a university would make available useful facilities, such as a department of engineering. As usual, he advocated high standards, insisting that an M.D. degree should be a requirement, although "men who are not physicians at all and who have excellent qualifications . . . should have an opening into the career." Trained hygienists, he was sure, would have no difficulty obtaining positions commensurate with their abilities. "The present demand exceeds the supply, and with an increase in supply, the demand would increase."

Rose then outlined a plan by which a central institute of hygiene would be established in connexion with a university, but having a separate building, endowment, and nucleus of full-time professors. Embracing the essential subjects mentioned by Welch, it should combine opportunities for research and teaching, using the state and city health organizations for field work. But this school would be only the beginning; smaller, local schools should be created in geographic centres all over the nation, "the central institute becoming the great directive force which influences all the smaller units, the teachers for the smaller units coming from the central institute. The influence of the central institution will thus permeate the whole land. . . . Such an institution I would conceive to produce a larger effect than anything else on the public health service of the United States."

The impression made by Rose's proposal on all present was profound. Biggs approved it as covering all he had in mind, and more. And Welch was "deeply stirred." The main thing, he said, was the central institute, which would not only train health officers, but would "react on the medical school [of the university where it was placed] and contribute much to the training of physicians going into general practice." [15]

Welch and Rose were appointed a committee to prepare a report on the subject, and on October 27 Rose wrote Abraham Flexner that Welch "is going to get together some literature on the experience of Germany and England in public health training. He will then prepare a statement of this course of study. After he has prepared his statement we shall then call into conference a number of the other men who were present at our conference in New York."

This was an excellent plan, but somehow it did not seem to get done. Before leaving for the war zone as a member of a commission on relief for non-combatants, Rose wrote Welch that he expected the report would be prepared and acted on before he returned. Home again early in 1915, he learned that nothing had been accomplished, and hurried to Baltimore, where he found Welch full of ideas as usual, but with nothing on paper. Docilely Welch promised to write the report immediately, and even went so far as to consult Ford. A month later, Rose pushed Welch with a tactfully urgent note. Welch replied that he would be "tied up" until May 3, but after that "I shall put every minute of time I can spare into our report. . . . Of course I am more interested in this matter than in anything else."

Persuasion was still needed; Rose wrote Welch again on May 12: "Mr. [Abraham] Flexner has just been in to ask me about our report on the school of hygiene. The meeting of the General

Education Board is set for May 27th. He is again expressing keen desire for this report, at least in tentative form, to be presented at this meeting. . . . He suggested that I ascertain about what time we might expect you so that we may make our plans accordingly."

Then at last Welch completed the report, which was presented to the General Education Board on May 27, 1915, and to the Rockefeller Foundation on January 12, 1916. He argued that the greatest need was for the central institute of hygiene Rose had suggested, housed in its own building, staffed by full-time men, and offering opportunities for scientific training. "It would be a misfortune if this broader conception of the fundamental agency required for the advancement of hygienic knowledge and hygienic educàtion should be obscured through efforts directed solely toward meeting in the readiest way existing emergencies in public health service."

Information which he considered disturbing began to reach President Eliot of Harvard, inspiring him to write Abraham Flexner on February 1, 1916: "The more I consider the project of placing the proposed Institute of Hygiene at Baltimore, the less suitable and expedient I find it. . . . In comparison with either Boston or New York, it [Baltimore] conspicuously lacks public spirit and beneficent community action. The personality and career of Dr. Welch are the sole argument for putting the Institute in Baltimore—and he is almost sixty-six years old, and will have no similar successor. . . . My life-long interest in the great problems of public health and sanitation will account in your mind for this frank statement."

Abraham Flexner replied that the argument for locating the school in Baltimore was based not on Welch alone, but also on the medical school, and he ventured to prophesy that the medical school would endure even after Welch's days were over. However, Eliot was not appeased; he wrote that the Hopkins school was "one man's work in a new and small university made comparatively independent of community action by large bequests from one benefactor."

Undaunted, the Rockefeller Foundation appointed on April

11, 1916, a committee to proceed with the plans for a school of hygiene at the Hopkins. The committee reported: "The first essential to the successful inauguration of the proposed Institute would be the selection of a man of sufficient breadth of vision, interest in the project, and national prestige to assume the leadership in the undertaking. If Baltimore should be decided upon as the location, these qualities would be best embodied in Dr. William H. Welch. . . . If Dr. Welch should accept an offer of this kind, it would be necessary for him to retire from all other labors and responsibilities, to devote himself exclusively to the organization and inauguration of the Institute." The committee implied that he was not eager to do this, but could be persuaded.

Thereupon the foundation appropriated $267,000 to found "a school or institute of hygiene and public health" in Baltimore. This momentous action came thirty-two years after Welch had written President Gilman from Munich about the value of such a project. In the long interval Welch had not given up hope or relaxed effort to bring into existence a teaching and research body of the kind he envisaged. And if, in the end, success came from an unpredicted direction, it was after all implicit in the things he had done and was doing to advance scientific medicine.

Some anxiety was felt lest the Baltimore school harm already existing courses in hygiene which now would be so greatly overshadowed, as is shown by a letter Welch wrote Abbott on June 18: "I do not think the establishment of the School of Hygiene at Johns Hopkins will have any except a beneficial effect upon other efforts in the same line. It should stimulate the development of the subject and open wider the opportunities for careers in public health work throughout the country. In fact I think that the influence which the Johns Hopkins has been able to exert in improving conditions of medical education in general was one of the considerations in locating the school here, in the hope that we may be able to do something like this for hygiene. . . . Of course I appreciate your work for developing hygiene in Philadelphia, and I wish to get the benefit of your advice about the plans here."

At an age when many other men laid their affairs aside to warm themselves quietly in the thin sunlight of life's winter, Welch, as he told his Yale classmates in 1920, "retired from my chair of Pathology in the J.H.U. to assume a new kind of work, and one which is to me extremely interesting and somewhat novel. . . . Laboratories and institutes of hygiene have existed as parts of medical schools, but the conception here is an independent faculty, an independent school, a part of a university existing side by side with the other faculties of the university, particularly the medical faculty, closer linked with it than a hospital, but still a conception based upon the view that the time has come for specialized training for those who desire to enter into that field of work, perhaps as health officials connected with state and municipal boards of health. The great opportunity in industry, so-called industrial medicine, industrial hygiene, and this whole field in preventive as distinct from curative medicine, rests now upon such a body of scientific knowledge that the feeling is that the time has come to recognize it as a profession somewhat apart. . . . We shall have opportunities there leading to degrees of Doctor of Public Health, Doctor of Science in Hygiene, certificates in public health, and eventually opportunities for training women nurses who desire to take up public nursing, social service and all that sort of thing."

III

Welch resigned his professorship of pathology in 1917, although he kept his connexion with the medical school as a member of the faculty advisory board. President Ames writes: "It was always amusing to see Dr. Welch come in late, as he generally did, to the meetings of the Medical Advisory Board, and walk down to the end of the table and wait patiently behind the chair of the man sitting at the corner until he got up and gave him this seat."

On October 1, 1918, the School of Hygiene and Public Health opened. The faculty, which Welch selected with Howell, the assistant director, as with Gilman he had gathered the staff of the medical school, was like that first group chiefly made up of ardent young men fired with enthusiasm for the new horizons they saw before them. And the School of Hygiene started with seventeen students as the medical school had done. Old patterns were repeating themselves in the life of the sixty-eight-year-old man who was once more embarking on the adventures of youth.

In 1896 Welch had been called on to edit the first scientific medical magazine in the country; now, in 1921, the *American Journal of Hygiene* was launched, again under his editorship. But there were differences here as well as parallels; where the *Journal of Experimental Medicine* had dangerously lacked funds, the newer periodical, appearing in an environment which had become convinced of the importance of science, was amply supported by the De Lamar bequest. The details of editing the earlier magazine had of necessity fallen on Welch, who was personally struggling to raise scientific standards; now his importance to the journal was as a leader of the many fellow-workers who had grown up around him. Welch gave to the new undertaking the prestige of his great position, while the actual labour of editing fell on the managing editor, Dr. Charles E. Simon. Furthermore, the *American Journal of Hygiene* was international in scope; workers from other nations were publishing in America, as once Americans had been forced to publish abroad.[16]

Welch, as he set out in new directions, enjoyed reviewing his past. To celebrate his seventieth birthday, his pupils determined to publish, under the editorship of Dr. Walter C. Burket, a collection of Welch's writings. In this project the old gentleman enthusiastically took part, going over, as Halsted writes, "each paper—I might say each leaf. . . . He not only rejected none of those approved by us, but even expressed the desire to have included a considerable number which we had discarded or marked doubtful." The resulting three volumes, entitled *Papers and Addresses by William Henry Welch*, contained all together 1963 pages; they were a startling indication of the industry of the scientist for whom writing was only one of many occupations.[17]

During a short time the School of Hygiene was supported by annual gifts from the Rockefeller Foundation, but in 1922 that body endowed it with $6,000,000. Three years later a separate building, richly provided with every facility for teaching and research, was opened beside the medical school. Things moved faster now than they had when Welch was a young man, but the vision which was now so solidly substantiated in brick was the old vision which Welch had experienced long before when he visited von Pettenkofer's institute. Some changes, of course, had been brought about by the steady advance of scientific medicine in the intervening time. To the main props of the Munich institute, physiology and epidemiology, the Baltimore school added bacteriology and immunology. Medical zoology and protozoology were also included for the part they played in the study of the parasitic origin of disease, and the chemistry in Baltimore was based not only on the classical principles of that science, but on the newer, exciting knowledge developing in relation to accessory food factors, or vitamins, as they afterward came to be called. A further innovation was the setting up of separate divisions for vital statistics and virus diseases.

The School of Hygiene had a double purpose: it prepared students in the scientific as well as the practical aspects of public health administration, and it instructed active public health officers in the foundations of their calling. The one may be compared to the medical school's purpose of training practitioners while producing teachers and investigators on the side; the other to the courses offered during the early days to graduate students who wished to extend the training they had received before higher opportunities for professional education had become available in America. Indeed, it is remarkable how closely the plans of the School of Medicine and the School of Hygiene paralleled each other. This parallel was to continue for many years and bring about like results in both cases, for the practice of public health, like the practice of medicine, was lifted to a more scientific plane, and in both fields there was a harvest of new knowledge.[18]

As director of the new school, Welch determined its policies in collaboration with Howell and took part in the handling of administrative details. There was no occasion for him to conduct laboratory courses or directly promote research, as he had done in the early days of the Pathological, since the organization of the new school was on a far ampler basis than had been possible when the university had been struggling under heavy financial burdens. The several departments were adequately staffed and organized to give systematic courses in a competent manner. Since the head of each division was a trained investigator, research went on independently of the director's special care, strong as his indirect influence may have been. Welch was therefore free to follow his own inclinations in the lectures which he proposed to deliver. The time had gone by when he might be expected to give a series of rounded, encyclopædic talks on varied topics in the newer pathology, bacteriology, and immunology related to hygiene as he had done with such distinction in the 1880's and 1890's; too much of his energy was being absorbed by his extramural duties as the recognized leader of American medicine.

We can follow, if imperfectly, the lecture courses on "selected topics in hygiene" which he gave at four-thirty on Wednesday afternoons.[19] He did not repeat the same talks from year to year; indeed, we gather that he never used a set of notes twice over. This may have been due to his lack of system in filing away papers, but it is more probable that he wished on each occasion to follow his interests and inclinations of the moment; he drew more on his accumulated learning and experience than on any pedagogic formula.

Welch found so much intellectual pleasure in studying the history of medicine, including hygiene and sanitation, that this interest constantly obtruded itself. Furthermore, he could be sure he was not treading on the ground of other teachers when he dealt with the importance of the historical method, as he did in the opening lectures of the academic year 1920–21. His purpose was to outline the bearing of philosophy and of political and social developments on health and disease. As Garrison says, "winding his way into the subject," he took examples from antiquity, asking, for instance, to what extent the ancient aqueducts, sewers, etc., are to be regarded as determined by sanitary considerations in Babylonia, Egypt, Greece, Rome. He examined also the Hebrew sanitary code and religious sanctions. Discussing the influence of views concerning the origin and nature of disease on medical practice, he came to the beginnings of rational medicine with Hippocrates, the Alexandrian school, Galen, the notions of miasm; [20] he commented on the small part which the idea of contagion played in ancient times. In the modern era, he moved from the first clumsy efforts to isolate and cultivate pathogenic bacteria, up to the astounding developments of our own day.

Some of Welch's preserved work sheets contain thumbnail sketches of early sanitarians from, say, Stephen Hales (1677–1761) to Sir Edwin Chadwick (1800–1890), or of statisticians from John Graunt (1620–1674) to William Farr (1807–1883). The influence of the Industrial Revolution is emphasized in discussions of Adam Smith (1723–1790), James Hargreaves (d. 1778), and such inventions as the spinning jenny.

Probably Welch told his students, as he told the National Conference of Charities in 1915: "It is a well-known fact that there are no social, no industrial, no economic problems which are not related to problems of health. The better conditions of living, housing, working conditions in factories, pure food, a better supply of drinking water, all these great questions, social, industrial and economic, are bound up with the problems of public health. The humanitarian movement has been one of the great agencies in promoting the better health movement. . . . Anyone who is informed as to the influences which were operative in the last century, from 1830 to 1850, which initiated the modern public health movement and culminated in the passage of the public health act in 1848 in England, knows that it was less a movement on the part of the medical profession than it was on the part of philanthropists. . . . But, after all, that impulse [benevolence] alone would not have been sufficient. It is of vital importance that health activities should be based upon accurate knowledge of the cause and of the spread of disease."

Able to leave daily, systematic teaching to his younger associates, Welch was looking at life and learning from another altitude, less directly instructive in the daily affairs of the laboratory, but no less important for an understanding of the broad principle of medical education and practice. Indeed, the wide view which Welch was now trying to give his pupils had in Welch's own case enabled him to see early in his medical experience the great future of pathology, and again ten years later the future importance of hygiene for America.

According to F. F. Russell,[21] the founding of the Hopkins School of Hygiene "marked the turning point in public health education not only in this country but throughout the world. As every one knows the early efforts of von Pettenkofer were for a time overshadowed by the advent of the bacteriologists and education in public health became, as a result of this, the education of the health officer in the control of infectious diseases, to the almost complete exclusion of all other aspects of public health. In Britain and on the continent and here at the University of Pennsylvania under Abbott, and at the Massachusetts Institute of Technology under Sedgwick the main subject was bacteriology. Dr. Welch appreciated the one-sidedness of public health education and went back to von Pettenkofer and introduced into the new Hopkins curriculum all the disciplines which had any bearing on hygiene, statistics, nutrition, administration, parasitology and physiology, and he provided a faculty that was competent in all these fields, in contrast with the institutions of hygiene of Germany and Great Britain where the education in public health was under the charge of the professor of bacteriology of the medical school. Of the new departments that dealing with vital statistics was perhaps the most important, and Pearl developed this field in such a way that it has influenced all the departments."

As a result of Welch's efforts, Russell continued, "the entire personnel of our public health services is now being built up with men who have graduated from the new schools, and the day of the self-educated health officer has already passed. While it is too early to say that the new schools have eliminated politics from public health, it is fair to say that political appointments are now the exception rather than the rule. The papers presented at public health officers' meetings have radically changed; formerly the best dealt with methods of administration, at present more and more papers deal with the scientific basis on which administrative practices can be made more effective. Gradually a better class of men is being attracted to careers in public health. . . . This change in the whole question of public health is, I believe, due to Dr. Welch, and he foresaw the entire development when he planned the Hopkins, which in turn influenced other schools."

After the organization of the Hopkins school, Welch did not cease propagandizing on a national and international scale for the scientific teaching of hygiene; in a sense he returned to the role he had played in the last two decades of the nineteenth century as exponent of higher medical education.[22] Partly because of his arguments and the example of the school he led, institutes of hygiene that attacked the subject from a broad, university point of view were established in many places. Although Rose's dream of founding regional schools throughout the United States was never realized, the Rockefeller Foundation assisted Harvard to expand its department. Furthermore, the foundation helped to build schools of hygiene all over the world, bringing Welch's influence to bear in such diverse places as São Paulo and Bahia, Brazil; Trinidad; Prague; London; Toronto; Warsaw; Zagreb; Copenhagen; Oslo; Budapest; Belgrade; Tokyo; Angora; Sofia; Rome; Bourgas, Bulgaria; and Cluj, Rumania. Welch, as we shall see, took an active part in planning many of these institutions, and in most instances their directors were sent to Baltimore to study at the Hopkins school.

But before these things could take place, before international public health standards could be raised, the world conflict which America entered had to be won. Welch, the conciliator, the master of peaceful change, soon found himself clad in the khaki uniform of war.

CHAPTER XVII

War and the Building of Peace

I

"WE have arrived in the midst of a great war excitement," Welch wrote from Munich on July 27, 1914. "The German masses are apparently eager for war with Russia. The streets, restaurants and cafés are crowded with people; the bands play only national airs, and the air everywhere echoes with the modest shouts of 'Deutschland über Alles.' It is all quite thrilling, but a general European war is too horrible to contemplate, and it seems impossible that it will occur. The German emperor probably has the decision in his hands, and although a great 'war-lord' he has hitherto stood for peace.

"We were in a café last night filled with a shouting multitude, and soon after we left, the interior and the windows were completely demolished because the proprietor forbade the band to continue playing the martial airs, after several had been thrust into the streets for not showing enough enthusiasm. We had sense enough to get on the chairs and shout 'Deutschland over everything.' "

Thus the holiday planned by Welch for rest and another cure at Carlsbad plunged him into drama. On August 12 he wrote his nephew: "The war developments proceeded with such incredible rapidity that we found ourselves trapped in Switzerland without immediate prospect of escape." Letters of credit were almost useless, and a complete lack of information about trains or boats made it impossible to find out whether London or Italy offered the best chances of escape to America. "There are said to be 100,000 Americans over here eager to get home—some 10,000 in Switzerland and as many more in Italy. Some are destitute, and their situation is pitiable. Passage is engaged on all boats from Italy to their full capacity, and I do not see much chance of our leaving for home very soon. . . .

"What a horror and disgrace to civilization this general European war is! Probably you are getting more news and more important comments than we do here, notwithstanding our proximity to the Franco-German border. There are rumors of a battle to-day not far from Basel, but I place no credence in such rumors.

"I am in excellent health, and there is no occasion for any apprehension about us. This is an excellent hotel. . . . I am not worrying—indeed I am enjoying my vacation."

After a trip through France which he found both trying and exciting, Welch managed to sail from Folkestone on the *Rotterdam*, arriving in New York on September 7. Winternitz tells us: "That he was an incurable optimist became evident when he returned in 1914; we were all depressed over the war, and he took the attitude that much good would come out of the conflict."

As president of the National Academy of Sciences, Welch was soon urged to action by George E. Hale, the astronomer, who telegraphed him on July 13, 1915, that the academy "is under strong obligations to offer services to President [of the United States] in event of war with Mexico or Germany." Hale regarded America's neutrality as a disgrace. Welch, however, put Hale off by stating that, although he could "imagine no objection to the Academy offering its services to the President in the event of war," he considered war improbable "while Wilson is president."

Nine months later, on April 19, 1916, Welch presided at a meeting of the National Academy which by a unanimous vote resolved that "the President of the Academy be requested to inform the President of the United States that, in the event of a break in diplomatic relations with any other country, the Academy desires to place itself at the disposal of the Government for any service within its scope." Explaining this action in a letter to President Wilson, Welch wrote: "As you know, the National Academy of Sciences is designated in its act of incorporation by Congress as the adviser of the Government on questions of science. . . . The Academy now considers it to be its plain duty, in case of war or of preparation for war, to volunteer its assistance and to secure the enlistment of its members for such service as it can render." [1]

Hale tells us: "A committee, headed by Dr. Welch, was appointed to call on the President, who doubtless received us because of his respect for our Chairman. After some discussion President Wilson asked us to proceed with our plans of organization, but on no account to make his request public." The academy thereupon formed the National Research Council to prepare for war by promoting relevant research and securing cooperation among investigators in all fields. The thirty to forty members of the new body were not to be confined to members of the academy, but were to be "fully representative of the great national societies and all phases of research, both scientific and industrial."

Appointed chairman, Hale was obliged to proceed warily until July 1916, when President Wilson made the matter public, and wrote Welch: "The Departments of the Government are ready to co-operate in every way that may be required, and . . . the heads of the Departments most immediately concerned are now, at my request, actively engaged in considering the best methods of co-operation. Representatives of Government Bureaus will be appointed as members of the Research Council as the Council desires." [2]

Jubilantly Hale sailed for Europe to consult Allied scientists who were studying problems raised by the war. Since Welch had already projected a trip in connexion with the newly endowed School of Hygiene, the two friends embarked together on August 5, 1916. Their reactions to the crossing were very different. Hale was outraged that their American steamer "was kindly 'permitted' by the Germans to pass unmolested. I shall never forget my chagrin at the ignominious necessity of accepting such a passport at a time when we should have been assisting the Allies in resisting German domination. It was far more satisfactory to sail homeward on a French liner, showing no lights and zigzagging its way through the danger zones." Welch's letters and diaries contain no such passages; he spent most of his waking hours, as Hale remembered, sitting placidly in his deck chair with "a vast pile of detective stories beside him"; he was "always cheerful and full of jokes."

Welch's principal mission was to discuss his plans for the organization of the School of Hygiene with the leaders of the English public health movement, and to secure the advice of the English physiologists, whom he considered the best in the world, about a successor to Howell as professor of physiology at the medical school. To these objects he added, now that the National Research Council was really under way, the study of military hospitals and of medical problems created by war. Each of his days was crowded with interviews and visits of inspection which might easily have tired a much younger man, yet he found time for two delightful visits to Osler at Oxford. The old cronies renewed their intimacy, going on excursions together and fervently discussing rare medical books. There is no hint of tragedy in Welch's notation: "Revere Osler is a very fine fellow—about 20, in artillery, soon to go to front. Has taste for architecture—draws, etches—also love of books—good collection of Isaac Walton's Lives—a devotee of angling." *

Welch's comments on the war activity were those of an unimpassioned observer. "Hale and I," he noted in his diary, "walked back through Leicester Square and Piccadilly to hotel—stood for a while in Piccadilly Circus watching the searchlights in great numbers streaming over sky from all directions. Darkened London at night with the searchlights (which play only for a short time) is wonderful, mysterious, unforgettable sight."

He spent thirteen days in France, conferring with French doctors and scientists. Twice he approached the front; first to inspect Alexis Carrel's hospital at Compiègne, and later to visit Sir Almroth Wright's hospital at Boulogne. "We were talking in the laboratory about 4:30 p.m.," he noted while in the Channel port. "A transport with troops came in—a large boat loaded with

---

* A year later Welch wrote Hale: "I suppose you have seen that Osler's only child, Revere, was killed at the front last August. It is a terrible blow for them, but Osler writes bravely."

troops, who completely covered the decks, which seemed a mere mass of human beings. They were singing and cheering and all was gay enough with the poor fellows on their way to the trenches, many to be 'cannon-fodder.' It is a bright, balmy day, and they had evidently had a good crossing." After his return to England, he wrote Hale, who had accompanied him: "What a wonderfully interesting time we have had."

Back in America after six weeks abroad, Welch soon found himself in his usual role of mediator. The officers of the National Research Council told him of a newly arisen danger that President Wilson's Council of National Defence would set up a scientific committee of its own under one of its members who, as Welch agreed, was inadequate to the position; the result would have been a jurisdictional tangle that could only have led to inefficiency. While he resisted frenzied appeals from members of the Research Council that he make an issue of the matter before President Wilson, Welch worked quietly behind the scenes with sympathetic members of the Defence body. Careful never to allow the issue to be raised in a conspicuous form, he manœuvred the Defence body into officially resolving that the mobilization of America's scientific resources be entrusted to the Research Council. Then, to the horror of some of his more hotheaded supporters, he insisted that the offending member of the Defence body be appointed to the Research Council. "We have won out and must secure harmony."

Welch had never lost his good humour, though many others had. In the middle of the passionate disagreement he wrote Hale: "Thanks for the return of the collar. My faith in human nature is restored. Although I have suffered great inconvenience by the absence of that collar, I am consoled by the thought that it must have been of the greatest service to you during these many months."

Once the National Research Council was firmly established, Welch, who had refused to consider succeeding Hale as chairman, ceased to take an active part in its business. He gave all his attention to new problems.

II

"I knew General Gorgas, the Surgeon General, intimately," Welch told his Yale classmates at their fiftieth reunion. "He had been a pupil of mine when I first started out in New York running that very demoralizing thing called a cram quiz. . . . I knew him well enough to go over there right after the war started and tell him to put me to work, if he thought he had anything I could do. From that time until the end of the war . . . I was actively at work there in the Surgeon General's office."

On July 16, 1917, Welch was appointed a major in the Medical Section, Officers' Reserve Corps. "I do not like the idea at all of being commissioned a medical officer in the army," he wrote. "If I have to put on a major's uniform, I think that I shall drop out." Later he was to tell his niece: "I have been a kind of privileged person all of the time, and they have let me infringe regulations about a number of things. For months I did not even get into a uniform, which I realize now was the most irregular thing imaginable, and I wonder they winked at it."

Welch served as liaison man between America's medical laboratory men and the army. Assisting in the mobilization of the profession, he worked to place scientifically trained doctors in positions of influence, a task requiring great tact, as he soon discovered. On October 25, 1917, he wrote: "I am going to urge upon the Surgeon General the desirability of appointing a consulting staff for the office of the commanding medical officer in France. There are many excellent men over there like Cannon, Cushing, Finney, Boggs, etc., whose services could be commanded. A difficulty, as Strong says, is getting regular army officers to avail themselves of the services of skilled men from civil life. The same difficulty exists here, but with General Gorgas it can be overcome. Over there there seems to have been no effort to meet this rather natural reluctance of the regular army men."

An example of the type of difficulty Welch faced was the case of C. G. Bull, who had developed an antitoxin for Welch's gas bacillus, which was being very destructive on the western front. Eager that this promising discovery be tested and widely used if found efficacious, Welch wanted Bull sent to France at the head of a special commission; experience had shown that when scientists were placed under the command of the chief surgeon of the A.E.F., they were not allowed to carry out their work, which the regular army doctors considered visionary and impractical. Although, as Welch wrote me, "General Pershing has been much annoyed by the number of men who have been sent over on various special missions and . . . has cabled over not to send any more 'experts' over," Welch expected little difficulty about Bull, because he would have the support of General Gorgas. Five days of negotiation, however, forced him to resort to subterfuge. Securing the Rockefeller Institute's agreement to pay all expenses, he persuaded the British ambassador to persuade the British Surgeon General to ask that Bull's commission be sent abroad. When the request arrived, Welch argued blandly that it would be discourteous to refuse the desires of our distinguished ally. Bull's commission sailed triumphantly, and reported first to England, where they were formally requested by the British to carry on their work in France.

Another aspect of the Bull matter contained even wider implications; in June 1917 Welch wrote: "Gorgas is entirely opposed on general principles to withholding the publication of Bull's discoveries, but he wished me to lay the matter before the Secretary of War, so we both saw Secretary Baker. The Secretary took at once the humane view and said that we should not consider for a moment holding back such a life-saving discovery on the ground that the enemy could also make use of it. I was very glad that both the Secretary and the Surgeon General without any hesitation took this position, for on thinking over the matter I had reached the same conclusion."

At my suggestion, Welch secured Gorgas's agreement to making the Rockefeller Institute a training unit. "Unless some such arrangement is effected," he wrote me, "and those on your staff who are commissioned are definitely assigned to duty with the laboratory unit, I fear that it may be difficult to hold them permanently with you. . . . It is, I think, a novel idea, but I do not see why it could not be made a very practical one and would give you and your staff a regular status in active service where you could do just the things which you are best fitted for."

Intent on improving the conditions under which trained nurses worked in military hospitals, Welch argued for a bill giving them official rank such as army doctors had. "I have always sided with the nurses in almost everything they wanted," he wrote, "and they have got most everything in spite of the opposition of the majority of the medical profession." [3]

Welch was assisted in agitating for such reforms by his membership in the executive committee of the medical advisory board of the Council of National Defence. The historian of that body remembers: "Dr. Victor C. Vaughan, of Ann Arbor, and Dr. William H. Welch, of Baltimore, we dubbed the 'Gold Dust Twins.' . . . They were inseparable companions, and always appeared together at our meetings, sauntering down the long corridor, nodding friendly greetings to all the staff, their rotund bodies radiating cheer and good nature." Although Welch attended many meetings of the council and was appointed to several committees, he could not give much time to this activity; his role was primarily that of adviser and critic.

Often Welch's administrative duties were interrupted by problems of practical hygiene; epidemics, not only of meningitis and pneumonia, but also of measles and mumps, became a serious problem in the training camps where recruits from many regions were brought together. It was as if the men had pooled their diseases, each picking up the ones he had not had, and the process of transfer was greatly assisted by faulty laying out of camps, poor administration, and lack of adequate laboratory facilities.

In July 1917 Welch began visiting stricken training camps. "It was no compliment for a camp for me to appear there, because it indicated that there was trouble, that there was an undue amount of sickness there." Six months later, on January 12, 1918, he wrote that "none of the hospitals are even yet complete, and most are lacking in running warm water, sewerage and other necessities. It was a great mistake to send troops to the camps before the hospitals were ready, and a mistake to leave the hospitals to the last. . . . At Camp Jackson meningitis overshadows everything else, although there is a good deal of pneumonia—155 cases in all. They have had 1950 cases of measles, but the epidemic of this is subsiding. They are at the height of a mumps epidemic—about 600 cases during the last months."

On another occasion, he recorded: "While there are serious deficiencies, some indeed very serious, I do not feel like criticizing after seeing the magnitude of the undertaking assumed by the government and realizing how much has been accomplished in so short a time. Of course the fundamental criticism is that preparations should have been started long before anything was done. The medical and sanitary problem of the camps is the control of communicable diseases, especially those of the respiratory tract and conveyed by contact. . . . There is overcrowding and only quite recently have there been sufficient warm clothing and blankets. Some of the camps, especially Funston and Doniphan, are at times subjected to frightful storms of dust or sand. Funston is badly located, but most of the camps are well situated. Measles, pneumonia and meningitis are the chief diseases to contend with."

All during the war Welch's trips of inspection continued; sometimes they involved great exertion for a man approaching seventy. "We had a hard journey of 30 hours from San Antonio to Deming [New Mexico], arriving at 2:30 in the morning," he wrote. "We were extremely lucky to secure one bed [over the railroad tracks] which Col. Ashburn and I shared in common with a third man in the room and fortunately in another bed." Since the railroads were disorganized, they often missed their connexions. "This is only the third night since we left Washington that I am sleeping in a bed instead of a sleeping car, and it is an agreeable relief to get a bath. The journey of twenty-four hours from El Paso to Fort Worth through western Texas took us through the most arid, dusty country I have ever seen. . . . Ashburn seems to have contracted the prevailing camp bronchitis, but I am in good shape and not fatigued." Always Welch found comfort in boasting that he withstood hardships better than his younger companions did.

Four notebooks filled with records of his visits to the training camps show that in trying to trace the causes of disease he studied every detail of the environs and the personnel for clues. He examined the living sick and supervised autopsies on the dead; he interviewed the commandant and the other line officers; he questioned the doctors to get information on the sick, and also on the competence of the doctors themselves; he examined the tents, the laundries, the sewerage system, the kitchens, and the recreation rooms; he weighed blankets in his hand and scrutinized clothing; he shuffled his feet in the soil to see if there was likelihood of sandstorms to increase respiratory ailments; he looked into dance halls to see if there were women who might spread disease, and pondered the ventilation of the motion-picture theatres. The infirmary, of course, was especially examined; he even peered about the shelves to see what medical texts they contained, and he studied the laboratories with care. Finally he wrote a report to the Surgeon General recommending every kind of improvement.

"I have been kept on the go at a pretty lively pace; up at six o'clock every morning and a pretty strenuous day going around the camps, but I am standing it all right. I think that I am of some help, especially in improving the laboratory side, which sadly needs it in every respect—men, space and equipment. There is a great lack of competent bacteriologists and Russell will be glad to know of any who are available. Another urgent need is a supply of mice."

Not only did he have to work all day, but at night he had to take part in entertainments. Colonel F. F. Russell, who sometimes accompanied him, tells us: "The men in the base hospitals were of course delighted to have the visits, and usually staged a dinner for us in the evening, at which we all had to speak, and Cole and I soon learned that Dr. Welch in his address, which usually came first, would use a sort of synopsis of all that any of us had said the evening before, so that we were never able to make the same speech twice, but had to get up something entirely new for each evening. Although these evenings had a social setting, they were terribly earnest times, and had a very good

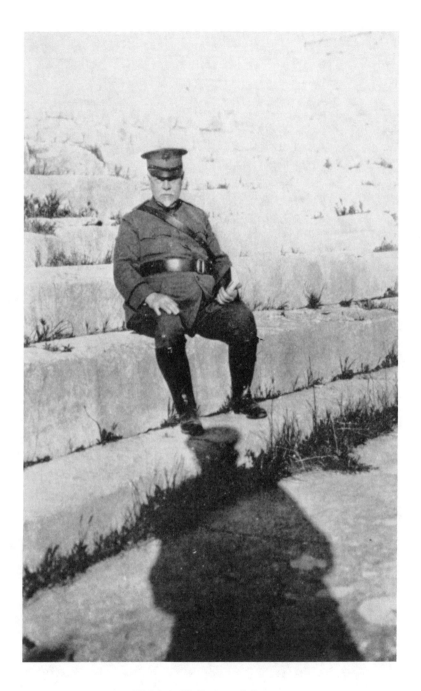

Welch in Uniform at Arles, 1919

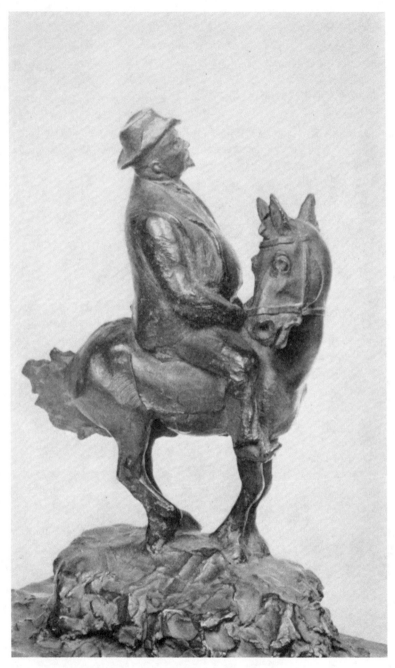

"Welch Rides in China"

A statuette by Mrs. Harriet H. Mayer and Miss Anna Hyatt

effect on the morale of the medical personnel in the camps. Dr. Welch had a way of understanding the local situation perfectly and of explaining it to the men on the ground who were often too near to it to know just what it meant. As always he encouraged the staff, stated the various problems so that they were relatively simple to grasp, and he also explained the medical situation in other camps that we had already visited."

Welch soon grew aware that he would seem to army officers to speak with much more authority if he discarded his much prized civilian costume. "We met and talked to all the doctors and also addressed all the line officers. I never supposed that I should be called upon to speak to line officers on medical and sanitary war problems. I really must get into a uniform, if I am to be on any more such missions."

How successful was his military masquerade is open to question. Despite the silver oak leaf of rank on his shoulder that turned to gold and eventually was transmuted into an eagle,[4] the stout old man, who looked even stouter in uniform, never gave off a martial aura. When he walked the streets of Washington in all the majesty of high rank, he replied to the crisp salutes of his inferior officers by lifting his hand vaguely in the direction of his hat and gently wiggling the fingers. But woe to the line officer who tried to oppose this lax-looking gentleman by promulgating some such rule as forbidding autopsies!

Little by little, conditions in the camps improved until the major object of Welch's inspections changed from solving crises to "stimulating the medical staff to better work and clearer thinking." As usual when one of his projects was well started, Welch wanted to resign and leave the carrying on to others. "The medical service of the army is now well organized," he wrote on July 23, 1918, "and conditions are very much improved in our camps. I do not feel that it is very necessary that I should continue, but as I am about to be promoted to a Colonelcy it may not look quite right to ask to be placed on the inactive list or to resign."

In the same letter, he said that General Gorgas wished him to go abroad for a congress which was to co-ordinate the scientific war work of the Allies. "It is hard to turn down such an opportunity, but I do not see how I can leave, as we are starting the new School of Hygiene the first of October." Welch urged me to attend; he wrote my wife: "Ever since my visit to the other side in 1916 I have been anxious for him to go over. . . . It is a great human as well as professional experience, something which reading and telling about it can not impart."

Concerning the soldiers of the expeditionary force he wrote: "It was an inspiring sight to see the crowd of fine fellows, and I gave them our blessing, love and best wishes for safe voyage and return. They are to be envied for having such an opportunity as awaits them on the other side." However, it was the opportunity of adventure he envied them, not the opportunity of killing Germans. All through his war correspondence there is not a single reference to hatred for the enemy from whom he had learned most of the science he knew. Although he worked as hard as anyone to win the war, he regarded it as a job that must be done, not as a holy crusade against subhuman "Huns." [5]

Shortly after Welch had convinced himself that the camps were in such good condition that he might retire, he was called to investigate a mysterious epidemic. Cole tells us: "The only time I ever saw Dr. Welch really worried and disturbed was in the autumn of 1918, at Camp Devens, near Boston. . . . It was cold and drizzling rain, and there was a continuous line of men coming in from the various barracks [to the hospital], carrying their blankets, many of the men looking extremely ill, most of them cyanosed [blue] and coughing. There were not enough nurses, and the poor boys were putting themselves to bed on cots, which overflowed out of the wards on the porches. We made some inquiries about the cases, went to the laboratory, and then on down to the autopsy room. Owing to the rush and the great numbers of bodies coming into the morgue, they were placed on the floor without any order or system, and we had to step amongst them to get into the room where an autopsy was going on. When the chest was opened and the blue, swollen lungs were removed and opened, and Dr. Welch saw the wet, foamy surfaces with little real consolidation, he turned and said, 'This must be some new kind of infection or plague,' and he was quite excited and obviously very nervous. . . . It was not surprising that the rest of us were disturbed, but it shocked me to find that the situation, momentarily at least, was too much even for Dr. Welch."

Thus the great influenza epidemic, which must rank with the most destructive epidemics of military history, got under way. There was, however, a comic side to that first hectic day. When Dr. O. T. Avery, who had been rushed from the hospital of the Rockefeller Institute, searched the lung sections for influenza bacilli, he used for the crucial "Gram" test the bottles labelled "alcohol" which were already in the laboratory. To his amazement, the expected reaction did not take place. Lung sections kept being piled up before Avery until at last he had used up all the alcohol and was forced to send to the storeroom for a fresh supply. Instantly the correct reaction appeared. Investigation showed that someone had drunk the alcohol in the laboratory bottles and refilled them with water.[6]

Welch undertook his trips to the camps with new vigour, trying to fight what he admitted was the most serious situation that had yet arisen, but science was largely helpless and the epidemic continued to rage long after the camps were disbanded. The return of peace enabled Welch to write: "I finally secured my release from active service in the Army dating from December 31 [1918], so that I have donned again civilian clothes and am trying to resume my normal existence." But he was soon to be in uniform again.

III

During the war, the American Red Cross had collected a record-breaking sum of money, and the return of peace left them with a large amount unspent. Eager to use the remainder for the advancement of humanity, Henry P. Davison, chairman of the American Red Cross War Council, conceived the idea of organizing the national Red Cross Societies into a world-wide agency for fostering public health. This would enlarge the scope of the International Red Cross, which had up to that time specialized in dealing with the medical problems created by war. Naturally Davison consulted the dean of American medicine, and on March 15, 1919, Welch sailed on the *Leviathan*, then being used as a troop transport, to attend the organizing conference at Cannes.[7]

On April 1, delegates from the five principal Allies—France, Great Britain, Italy, Japan, and the United States—were called to order in Cannes. Officially Welch was chairman of the executive committee, but the president, Emile Roux, of the Pasteur Institute, was forced by illness to leave after a day or two. Welch was the actual president of the conference.

At the first meeting he said: "We who have been joined together in close association during this war in fighting the common enemy, an enemy of civilization, are to continue in closer bonds of friendship, because we are joined together not to forge weapons of destruction, but united to consider what we can contribute for the healing of the nations. There are assembled in Paris delegates to consider the formation of a League of Nations.[8] We are assembled here to confer upon the formation of a League of Health. And I venture to say that what we negotiate here will signify to mankind fully as much as the result of the deliberations in Paris."

Even before the conference opened, however, an ominous note was struck. "The French," Welch wrote in his diary on March 31, "inject a bombshell by determination to record their decision not to have anything to do with an international organization which includes Germans." Welch's method of dealing with this outcropping of the old Adam was to ignore it. "Arranged to have meeting of Executive Council to-morrow morning . . . to permit Roux, Widal and Rist to record their reservation, which it is hoped will permit the conference to proceed without further consideration of this feature. . . . He [Davison] is disturbed by the attitude of the French delegates but I think he exaggerates its importance." Welch was proved right. The objection having been noted, it was forgotten, and when the League of Red Cross Societies was eventually organized, the Germans as well as the French were members.

This difficulty side-stepped, the conference proceeded to draw up a tremendous programme which reflected the optimism of those first ebullient months of peace. A permanent League of Red Cross Societies maintaining a Bureau of Health in Geneva was to be financed by the national societies and to act through them for the establishment of a unified programme of public health; where no national societies existed, they were to be established. The conference stated: "Recognizing the prevention of disease and the protection of the health of the people as a primary responsibility and function of government, a non-political organization, such as that of the Red Cross, will be able by the education of the people and in many other ways, to stimulate, support and aid a government in its health work."

Resolutions, in the drafting of which Welch had played a major part, were adopted "for the purpose of indicating in a general way some of the lines of activity which the new organization may wisely follow." They provided for an immediate campaign to fight typhus fever; for "the promotion of a wide extension and development of Child Welfare Work"; for the encouragement of wise public health legislation, its efficient administration, "and particularly that the accurate and full registration of Vital Statistics be urged as forming the fundamental basis for definite and permanent improvement of health conditions"; for a campaign to standardize vital statistics; for the encouragement of scientific investigation in hygiene and sanitary science; for "the establishment of Public Health Laboratories or the provision for laboratory service for every community"; for "the extension of the employment of Public Health Nurses or Health Visitors" and the development of "standardized educational centers for training" them; for a programme to control tuberculosis, malaria, and venereal diseases; for the international dissemination of educational propaganda through "scientific publicity methods"; for the placing of properly trained teachers of hygiene in all the schools of the world; for directing special attention "everywhere to the importance of town and city planning and proper housing for workingmen"; and for the establishment of community health centres as the best possible war memorials. Suggestions on how to implement many of these resolutions were set forth in special committee reports. The scale on which everything was conceived was grand in the extreme; one incidental detail of the plan for fighting tuberculosis involved, for instance, raising the standard of living of the poor all over the world. Welch commented in his diary: "Remarkable agreement on the tuberculosis program."

The conference had laid down a comprehensive plan for world health improvement which entirely overlooked the question of feasibility. It is clear that Welch regarded it as a Utopian scheme which it would take years to accomplish. "The future developments," he said, "are obviously dependent in no small measure upon the successful initiation of the plan upon relatively simple lines." Underneath the thinking of some of the sponsors, however, lay an emotional feeling that Utopia was right around the corner. Dr. Stockton Axson, then acting secretary general, wrote Welch in June: "It is confidently believed that the League of Red Cross Societies . . . will prove to be one of the most significant of modern institutions for the advancement of civilization." He added that the Cannes conference had "made it possible to translate an altruistic impulse into a scientific achievement." The societies were not only publishing the proceedings of the conference, but an album of photographs of its deliberations, so that, we gather, posterity would be able to visualize this turning point in the history of mankind.

To one of his friends, Welch wrote: "I am enthusiastic over the possibilities and believe that a really great movement for the world's health will result provided the right men organize and direct it." He added to a critic who considered the plan impractical: "I infer that you are dubious about the medical or sanitary future for the Red Cross League. It is just one of those ventures where everything depends on getting the right man in control." Welch wanted Wickliffe Rose and Hermann Biggs to collaborate on starting the central agency in Geneva, but neither was available. Only Americans were considered for the position, although there was great difficulty in getting a suitable person to accept it.

Maybe Welch doubted more than he was willing to say the

possibility of carrying out so vast a programme, for he departed from his usual behaviour in connexion with new ventures by failing to take an active part during the crucial period of organization. Although in 1920 he accepted appointment to the advisory committee, he did not attend the meeting that year, preferring his fiftieth reunion at Yale, and thereafter the League of Red Cross Societies is rarely mentioned in his correspondence. He watched without recorded comment while the already broad scope of its work was expanded by founding a monthly review, the *World's Health,* to be published in three languages, and by planning the establishment of independent hygienic laboratories in backward countries. Many Red Cross Societies enrolled, and all was optimism as long as the original American donation remained unspent, but when funds dwindled and other national groups were asked to contribute, they demurred on the ground that the programme was too vast to be effectively applied and had little bearing on the basic purposes of the Red Cross. A paring-down process, begun in 1921, continued until the League was keyed efficiently into the Red Cross structure.[9] Since the International Red Cross Committee was concerned solely with relief in wartime, the League came to concentrate on disaster relief in peace, serving as a clearing house for information on such matters as nursing, the use of airplanes in first-aid work, highway accidents, etc. Occasionally, however, more general matters such as rural hygiene were discussed at periodic international conferences, and the League carried on the work of international health education through strong support given to the Junior Red Cross. Acting efficiently in this more specific field, the League of Red Cross Societies goes on today, a major agency for world betterment. Its membership in 1926 included fifty-four nations.

IV

In April 1919, after the organizing conference at Cannes was over, Welch motored through France, sightseeing and visiting American base hospitals, most of which were still intact, since the bulk of the army had not yet returned home. He recorded interesting cases of wounds and diseases in his diary, and commented on the medical personnel, noting that such and such a man might be useful in the School of Hygiene or the Rockefeller Institute. His dislike of appearing in uniform had vanished with usage; on his discharge from the active list some months before, he had been recommissioned in the Reserve Corps, "so that I could wear a uniform while in the military areas where our troops still are in France and Germany."

His diaries deal voluminously with two trips through the devastated areas. "As we drove beyond this evacuation hospital and on far beyond Verdun we traversed scenes of indescribable desolation, villages with not a house standing, only a few walls left, all else heaps of stones, ground full of shell holes, miles of barbed wire netting, pill boxes for machine gun nests, human bones from graves opened by shells, unexploded grenades and duds in fields (most dangerous to handle or tread on), soldiers engaged in clearing ruins, making roads and in salvaging, here and there a family in a house partly wrecked—all too horrible to imagine or describe—the very hell of war. It was a most wonderful opportunity to see the devastated area, and to pass through places like Secheprey, Mont Sec, Verdun and its hills, whose names were so familiar. . . . We drove—preceded by Col. Thornburg's car—to the most desperately assaulted and defended part of the fortressed hills East or N.E. of Verdun. Here stood a village called Fleury, where not a stone is left. As far as the eye reaches the ground is upheaved with innumerable shell holes. Here lay human bones mostly of buried French upheaved by shells. I picked up an astragalus as a souvenir. We were near Fort Douaumont. The place was once captured by Germans, then retaken by French. No scene of war can surpass this terrain. We picked our way carefully among grenades and duds, which lay around, partly buried, in great numbers. We saw a shoe full of the bones of the foot, an entire corpse, in a shell hole, whitened loose bones of entire skeletons. The French said to have lost 600,000 lives around Verdun, Huns probably more."

His use of the word Huns in this moment of emotion seems to mark a change in his attitude toward Germany; never before had the excitements and anxieties of the war elicited from him any insulting reference to the enemy. Now, however, as scenes of desolation burned themselves into his mind, the word Huns fell more and more often from his pen. When he crossed the frontier into the occupied areas on the Rhine no word of pity escaped him for the German population, which, during months of armistice, was being forced to starve by the continued blockade. With no emotion, only intellectual curiosity, he reported: "While soldiers are ordered not to fraternize with Germans, and one is arrested if seen with a German girl, when the 42nd (Rainbow) division left they were surrounded at the train by weeping German Fräuleins, who pinned flowers on them, so that there must have been a good deal of sororization in their billets and clandestinely. The French in their area are seen with the German girls, and are apparently not restricted in this intercourse. The French are trying to win good will of the Germans, feed them, contrary to the allied agreement, etc. Food is just beginning to be distributed, but there was an interallied conference here to-day on the subject. The German children are undernourished, flabby, pale, underweight."

On his return to Paris, so great a military ardour filled him that he refurbished the uniform he had once refused to wear; he had his Sam Browne belt refitted and went to a shop "near the Champs Elysées to have maroon tape and colonel's insignia put on my overseas cap." Then he set out for a two-day trip through the Soissons area. Here real hatred of the Germans overwhelmed him. He speaks of their "barbarism," repeats tales of how, when they retreated, they left bombs in the pillars of churches to kill the returning parishioners, and concludes: "Notwithstanding the bad weather and the bad roads the trip was most interesting and has filled me with horror at the devastation, and a desire that the Boches, who started this war and are responsible for it, all be made to suffer and to pay the utmost possible, although no possible punishment can fit their crime."

V

When Welch went abroad again in the summer of 1923, he attended ceremonies commemorating Europe's glorious past and had glimpses of Europe's future, a few hopeful, many profoundly disturbing.

One thing was clear: Welch's reputation had leaped the Atlantic. As he moved from nation to nation, he was recognized everywhere as a scientist of wisdom and power. He received an honorary degree from Cambridge University at the same ceremony with Stanley Baldwin and with two Nobel prize-winners, Hendrik A. Lorentz of Leiden and Niels Bohr of Copenhagen. Welch and Baldwin spoke for the recipients before a commemorative luncheon at Corpus Christi College.[10]

First, however, Welch took part in two weeks of celebrations in honour of the centenary of Pasteur. Sitting on platforms with cabinet ministers and the great scientists of the world, he was called on again and again to speak for the foreign delegates. When the progressive celebration moved to Strasbourg, where Pasteur had been professor of chemistry, Welch came face to face with memories of his youth; in this city he had begun his scientific career. Often he left the conferences of the important to walk the streets and try to recapture the eager young man who had been homesick at first and then enraptured by the learning of an older world. But though the streets were the same, Welch had changed; his slower, heavier footfalls echoed with a different sound from the medieval buildings. Searching the Kalbsgasse, now renamed Rue de Veaux, he could not find the boarding house where he had lived. Only the minster, that pile which had seemed the symbol of his first European adventure, came back to him with emotion; again he admired the warm colouring of the stone and decided that it was the finest of cathedrals.

Soon the present, that glorious present which had realized the wildest dreams of his youth, called him to London to help celebrate the eight-hundredth anniversary of the founding of St. Bartholomew's Hospital. He was deeply moved by a pageant which brought back the times when William the Conqueror was a memory in the minds of the living; he heard the Prince of Wales say that it was not at all impossible that "a few aged men, troubled with old lance or arrow wounds from the battle of Hastings, came to pass their last days in this house of healing." When the hospital was founded, London was still a walled city and the Magna Charta had not been written. And there sat Welch representing a continent that was not to be discovered for hundreds of years. Twice during the celebration he was called on to speak; he dwelt on America's debt to British medicine, and rejoiced that the scientists of the New World were at last in a position to pay back what they owed by making discoveries of their own. He was one of the few delegates received by the Prince of Wales.

Then Welch prepared for a trip to Germany. Since the war he had done what he could to help German and Austrian science, whose continuance he considered of the greatest importance for the good of the rest of the world,[11] but his reactions to the consulate where he obtained his visa showed that he had not completely lost the hatred that had overwhelmed him in the devastated areas. "General impression I carried away not pleasant," he wrote. He found the Czech consulate "a contrast in surroundings and courtesy to that awful German place."

On the train to Berlin, his dinner cost 55,000 marks and he left a tip of 5000, for one dollar was worth between 130,000 and 145,000 marks. After looking out the window of the train, he wrote: "Somehow I felt there was a general air of depression, but not very tangible—crowds quiet, rather smaller than usual, I thought, and country-side and towns seemed less populous than I recall of old." Although Germany was the enemy for whom he had said no punishment could be severe enough, memories of his former happy days there would not down. He found his walk along Unter den Linden depressing, and before he had been in Berlin forty-eight hours he wrote: "In the afternoon from four on and late in the evening the café of this hotel is crowded with Americans; living luxuriously on nothing and chattering away —a most unpleasant impression when one considers the misery outside, the pinched, poorly dressed natives on the streets, the unattractive and bold young girls forced to street-walking, the poor professors—I could not stand remaining here with such contrasts before my eyes."

And when he discovered at first hand what had happened to German science he was horrified. Professor Wilhelm His told him how inflation had wiped out the funds of the hospitals and the universities and destroyed the middle class, "from which were recruited the scientific men and the intellectual leaders." The students' fees, which once made up four or five times the salaries of the professors, now were almost worthless. " 'Mine,' His said, 'for a year would not buy these two cups of coffee and glasses of cognac.' (I paid for these 44,600 Mks., about 32 cents)—Young men cannot turn to science and medicine any longer for a living; they must go into some other kind of work. . . . Those dependent on salaries are suffering actually from insufficient food." Welch noted His's statement that men who wished to carry on scientific investigation "have to engage in practice, give courses, teach, do anything to earn enough to feed and clothe them, and in spite of all it is fine to see their eagerness to snatch scraps of time, perhaps at night, to pursue some research. Animal experimentation is greatly hampered both by cost of the animals, and as much also by the cost of fodder. . . . He [His] could not afford animals and their fodder for his experimental work if it were not for some Japanese students, especially one who is working with him, who pay for the animals."

As he listened to this story, how could Welch help remembering the marvellous German laboratories that had inspired his youth, and the depression he had then felt in returning to America, where a man could not make his living by research? Now the situation was reversed; he noted in his diary that the Americans should rescue His by calling him to the United States, where laboratory work flourished. Welch, however, was not exhilarated that his own handiwork now overshadowed the handiwork of his teachers; his German diary breathes a deep sadness.

Welch agreed with His that the French reparation demands should be relaxed lest they father calamity. Since the middle class was being destroyed while labourers were comparatively well paid, the power of the ignorant, anti-intellectual masses was increasing; there was danger that they would rise and tear down the structure of German intelligence Welch had once so admired. He recorded His's belief that the saving of German civilization depended on a race with time. No effort had previously been made to give the working classes "an appreciation of the methods and value of science." Although a frantic attempt to remedy this deficiency was now under way, probably it was too late. Welch wrote: "There is apprehension of Bolshevism if the economic situation becomes intolerable through the determination of France to render Germany prostrate and ruined, although the natural inclination of the people is against Bolshevism."

Welch called on his old professor, Flügge, whom he found presiding at a birthday party for his son. "There was a large cake, for which Flügge apologized as unwonted luxury. . . . Flügge seemed most appreciative of my calling to see him. He recalled that I had spoken when I saw him last (I think in 1913 again on my way to Carlsbad) of his coming to America to give the Herter lectures. I explained that the war had prevented. He is 76 years old. I mailed him my personal check on my Baltimore bank for fifty (50) dollars, with a friendly letter, hoping that he would use money for himself and family or however he may desire."

After four days in "a changed and depressed Berlin where I should not care to stay long," Welch set out for Carlsbad, now in Czechoslovakia, to take the cure. During the journey he wrote: "There was also a Pole in the compartment, who is ardent for Poland and considers the future secure for Poland!" And a day or two later he added: "I learned a great deal about the German side in Czecho-Slovakia. Feeling between the two races is extremely bitter, and there seems no doubt the Czechs are treating the Germans badly. . . . Masaryk is a good man but with little influence. Benes, the premier, able and liberal, but even he cannot offend the extreme anti-German, chauvinistic leaders, who seem to be a terror and doing everything to destroy prosperity of German population. . . . Of course there may be another side, but it is evident the hostility between the races equals that between English and Irish, and no chance of amalgamation." Even in the new nations created by the treaty of Versailles strains were evident.

His cure over, Welch moved on to Prague, the national capital; he had been asked by the Rockefeller Foundation to examine the plans of an institute of hygiene it was helping to erect there. At the station he was met by President Masaryk's car, which remained at his disposal during his two days' visit, while he conferred with the ministers of health and state, and with numerous members of the Health Department whom he considered "enthusiastic, fine young men." After several sightseeing junkets, he had lunch with Masaryk himself. "It was an intimate, family luncheon. . . . The President has a winning personality, very pleasant and courteous, playful with the little boy, not much of a talker, but sensible and with impression of restrained power, but not of a dominant personality—perhaps 50 to 60 years old, good looking, carries himself well, quiet, inspires confidence in his goodness and sincerity. He was in Chicago, also visited Baltimore, but did not lecture there. We chatted familiarly together over our coffee. The view from his rooms at the Hradschin over the city is superb, unsurpassed. Altogether the occasion of this intimate luncheon with the family was more to my liking than a big, formal luncheon would have been."

Welch's next visit was to Vienna, which he found a great contrast to Berlin, since a loan sponsored by the League of Nations had stabilized the currency and "brought a spirit of hopefulness and even gaiety and cheer to this light-hearted, attractive people —not, however, in equal degree to the university professors. The Rockefeller aid given the three Austrian universities is of incalculable benefit and they are most grateful." Welch made the rounds of the pathological institutes, had good talks with Paltauf and the newer and younger pathologists, Sternberg, Erdheim, and others. But he most enjoyed his conversation with the political historian Joseph Redlich, who said that the premier, Seipel, a Catholic priest, had wakened the rest of the world to Austria's plight when he went to Rome and offered his country to Italy. As a result, the powers lined up behind Austria and stabilized the crown. But not at a very high figure; in five days Welch spent 4,148,000 crowns, or $60.

In Geneva Welch hoped to have a few quiet days, provided "no one discovers my presence." He started out bravely, lounging in his dressing gown till noon, admiring the view of Mont Blanc from his hotel window, writing long letters, reading Henri Béraud's *Le Martyre de l'Obèse,* which he noted was "dedicated to 18 presumably corpulent men and women." Soon, however, he could not resist visiting the League of Nations and the Health Section; then the usual round of visits and entertainments began. When his grandniece and her husband, Philip Jessup, came to attend lectures at the League, Welch felt that he "must take some of them." He had a long talk with Ludwik Rajchman, the medical director of the Health Section, who gave him a statement of the organization of the League which he found satisfactory. Welch had long felt that the hope for the future of the world lay in international co-operation; he was president of the Maryland branch of the League of Nations Non-Partisan Association and a convinced advocate of America's entry.

Leaving Geneva, Welch followed his usual custom when in Europe by going to a seaside resort; on this occasion he chose Dinard, and in a day or two he wrote typically that the bathing was "good enough of the kind, but not comparable with our Jersey coast." He always found European bathers and European surf tame. In 1909, when he was almost sixty, he had proved too adventuresome for the German laws at Norderney, on the North Sea. "I was startled when my first swim out into the ocean was greeted with the frantic shrieking of horns from the shore. I was over my head and this is prohibited by law and fined. . . . The surf is considered fine by those who know nothing better, but would be considered a calm on our Atlantic coast."

In Dinard, Welch had dinner with the Queen of Rumania; he complimented her on her success in making royal marriages for her daughters. "She said that her daughters were so good-looking that there was no difficulty in their making desirable matches, and I replied that the established laws of heredity ensured their beauty, etc., etc. The Queen wore a magnificent chain of pearls two or three times around her neck and hanging down to her corsage, and a crown-like broad silver band, cut into spoon-like or laurel-leaf-like parts—quite remarkably queenly and effective, I thought."

During his return voyage to America, Welch, as he wrote in his diary, spent a large part of the voyage "summarizing, balancing and analyzing my accounts of expenditures, for which I have kept full daily itemized statements. . . . I might have been more profitably employed, and do not think it worth while to keep such minute accounts, as it takes much time and becomes a kind of monomania, after one has started on it and determined to see it through to the bitter end."

One of the strangest peculiarities of Welch's later years was his financial records of his European trips. They run for pages and pages; no expenditure is too small to be carefully noted; indeed a single penny paid for a postage stamp may appear a half-dozen times, for he was continually breaking down his accounts, summarizing them, changing them into different currencies, and even entering items for no obvious reason in his diary as well as in his account book.[12] When in Yugoslavia, he was concerned at being unable to account for half a dinar that was missing from his pocket; nine days later he found the coin on the floor of his hotel room, and turned back to balance the entry.

The type of minutiæ he recorded is shown in the following summary headed *Cigars:* "I arrived in Europe with a fair supply of cigars, Jaccaci (August 15) gave me a box of 25, Marburg gave me several cigars. I probably had about 680 cigars, after leaving New York May 12 [in 125 days], including those which I purchased in Europe, those brought with me and those presented to me. A box of 25 Romeo and Juliets, given me by Fred Walcott, I reserved for special occasions. My itemized accounts show that I paid *$54.22 for 573 cigars and 1 box of cigarettes,* the last costing *16 cents.* I thus paid just about *9½ cents per cigar.* The quality and price varied, but in general I did not buy many expensive cigars. On the whole they were inferior to American

cigars at corresponding prices. In Berlin cigars were one cent
or less apiece. 'Graciosa,' 'Regalia' and 'Brittanika' cigars were
the principal brands in Czecho-Slovakia and Austria—the best
about 10 cents a piece or a little more. 'Romeo and Juliets' and
'Henry Clays' were to be had and were not very expensive except in England."

VI

The next summer, that of 1924, Welch had a glimpse of a
part of Europe that had not been ravaged by war; and he was
deeply impressed with what he found. With Dr. Allen W. Freeman of the School of Hygiene and Mrs. Freeman, Welch sailed
at the request of the Rockefeller Foundation to attend a meeting of a subcommittee of the League of Nations on health education and social medicine; but first he prepared for the meeting by making a hurried trip to Norway, Sweden, and Denmark.

His two young friends had never been abroad before—"the
delight of the Freemans in everything is worth the trip"—and
he teased them unmercifully. Although he admonished them to
cut their baggage to the smallest possible compass, when they
asked him how many bags he had, he replied, "somewhat sheep-
ishly," Freeman thought, that he had ten, which was a great exaggeration. He told Mrs. Freeman that he did not expect to wear
a top hat on the trip but that the hatbox was an excellent place
in which to keep his passport.

Freeman remembers that Welch was "interested in teaching
us the technique of life on shipboard." During long evenings
on deck, he "recited poetry, composed limericks, set us puzzles
to work out [he had been sent a vast number to the boat, his
weakness being well known], and told us stories of every period
of his life. . . . One evening he was telling us about the adventurous things he had done; how he had been one of the first
people to go up as a passenger in an aeroplane, had been the first
down the chute the chutes at Coney Island, etc. He remarked
that he liked to do adventurous things. I tried to tease him by
remarking that after all there was one adventurous thing which

he had never tried, meaning matrimony. There was quite a long
pause, and then he remarked, somewhat drily and finally, 'Perhaps I tried to try that too.' I did not pursue the subject." Undoubtedly Freeman had failed to catch a twinkle in Welch's
eye.

During the crossing, Welch read an "admirable" report made
to the Rockefeller Foundation by S. M. Gunn on Scandinavian
public health activities; it gave the necessary basis for his observations, so that it merely remained for him to see the work in
operation and meet the important officials. In Copenhagen Welch
wrote that although the United States might be ahead in laboratories, public health nursing, and popular education in hygiene, "we are behind the Scandinavian countries in our institutions for care of the sick and in provision for university teaching
and clinics, and we have no such beautiful grounds and spacious
accommodations for the staff as they have. Moreover, our hospitals for teaching are comparatively small affairs, whereas they
have 600–1000 beds. . . . One may even inquire whether Denmark has not overdone its social program. It is to be noted that
patients when sick practically always are treated in hospitals. The
whole system is linked with the sickness insurance policy, with
which those with whom I have spoken are entirely contented."

Denmark, he added, "certainly stands foremost in health protection and disease prevention. The health insurance system is
largely responsible. . . . Madsen [13] says that Denmark has so
much social legislation and the government now makes such
ample provision, that there is not much need of private charities
. . . and they have now difficulty in getting enough inmates."

Welch had no intention of allowing business to keep him from
sightseeing. He visited all the art galleries and museums he could
find, seriously studying modern Scandinavian art, and he viewed
innumerable fjords. Despite Freeman's pleading, he climbed "a
cliff that rose some 1200 feet almost straight up. . . . Mrs. Freeman and I wanted to wait for him, of course, but he insisted that
we leave him alone to take his own gait. 'You worry me hanging
back this way,' he said, and there was nothing to do but to obey,
although we kept him in sight. He walked the whole way up and

arrived at the top, after a climb that made the rest of us pant, in as good shape as any. It was a severe physical test for a man of seventy-four."

Welch comments on the same incident in his diary: "The climb up this mountain road with numerous curves (17) of the road took me about 1¼ hours, as I took it at a very slow pace on foot. The horse and cart followed or rather passed me and waited at the top. It is a longer climb, but not so steep, I think, as that at Stalheim [another Welch had taken]. I think an automobile could make the ascent with passengers. It requires a sound heart to climb up, as it does at Stalheim, and undoubtedly not every one is fit to go up the long climb on foot."

It gave the septuagenarian pleasure to seem more energetic than the younger Freemans. One evening in Copenhagen, Freeman remembers, "we went out for dinner at the Vivel Restaurant, just the three of us, and afterward into the Tivoli amusement park. We had had a long day of libraries and hospitals, and I was rather fatigued when we started out. After dinner we did the amusement park, walking about for a couple of hours, and when the time came to start back to the hotel, both Mrs. Freeman and I were pretty well exhausted. Dr. Welch insisted, however, that the hotel was not far, only a mile or two, and we walked instead of taking a cab. Just before we got to the hotel Dr. Welch said, 'Now you children run off to bed because you are tired. I want to poke around a little bit. The only way to know anything about a city is to walk about at night.' "

For years Welch had enjoyed Turkish baths; Garrison tells us that in Baltimore he sometimes spent the night in such establish ments to hide from importunate visitors. When he announced in Stockholm that he was going to take a Turkish bath, "Mrs. Freeman and I smiled at each other," for they knew that the attendants in Sweden were women. Welch went off gaily. On his return, Freeman asked him whether he had enjoyed himself With a grave face under amused eyes Welch answered: "It wasn't a bit exciting. They were all old women."

In Copenhagen he called on Salomonsen, but found his friend, with whom he had once dreamed youthful dreams, "much broken. He is so badly crippled with deforming (?) arthritis and marked tremor from paralysis agitans that his condition is distressing. His mind seems clear and he talks, although hesitatingly, well. . . . Salomonsen talked of his close friendship with Ehrlich, whom he regards as a more original genius than Koch, and I agree."

In contrast with his old friend, Welch was very sprightly, but yet his Scandinavian trip had been too strenuous; he was completely exhausted when he took the train for Hamburg. A battle with the German customs officials over the vast number of cigars he was carrying reopened the old wound of his wartime feelings about Germany. "Catch me doing anything more for the Germans!" he wrote in his diary. Freeman remembers: "He was indignation itself. After all he had done for the Germans, the money he had raised for German professors, his friendship for the country, to be treated like this was just too much, and he fumed about it most of the day."

He was amazed to find that, since the year before, living in Germany had become expensive even in American dollars, and that there seemed to be a great deal of money. "Hamburg," he complained, "typifies modern Prussianized Germany, with its colossal really Brobdignagian statue of Bismarck, its tasteless huge modern structures, and generally grandiose air of the newer parts." But German science still had the power to soften his heart. After visiting the Institut für Schiffs- und Tropenkrankheiten, he wrote: "I am glad to have had an opportunity to see this great institute. The experience corrects in a measure the bad taste of my disagreeable experience with those outrageous customs officers."

After spending four days in Amsterdam studying the Dutch public health service, he hurried to The Hague for a rest, arriving, as he wrote, in an exhausted condition; his gout was giving him much trouble. "I took a sea bath and did not enjoy it particularly, as I had difficulty in getting a bathing suit large enough, which was said to be the largest they had. It was a poor kind of striped red and white suit with sleeves."

On August 30 he reached Geneva, after a trip in a compartment with a crying baby: "not at all [a] pleasant situation"; he had omitted the cure he needed at some health resort in order to be an onlooker at the meetings of the Assembly of the League. "If Carnegie were alive I agree with Wickersham that he would give 10,000,000 dollars at least to the work of the League," Welch wrote, adding a few days later: "I should say that now the League is not so much in need of America, as America is of the League, and that there is a growing feeling that we should not at the present stage be particularly helpful in developing the traditions, ideals, and methods of the League."

Provided with a permanent ticket to the floor of delegates, Welch attended meetings of the Assembly, hearing a critical debate on security between Ramsay MacDonald and Herriot. Although he considered the English prime minister an excellent orator, he felt that he did not suggest "a definite solution of the problems." Herriot, on the other hand, "stood by the Covenant completely. . . . This matter of arbitration is the common ground on which MacDonald and Herriot agree, but they stand apart when it comes to security and disarmament. MacDonald's position here is that of pacifism—no force—; Herriot will not hear of the abandonment of military sanctions for security as a necessary prelude to disarmament." A great subject was that of the admission of Germany to the League. MacDonald would admit Germany "demain," Herriot "après-demain."

After the brilliant Assembly meetings, the subcommittee on health education and social medicine, which Welch had come to Geneva to attend, seemed pale by comparison. He worked to whittle the committee's programme down to something practical, urging that the project of educating all the peoples of the world in personal hygiene give way to considering "opportunities and methods of special training for those who engage in public health work"; he emphasized the "importance of training the subordinate or inferior personnel, especially sanitary inspectors (disinfectors) and public health nurses." Welch's suggestion that the first step should be an international survey was agreed to, but it was decided that the members should not report on their own countries. Welch was unenthusiastic when assigned England,

Canada, China, and Japan; he was amused when Siberia was added. Although he felt that one or two competent investigators could do the whole job, he agreed good-humouredly to carry out his assignment. Once he was back in America, however, he could not find the time; his report was never written.

CHAPTER XVIII

Across the Pacific

I

ONE of the early major undertakings of the Rockefeller Foundation was the promotion of modern Western medicine in China. After a commission sent over in the summer of 1914 recommended the creation of up-to-date medical schools first in Peking and later in Shanghai, the foundation established a subsidiary body, the China Medical Board, to carry on the work. Wishing to examine the ground for themselves, the board organized a second commission made up of Wallace Buttrick, its director; Gates, the vice-chairman; his son, Frederick L. Gates; and two medical members who happened to be Welch and myself. At the last moment the elder Gates was unable to go with us; his son represented him.[1]

The commission sailed for China late in August 1915, but Welch, enthusiastic over the prospect of seeing the Far East, had set out some weeks earlier. In the Hawaiian Islands his diary * bristled with superlatives. He wrote of "three wonderful weeks, full of delight and interest, abounding hospitality, luncheons and dinners." Though he listed his engagements and the many important people who paid him attention, and enumerated the health problems of the islands, it was the islands themselves that aroused his enthusiasm. He wrote his niece of "violets growing as trees five and six feet high! It seems quite contrary to the nature of that shrinking, modest flower. . . . The night-blooming cereus . . . thousands of blossoms, a foot long and a foot across,

---

* Welch first began to keep diaries on this trip to the Orient. Thereafter, when he was abroad, he always wrote down his daily experiences in a journal; the notations became more and more voluminous as he grew older. In two instances only did he keep such records while at home: once during the World War on visits to army camps in the United States, and again while working at the Huntington Library in Pasadena.

around two sides of the large square where the college of Oahu is located."

To his nephew he wrote: "Of course the volcano of Kilauea on Hawaii is unique and one of the greatest spectacles the world offers, worth crossing oceans and continents to behold. The seething lake of fiery lava, breaking into spray, is quite indescribable. . . . I was taken by auto about three hundred miles around the island of Hawaii and saw the marvelous old and recent lava flows, a terrible and awe-inspiring sight. By contrast the Kona coast of the island, celebrated by Mark Twain and Stevenson, is full of charm and delightful in climate, a veritable paradise. . . . These were the culminating events of my trip and of my experience in seeing the sights of the earth. There can be nothing like them or quite equal to them. . . . Altogether Hawaii will haunt me with a longing to return the rest of my days. There is a magic about these islands of delight."

When the remainder of his party joined Welch,* they all sailed for Japan. A delightful travelling companion, and to the ladies especially charming, he watched his friends with his usual dry amusement. "I think the members of our party will get along together very well, although our interests vary," he wrote. "Mrs. Flexner will go in for art. She is distressed to have the Rev. Buttrick call the great Buddha at Kamakura an 'idol' and thinks she could worship there as well as at such a service as one of the missionaries gave us this morning. Horror of Buttrick!"

Welch did not allow himself to be made a victim by the many fellow-passengers who tried to engage him in conversation. After exchanging a few words with him, somehow they vanished, or he himself left them, but he seemed never to give offence. Long years of practice had no doubt perfected his technique of self-protection.

At Yokohama we were met by some of the leading bacteriologists in Japan, comprising a delegation from the Kitasato Institute,[2] and in Tokyo, which became the centre of the commission's activities, we were given elaborate dinners in the Japa-

---

* The commission was accompanied by Mrs. Buttrick, Miss Caroline Buttrick, and Mrs. Flexner.

nese style. The entertainments opened with intricate and graceful pantomimic dances, after which everyone sat on the floor and ate course after course with chopsticks. Geisha were assigned to entertain each guest, and Welch as the most distinguished was at all times honoured with the most beautiful geisha according to Japanese standards, who was usually very young. As a less important personage I was assigned older entertainers who sometimes could speak a few words of English. While his ingenue got in his way by trying to feed him titbits, Welch enviously watched me as I talked and laughed with my companion. "Flexner," he asked me, "why do they always give me these children?" and he noted in his diary: "Very entertaining to Flexner, aided by Kitasato!"

We were invited to luncheon by Count Okuma, premier of Japan, about whom Welch wrote: "He is bald, oriental in appearance, looks something like Mr. Rockefeller, Sr., about 80 yrs. old, I believe—lost a leg from a bomb thrown at him when minister of foreign affairs years ago—talks very intelligently—rather reserved, but spoke freely and sympathetically of our mission and of modern medicine—spoke of China as a whole being a 'sick man.'" Recalling that the Occidental part of Japanese civilization had begun with the introduction of Western medicine, Okuma hoped for the same effect in China.

Welch noted that Baron Shibusawa expanded on the same theme; he "spoke of three phases of development of western civilization in Japan—first came medicine, the first or elder brother, second, improvement of government and political conditions, the second brother, and last development of industry, commerce and finance, according to western ideas, the third brother, to which class he belonged, but there had not been time for this brother to grow into a Rockefeller. Praised Mr. Rockefeller." [3]

Welch's reply was characterized by a newspaper the next day as "racy and pleasant"; he summarized it in his diary as follows: "Something of our mission—of the welcome accorded to us—of the need of mutual acquaintance and understanding, and gave considerable satisfaction by praising the Japanese exhibit in San Francisco." Although the premier had spoken of "strong nations absorbing the weak as their destiny," Welch's comment on the luncheon was: "It was most gratifying to find such sympathetic comprehension of our mission and expressions of good will and hope of success from such eminent representatives of the governing class."

To his niece Welch wrote that the three weeks spent in Japan "are all too short for the sights of this beautiful country. We have followed the regular trail of the tourist—Yokohama and Kamakura, Tokyo, Nikko, Tokyo again, Miyanoshita, Kyoto, Nara, Kobe, and now Miyajima. . . . I have become interested in the various forms of Japanese art—architecture, painting, sculpture, bronzes and porcelains, the gardens, etc., all quite fascinating in their way. We have visited a great many temples, the finest being those of Novu-ji near Nara; in fact Nara is a most fascinating place. Of course, the Nikko temples are the most splendid in decoration, but those at Novu-ji the finest in architecture. . . . It is wonderfully fine and interesting, when one throws off our conventions and realizes the beautiful achievements of this most artistic people. . . .

"It is hopeless to try to describe to you all that we have seen and experienced. In Kyoto I found my Yale classmate, Dwight Learned, the valedictorian of my class, who has been a professor in the Doshisha College since 1875, as queer as ever, but I have always liked him.

"I am very much impressed with the Japanese people . . . hardy, virile, able, with a devotion to their country and Emperor quite unmatched in Western countries. Much of the Western civilization here is only a veneer, and fortunately so, for the best of Japan is their own art and civilization, alien as it may seem to us. . . . The country itself is probably the most beautiful in the world, when one considers the variety and extent of charming scenery, the combination of sea and mountains."

On our sightseeing trips Welch and Buttrick, who was also very stout, were themselves regarded as a sight by the rural Japanese. As our commission rolled majestically down the narrow streets of country villages, Welch first in a ricksha with a coolie labouring fore and aft, Buttrick next, also propelled by two sweating coolies, the Japanese women working outside their frail houses looked, became alert, rushed off, and brought their children, even babies in arms, to see the strange sight. It was as if the god of good luck, Hotei, in twins, had appeared and passed before them. Welch and Buttrick saw the resemblance, of course, and enjoyed the scene. Whenever it occurred, Welch would say that he felt sorry for the unfortunate children who had missed the apparition and could not describe it to their children.

II

The commission travelled to China by way of Korea.

At Mukden, where we were met by Roger S. Greene, representative in Peking of the China Medical Board, and Dr. Charles W. Young, we began our task of inspecting medical schools and hospitals. The largest, best-equipped, and most adequately staffed medical college in China, operated by the Japanese in connexion with the South Manchurian Railway, was there. Welch noted in his diary that, although Chinese students were admitted free, most were kept away by anti-Japanese sentiment, following the recent political crisis arising from the demands of Japan. Later in Peking he heard that this resentment against Japan was so strong that the Chinese favoured the Germans in the World War, since the English were allies of the Japanese.

We also inspected the Mukden Hospital, a missionary institution which combined the treatment of the sick with the education of Chinese medical students. Welch wrote: "It has evidently developed around one fine personality—Dr. [Dugald] Christie. . . . Young says that we shall find many similar institutions in China, although this is superior in building and equipment to most, and Christie is one of the strongest men in the medical mission field. Another man of similar type is Dr. [Duncan] Main of Hangchow. . . . Christie is a remarkable man, evidently of great force, perhaps 55 yrs. old, a Scot, who has been here since 1883, when he started the medical missionary work in Manchuria. . . . Christie has been eminently successful in establishing cordial, even intimate relations with Viceroys, Governor Generals, guilds, and the Chinese community generally, and during his 30 yrs. here has done a really great work. The hospital has 140 beds, the wards are pavilions running alternately east and west from the corridor. They are plain, but clean and bright. Abundance of flowers in grounds. There is an x-ray department—a good operating room with evidences of antiseptic technique.

"Dr. Christie and the surgeon Dr. David D. Muir—(all the professional staff of hospital and college are Scot or English)—are the only members of hospital staff, although members of college faculty help—other assistance is by Chinese. No European nurses, only Chinese. The hospital as a whole is a much less costly and well equipped institution, and much smaller than the Japanese hospital, which we visited yesterday—few books or journals, still it is probable that the quality of clinical work may be as good, if not better in Dr. Christie's hospital. We really have little information as to the quality of clinical work in the Japanese hospital."

The commission's longest stay in China was its three weeks in Peking, where the Peking Union Medical College, the school of the London Missionary Society, was situated. This institution was to be made over by the China Medical Board into a complete school with hospital and laboratories along modern lines. Dissections and post-mortems, banned by the Chinese because of ancestor worship, were to be introduced, and a trained faculty assembled. This proposed merging of the religious interests of the existing missionary school with the scientific interests of the China Medical Board brought up many issues which had to be resolved. The missionaries in Peking and elsewhere, who were thoroughly familiar with the local conditions, and the scientists from the outside, who were perhaps in closer contact with the medicine of the Western world, both had important contributions to make to the projected school; it was the task of the commission to bring together their points of view. This involved visits to medical schools and hospitals as far south as Canton to ascertain the attitude of the teachers and physicians already in China, and to carry to them the most modern ideas on medical teaching. Welch was soon called on to exercise his long-practised abilities as a mediator.

A perplexing problem concerned the language of instruction. The prevailing system was to teach in Chinese, and many missionaries felt strongly that the remodelled school should continue this practice. The decision had a direct bearing on the character of the teaching body; if Chinese were decided upon, it would be much more difficult to make use of Western-trained scientists, but on the other hand the employment of English might conceivably open the doors to individuals out of sympathy with the missionary point of view. The commission set out to allay the fears of the missionary body about the use of English by convincing them that, although scientific qualifications would be the first requisite of the new faculty, great care would be taken to select men who would appreciate the religious side of the missionaries' work.

Very important was the fact that there was no medical literature in Chinese: textbooks had to be specially translated and were likely to become obsolete long before new translations were made; no periodical medical literature existed to bring new discoveries to the Orient; and the Chinese language itself lacked scientific terms, though some progress had been made to provide them artificially. Since the missionary body was as eager as the commission to raise medical standards in China, such arguments prevailed; English was agreed on as the language of instruction.

When, many years before, the Hopkins Medical School had been founded, Welch had been perturbed by the suggestion that it be coeducational; now he found himself arguing for coeducation against grave fears similar to those he himself had once felt. Women doctors, he was able to point out, already played an important role in China; there were special medical missionary schools for women, and at Canton a small beginning had been made in coeducation. Although the women students had in general not been satisfactory, this situation could be remedied, he and the other members of the commission argued, by admitting them only on the same terms as men and by giving them the same opportunities. Again the missionary body accepted the advanced point of view, and the mission schools co-operated by preparing women to meet the entrance requirements.

Planning pre-medical studies for both men and women presented difficulties. Fortunately, English was already taught in many of the "middle schools"—the missionary ones especially —and in the colleges. Opportunities to study the basic sciences of physics, chemistry, and biology, however, hardly existed, a situation that was gradually remedied by providing the necessary training in a preparatory school in Peking, and by the China Medical Board's assisting selected missionary colleges to establish laboratories and appoint trained teachers. The greater opportunities presented by the new medical school aided considerably in solving the problems of preparation they raised, since the school attracted a more educated class of Chinese than the old institutions had done. Indeed, by the time the remodelled Peking Union Medical College got under way in 1919, the gap in preliminary training had been largely filled.

As Welch told the student body of Yale-in-China at Changsha, where he took the place of the preacher at a Sunday morning chapel service, the China of 1915 was standing where the Western nations had stood at the beginning of the seventeenth century before development of the experimental method which enabled them so greatly to surpass the Orient in material progress. For generations the Chinese had trained themselves by reading and being told about things; they learned by committing texts to memory, page after page, sometimes being able to repeat whole books by rote. Indeed, the Chinese were just emerging from the Middle Ages into the modern, or experimental, period, where speculations and hypotheses are tested by experiment. "What you need in educational methods," he continued, "is in the first place the power of making and recording accurate observations, but that alone is not enough. The scientific mind is keenly alive to inquiry into the how and why of things. . . . You need the power of independent observation, to make experiments and draw inferences, to see with your own eyes, and touch with your own hands, and hear with your own ears. You need to go over for yourselves the processes by which natural knowledge was first acquired. This point of view I believe to be of fundamental importance for education in China. . . . That is the kind of knowledge that gives power and should bring some measure of wisdom with it."

The habit of learning from books was so deep-seated that doubt was expressed in Peking as to whether the Chinese genius was capable of mastering experimental science. Undisturbed by such gloomy prognostications, the commission expressed its conviction that the institution to be founded should regard its initial Western faculty as merely a stop-gap, serving until their Chinese pupils were well enough trained to take over. Chinese medicine would have to stand on its own feet if the vast population were ever to receive adequate medical care.

Welch himself was deeply impressed by the life and the art of the Chinese. During his first afternoon in Peking, he wandered alone about the streets, on foot and in rickshas. He found his way at once to the South Gate of the Imperial City, through which he was not permitted to pass. Then by following devious lanes he managed to circumnavigate the Imperial City as closely as possible. "Scarcely any of it was to be seen," he recorded in his diary, "except occasional glimpses of trees and yellow-tiled roofs and the beautiful pink walls. . . . At one place there was an opening through which I had a beautiful view of the wall, parapets and moat. . . . The streets were dirty and odorous and very dusty—street scenes not particularly interesting or lively. . . . I probably walked altogether about 4 miles." After a night on the train and an early morning arrival, this expedition through the deep dust of Peking streets was a notable proof of Welch's interest.

Whenever he could escape from duty he was off, either alone or with his associates. "After dinner Greene, Buttrick, Flexner, Gates and I had a short conference. . . . We then with Mrs. Flexner took a fascinating walk on the top of the wall separating the inner and outer cities until we were stopped by an Austro-Hungarian sentry guarding a tower. Beautiful moonlight night, enchanting effect." He often walked in the late afternoon on this wall, an activity which he regarded as "one of the delights of the stay in Peking."

On their second day the members of the commission, after inspecting a hospital, visited the Temple of Heaven, or Tientan, which happened to be near by. "Very interesting and much that is beautiful. The altar or Tien-tan proper, the most sacred place, where the Emperor came to pray, is now a deserted place. We ascended and stood on the central round stone—the centre of the Universe. This would have been impossible for us before the republic, and it seemed a sacrilege,—beautiful blue tiles."

Welch, Caroline Buttrick, my wife, and I together made the two-day expedition north to Nankou to see the Great Wall and the Ming Tombs. Concerning the inner wall Welch wrote: "The view of it is wonderfully fine, one of the great sights of the world, the most stupendous work of man, when taken in its entirety. We saw it winding like a serpent, climbing steep heights, dipping into valleys, stretching as far as the eye could reach on both sides of us. . . . Many flowers in the broad path along the top of the wall—bluebells, asters, pinks." The next morning the group went to the Ming Tombs. Welch complained of his "pony with a sharp saddle. An uncomfortable and fatiguing also chafing ride on the backs of these most uncomfortable beasts over a rough road and paths for seven hours. . . . Still the sight is not to be missed. The magnificent five-span pailow—a beautifully sculptured monument—some 50 feet high and 75 broad, makes a truly splendid entrance. The distance of the Yung-loh tomb from this gate-way is about 3 miles. The holy way is lined on each side with elephants and fabulous animals, horses, warriors, sages, priests, a most remarkable sight." We visited only one tomb (that of Yung-loh), but Welch found the courtyards with their fine pines and other trees delightful, the pavilions beautiful, and the whole effect enchanting. "Our two days at the Great Wall have been full of wonder and delight."

The summer palace near Peking aroused Welch's particular admiration. He noted that the old palace having been ruth-

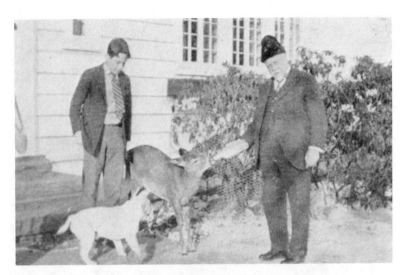

Feeding Time:
Welch and Alex Walcott

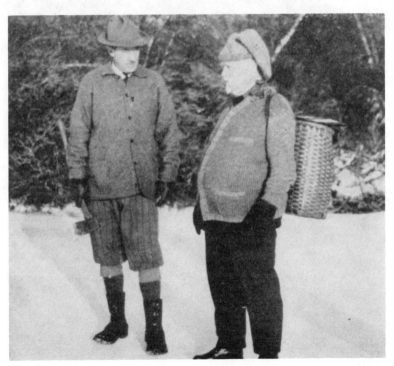

The Woodsmen:
Welch and Frederic C. Walcott

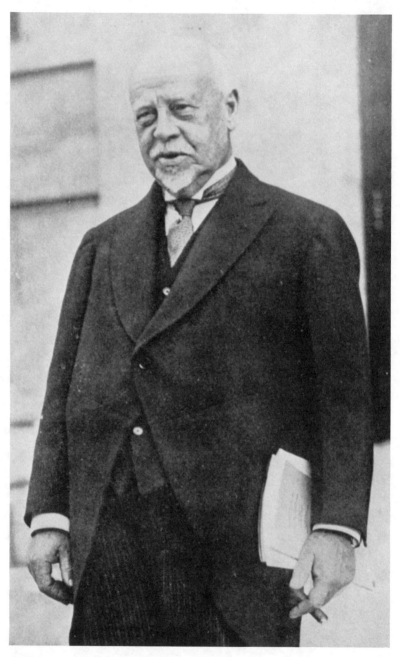

Welch at Seventy-Six

lessly destroyed by the British and French in 1860, the present one was largely the creation of the Empress Dowager. He delighted in the two bridges connecting the artificial island with the lake shore: the 17-span bridge with its fine curve, and the famous camel-back bridge, both of marble. "There are numerous courtyards and halls and pavilions, and there arise from the shore of the lake up the hillside the most beautiful series of pavilions with golden yellow and green tiled roofs culminating in the magnificent temples at the top."

There were some disappointments, however: the Lama Temple which Welch visited with Buttrick disturbed his usual equanimity. "Nothing could exceed the irritation and annoyance caused by these predatory rascals, dressed in brown robes of Lamaists, who guard every gate and door to be opened only upon payment of as much as can be extorted, of the crowd of loafers, alleged guides, beggars and boys who surround the visitors. . . . We dropped $2.20 altogether before escaping from the temple." But calm returned with the prayer wheels and the Confucian temple, "impressive and serene," which they next visited. The Hall of Classics was another compensation, with its ancestral tablets of Confucius and various sages, its magnificent marble and tile pailow, and "the stones on which the thirteen classics are inscribed so that they may be imperishable and serve as the authorized text." Welch recorded that the mad emperor, Chin-Shuh-Huang, who began the building of the Great Wall, had burned all the books.

When he was a medical student in New York, one of Welch's most enjoyed diversions had been to visit art collections, especially with his sister when she came to visit him. So he took great pleasure from the works of art in Peking. The first opportunity he had to see them was when the Minister of Foreign Affairs, Lu Ching-hsing, entertained the commission and the ladies formally at tiffin at one of the beautiful old Chinese pavilions within the Forbidden City. The long table for fifty guests and the walls of the pavilion were decorated with national treasures, some of them recently brought from the palace of Jehol. Welch enumerated in his diary the bronzes, lacquer boxes, jewelled artificial flowers, tapestries, embroideries, and paintings, regretting that he had been given no opportunity to examine them. Later with my wife and me he visited the museum. "I should love," he wrote, "to spend more time and really study Chinese art in this exhibit."

With delight Welch entered into the gaieties of the Chinese people. He visited the theatre and hugely enjoyed the native food. I remember well one dinner of thirty-seven courses by actual count. While I picked my way carefully through the menu, searching for innocent dishes, Welch, as he wrote in his diary, "tasted everything—nothing really distasteful and many things I liked. I really enjoyed the '4000 year eggs,' the bird's nest and sharks' fins, the duck's liver and the roast Peking duck, dipped with chop-sticks into a brown sauce and then rolled within a pancake—really delicious." He found much of refinement and subtlety in Chinese sauces and dainty dishes; the Mandarins, he decided, must be great epicures. Sir John Jordan, the British ambassador, watched Welch with amazement and not without anxiety. "I think," noted Welch, "that he expects me to be prostrated." Indeed, I myself was worried for Welch, and this fear increased when on my return to the hotel I felt far from well despite the caution with which I had eaten; if a few simple dishes had this effect on me, what would sharks' fins and eggs of guaranteed antiquity do to Welch? The next morning I kept to my bed; Welch was never more blooming.

The Peking experiences closed with an audience with the President of China, Yuan Shih-kai, who "beamed and expressed his gratification and welcome and [spoke] of the need of China for improved medical education and practice." Welch noted that the President gave his approval to the plan "to establish a few first-rate schools to serve as models for the country," and was delighted that "the ultimate aim was to hand over the work, when it became possible, to the Chinese themselves."

From Peking the commission travelled via Changsha, where we visited Yale-in-China, to Shanghai. In this metropolis there were again fascinating sights to see and interesting people to meet: American, English, and Chinese. Having visited the mission schools and hospitals in the region, the commission approved the project of eventually making the Red Cross Hospital into a second modern medical school. We then went south to Canton, from which place we returned to Japan on our way home.

Welch, my wife, and I could not resist making a brief side trip together through the Inland Sea. When we started from Kobe, the day was overcast; my wife and I put on rubbers and carried umbrellas. Having taken no such precaution, Welch was delighted when the sun came out. "Flexner," he asked innocently, "do you always wear rubbers?" He enjoyed the joke hugely for a while, but by the time we reached the station, the rain was coming down in torrents. I offered him a share of my umbrella, which he spurned. With a resolutely casual air, he walked through the downpour to a little Japanese tea shop; the proprietor bowed almost to the ground to receive him. "Have you got an umbrella?" Welch asked in English. The man bowed even deeper. Welch repeated his question, spacing the words and enunciating with great clearness. I ventured to whisper in his ear that the Japanese probably did not understand English, at which Welch nudged me impatiently with his elbow and repeated his question even more slowly and with greater emphasis. Another deep bow was the only answer. Welch again spurned a place under my umbrella as we walked through the rain to the little boat that was to take us to the island of Miyajima.

On the island, my wife and I took shelter in the station, waiting for the hotel launch, but Welch walked off up the steep street, saying that now he would get an umbrella. Ten, fifteen, twenty minutes passed. We were beginning to be anxious when suddenly the dean of American medicine appeared at the top of the slope, a many-coloured Japanese umbrella over his head, and his bulk balancing precariously on high wooden sandals that kept his feet above water; they were tied to his shoes with cord. Gravely, deliberately he came down the flowing incline, on his face a smile of triumph.

The boat that was to take us through the Inland Sea was to pick us up at six in the morning, and I so informed Welch. He said I must be mistaken; that no boat ever landed anywhere at six in the morning. He also said that he could not possibly wake up, and that I would have to wake him, adding: "You know, Flexner, I don't sleep. I simply go into coma. When you come into my room, wake me up, which you will do with some difficulty. And then I will say, 'All right. I am awake. I will get up.' But don't go out of the room; stay until I am on my feet, or I will go to sleep again." I carried out the instructions to the letter.

Fortunately, the rain vanished before we got on the boat. "No words can describe the entrancing beauty of the scenery through which we passed," Welch noted; "the larger and smaller islands, all mountainous, the narrow passages between the islands, the wonderful and ever changing shapes of islands, mountains and stretches of water. We had a glorious sunrise." In fact he was so enthralled that he refused to turn back with my wife and me; he went on alone to the famous temple at Kotohira, although this involved spending the night at a native inn at Tadotsu.

Welch was met at the door not only by the landlord, who spoke hardly any English, but also by "three maids with something of the manners and appearance of Geisha of the giggling sort." Removing his shoes, they escorted him to "a good-sized room with fine, soft mats, an alcove with a pretty Kakemono and a vase of chysanthemums, and not a single piece of furniture in it. . . . The girls were much too attentive. A chair and a table were brought in to suit foreign tastes, and I ordered a dinner of chicken, rice, fried eggs and tea to be served at seven o'clock. The meal was good enough, but the girls flitted in and out, and knelt before the table as I ate." After they had laid his bedding on the floor, the girls offered to help Welch disrobe and had to be shooed from the room. Suspecting that they had not gone, Welch pushed back one of the screens and the girls laughingly scampered away. "It is apparent that the girls are there for other purposes than as maid-servants. . . . I wanted an experience in a Japanese inn, but once is enough."

Special performances of the ancient No dances were being given all over Japan at that time in honour of the national festival. In Tokyo Welch went to several with my wife and me; he was keenly interested by discovering a similarity between these dances and our Western opera, of which he was so great a lover. Unfortunately there is no reference to the No dances in the hasty notes of his last days in Japan.

On December 8 a representative of the Minister of Education came to the hotel to confer decorations on Welch and on me. "A room with fire and tea" had been taken, and here the commission, wearing Prince Albert coats, awaited the emissary. The record in Welch's diary is: "I received the Order of the Rising Sun, 3rd Class, and Flexner the Order of the Sacred Treasure, 3rd Class. Superb red jewel in center of gold and enamel star, with red button. Flexner has blue button."

III

By 1921 the new buildings of the Peking Union Medical College were ready to be dedicated. The younger Rockefeller, who planned to attend the ceremonies with his wife and daughter, insisted that Welch come too. "It is of the utmost importance that you should be there," he wrote. "It will mean more to the medical world than the presence of any other one man." Thus in August Welch found himself crossing the continent in Rockefeller's private railway car. His diary records in his accurate way: "The car has five private rooms, kitchen, dining room, sitting room at rear and observation platform, shower bath, and is most comfortable. I have the front room to myself."

On his arrival in Peking Welch saw so great a transformation that he might well have thought some Oriental magician had been at work. In the six years since his previous visit the Peking Union Medical College had arisen full-fledged, a "Green City" rivalling in a way the Yellow, or Imperial, City which had taken generations to build. The fourteen buildings which comprised the main group were so designed as to harmonize with the great architectural monuments of Peking, their most striking features being the curved roofs of green tile, with conventional decorations of the eaves in colour; and the entrance courts designed after models of old temples and palaces, but adapted to the practical purposes for which the buildings were to be used. Welch wrote his niece: "The new buildings . . . are magnificent, one of the sights of Peking and indeed of all China, and are greatly admired by the Chinese for their conformity to their architecture. . . . They have cost between seven and eight million dollars, and there is nothing in America to equal them.

"The trustees," Welch continued, "had many difficult problems to solve regarding the future of the Medical School, and their meetings and many scientific conferences and addresses did not leave much time for sightseeing." Indeed, Welch was very busy during his two weeks in Peking before the dedicatory exercises. He familiarized himself with the new institution, inspecting every nook and corner of it, had conferences with the now assembled staff,[4] examined the laboratories with a practised eye, and made his own observations and drew his own conclusions on the qualities and personalities of the teachers, who had still to adapt themselves to the new conditions and to learn to work together. As in all such new organizations, there were personal adjustments to be made. The splendour of the school and the very excellence of the facilities placed before men who had previously worked with simpler and older apparatus raised wants which sometimes struck Welch as fantastic. Rockefeller remembers: "While in Peking there were daily meetings of the Trustees. . . . Dr. Welch was present one day . . . when an earnest plea was being made for more adequate equipment for one of the research laboratories. When asked for his opinion, with his customary modesty he said in substance: 'The research work, such as it has been, that I have done during my life, was carried on in quarters vastly less well-equipped than those which I have seen here. . . . It would hardly seem to me that they were inadequate or needed elaboration.'"

In the dedicatory exercises highest officials of government, foreign dignitaries, delegates from many countries participated. Welch recorded that the ceremonies were "simply perfect" and that everyone was "most enthusiastic." He referred especially to an account of the construction of the new building quoted by

Rockefeller in his address: "Master Chinese craftsmen have told me . . . that no other building erected in China in the past century was so profound an inspiration to Chinese artisans. They did not like the window-casings, they felt the lack of the massive deep-shadowed effect that columns would have produced and they thought the unsupported walls too frail for the roof, but, because the building was one in which the soul of a people could express itself, they travelled long distances for the privilege of working on it, even in the humblest capacity. Men who were master stone-carvers in their own districts were willing to work as coolies, if only they might say that they had been employed on the construction of this building. Farmers from the Western Hills, descendants of the architects that built the Peking palaces, were content to haul dirt on wheel barrows if they might have some share in this masterpiece. I once met an old artist, a painter of temples from his boyhood, who had painted certain of the figures near the roof of the hospital. From the ground they were barely visible, but he had put the training of a lifetime and all his soul into the work. 'It is,' he said, 'my monument.' "

Welch himself spoke several times, using the historical approach to emphasize again to his Chinese audiences the value of observation and experiment as compared to reliance on tradition. Eloquently he pointed out that modern scientific medicine began with the study of anatomy, which was still the basis of "real knowledge of disease." The meaning of these words was clear to his hearers: ancestor worship must not be allowed to interfere with human dissection and the performance of autopsies. At a pathological conference, Welch adjured the staff to study local problems of disease rather than to follow lines of research which could as well be pursued in Boston and Baltimore.

The exercises over, Welch sailed with the rest of the Rockefeller party in Standard Oil launches up the Whangpoo to Soochow and Wusih. "When we tie up for the night there are altogether six boats in our flotilla." This was another of the "not-to-be-forgotten experiences." It was delightful to sit in an easy chair on the deck, reading and watching the river. He saw men fishing with cormorants; he saw water buffalo, working stolidly in the fields or resting in the shallows with only their noses above water. And always there was the endless procession of junks, riding under brown rectangular sails, their decks teeming with the life of the Orient. This trip gave Welch an idea of the delights of house-boating on the streams and canals of China.

Since Welch had continually warned the Rockefellers of the dangers of unwashed raw fruit in China, Rockefeller was horrified one day to see him buy a persimmon from a vender on the street and immediately begin eating it. "Why, Dr. Welch," Rockefeller cried, "you should not do that!"

Welch looked up with benign surprise. "Why not?"

"You might get some disease."

"What, for instance?"

"You might get cholera."

"Yes, but what else?" Welch asked, calmly continuing to eat the fruit.

This incident was typical; once in London he ate unwashed cherries, explaining to Freeman that he did it to keep his immunity up. Welch, who continually advised a strictly hygienic life to others, loved to boast that he violated all his own precepts. Thus, after sending a friend a list of rules for health, he added: "I break every one of them and am perfectly well although my anterior-posterior measurement is large."

The work of the China Medical Board of the Rockefeller Foundation has done much to raise medical standards in China. As a result of the labours of the 1915 commission, of which Welch was the leading member, the missionaries became more conscious of the inadequacies of their own schools. A Council of Medical Education of the China Medical Missionary Society has been established, with a most salutary effect on the schools which continue to teach in Chinese.

The Peking Union Medical College itself has after twenty years almost reached its goal of preparing the Chinese to take over its teaching, its research, and the clinical duties of its hospital. The departments of biochemistry, physiology, bacteriology, and pediatrics are entirely in their hands. Although the departments of anatomy, pathology, medicine, surgery, gynæcology, neurology, and psychiatry still have European heads, their staffs consist entirely of Chinese. A beginning has been made, partly through Welch's influence, in bringing modern medical science to one of the largest and potentially most powerful nations of the world. The end, of course, lies in the future, but one need not be a visionary to foresee that as the vast reservoir of China fills with knowledge, new discoveries will arise there that will contribute to the well-being of the Western world, as Western science has contributed to the well-being of the Orient.

CHAPTER XIX

History of Medicine

I

ON New Year's Day 1925, Welch wrote: "It is more than time for me to resign from active academic duties. I shall be seventy-five in April. . . . I have always been critical of those who lingered on in professorial chairs, blocking the way for their eager successors. It was a good thing that I made way for Mac-Callum nearly ten years ago. The School of Hygiene is well launched and successful beyond my expectations within a remarkably short period of existence. The new building will be ready in a year, and Howell, who carries the heavier part of the load, deserves to be made full director and would carry on the work admirably. . . . The directorship could not be in better hands." [1]

Welch asked to resign at the end of that academic year, but was persuaded to wait until the following autumn, when the new quarters of the School of Hygiene would be dedicated and the university celebrate its fiftieth anniversary. "This will constitute a fitting termination of the great work you have done in building up the school," President Goodnow wrote, adding that he hoped Welch would not really retire, but rather change to another sphere of usefulness. "Your new title should be one of dignity and position. We cannot conceive of you as 'emeritus.' "

Indeed, Welch had just shown that he still possessed great energy. Intent on establishing on a full-time basis "a first class ophthalmological clinic, where young men could be trained and investigations in ophthalmology carried out," the university approached Dr. William H. Wilmer, who agreed to postpone accepting the offer of a new laboratory and hospital in Washington until October 1924, by which time the Hopkins hoped it could raise the necessary $3,000,000. The General Education

Board gave half the sum, but then the campaign bogged down. Although Wilmer postponed his deadline for three months, all seemed lost until Welch intervened actively. He made trips to New York and other cities, where he rose early day after day, getting interviews with wealthy people through their friends or through friends of friends. Wilmer tells us: "Mrs. Breckinridge presented him with the names of three persons to be interviewed. He first called upon P—— W——, and with his usual charm said: 'Mr. W——, I believe you are a patient and friend of Dr. Wilmer?' Mr. W. acknowledged the accusation. Dr. Welch explained the plan for the Institute and said with his disarming smile: 'If you could start us out with a little donation, say about $250,000, it would be very helpful in our undertaking.' This Mr. W. did without hesitation. Dr. Welch next called upon Mr. H., whom he also accused of being my friend. He then went on to say, 'I believe you sometimes match P—— W—— in his philanthropies.' Mr. H. acknowledged the impeachment, whereupon Dr. Welch explained the reason for his visit and said: 'Won't you match Mr. W. in this case?' Mr. H. replied that he would be very glad to do so. Then Dr. Welch called upon Mr. M., who had already given $30,000 to the Wilmer Foundation. Very ingratiatingly Dr. Welch expressed his appreciation of Mr. M.'s generous gift, but said: 'Don't you think that you should increase it a little?' Mr. M. asked: 'Would $100,000 do?' Dr. Welch replied that he thought it would do very nicely. Later Mr. M. told his partner that he was much relieved when Dr. Welch left, because Dr. Welch was so charming and beguiling that he could have gotten all of his possessions if he had remained a little longer. In the space of a portion of one morning Dr. Welch had secured $600,000." By the end of January he had raised all the necessary funds except $100,000, which the university agreed to assume. Thus the famous Wilmer Institute came into being.

No wonder his colleagues were convinced that Welch was still too active to retire; a plot was hatched to keep him in harness. Fielding H. Garrison, editor of the *Index Medicus*, wrote him on April 21, 1925, that he hoped "you will give favorable consideration to the idea Dr. Thayer broached—that you take up now the history of medicine and do something for it. Only you could do this in a country constituted as ours. . . . I mean there would be no intransigence if your suave, persuasive personality got these fellows going." Abraham Flexner, the secretary of the General Education Board, urged the creation of a chair of the history of medicine, with Welch as the first incumbent.

It was natural that these men turned to Welch, who had long recognized that American doctors, although better trained scientifically and technically than the physicians of previous generations, had lost touch with the cultural side of medicine and had little idea of the part medicine had played in the development of science. Welch, however, did not feel he was the man to inaugurate medical historical studies. He told Flexner that Garrison would be a much better choice,[2] and to Garrison himself he wrote: "The suggestion . . . does not commend itself to me for several reasons. The only consideration of the least weight is that an endowment for such a chair might be secured, if I would consent, and that thus the thing might be launched, which we have long earnestly desired. My dream has been a central library for the hospital, medical school and School of Hygiene, and in connection with this an endowed chair of the history of medicine. You are the one we have always thought of for such a chair. You and Streeter are the only serious students and representatives of the history of medicine in this country and there is no reason to look further. For me to take such a chair at my age would merely emphasize the spirit of dilettantism in which the subject is regarded and pursued generally in this country. I have a high conception of what a department of the history of medicine could be made—not merely a cultural centre, important as that is, but a real adjuvant of the development of scientific medicine."

Welch's suggestion that Garrison be given the position failed to take root, while the General Education Board made it clear that the money would be appropriated if Welch accepted. In May 1925 Welch gave in, for reasons which he later described to his niece: "The time is ripe and the opportunity splendid for getting the subject of medical history well established and properly recognized both on the research and the teaching sides in our medical schools, and I am quite enthusiastic over the prospects, although at my age I cannot expect to do much more than start the ball rolling. I should have insisted on retiring from academic work if it did not seem that my friends could get the money if I would undertake the job. Under the circumstances it seemed impossible to decline. I think they thought it would be a softer berth than I am inclined to make it." [3]

His friends went perhaps a little too far in their efforts to reassure Welch about undertaking a new project at his age. Thus Abraham Flexner wrote: "You should spend your loafing years lolling about in a chair of the history of medicine. I can't help thinking that you would find that a charming thing to do if no duties were attached to the post." Welch's letters reveal a little irritation at being thus considered an old man. "I wonder," he wrote Cushing, "if Weed has told you about plans to deposit me on a chair, litter or lounge of the History of Medicine." Yet he could not escape a sense of insecurity in tackling so big a job at his years; to Cushing he continued: "If I could hold it down for a year or two for you to come and really develop the subject, the thought and prospect would be a real elixir of life."

In February 1926 the General Education Board appropriated $200,000 toward the endowment of a chair of the history of medicine, and voted to co-operate with the university in establishing what was to be named the William H. Welch Medical Library. The necessary fund for the latter was completed two years later when Edward S. Harkness gave half a million.[4]

Goodnow formally notified Welch on November 2, 1926, of his transfer to the professorship of the history of medicine. Now that the chair of a humanistic subject had come to him, Welch must have felt that again he had realized an old ambition. Before he had been interested in medicine, he had wanted to be a professor of Greek, not because of a narrow interest in linguistics, but because he was fascinated by the history and literature of classic times. And when he became a scientist at last, he never lost contact with other aspects of culture. His delight in the classics continued. "I have lost most of my knowledge of the language," he wrote in 1907, "but I love to read about the Greeks, especially their literature." And to the end of his days he was convinced that "everything that moves in the modern world has its roots in Greece."

Of the arts, perhaps opera was his major love. Having admired Wagner while that composer was still anathema to conservative critics, he continued to glory in the "Wagner cult." Everywhere he travelled, he went to the opera, seeing not only established dramas but the work of local composers from Sweden to the Balkans. His tenacious memory was full of operatic lore; once he kept the singer Lawrence Tibbett enthralled until three-thirty in the morning, talking of debuts, and dead stars, and famous performances, all with dates attached. Afterward Tibbett said: "It is amazing the fund of knowledge that man has on musical subjects. . . . He told me many things which were absolutely new to me; and I shall never forget this evening." Welch's musical interest, however, does not seem to have carried over to concerts; he went to them only occasionally, and said little about them in his letters.

While abroad, he attended art exhibitions, reading them up in guide books; if his comments show no startling critical acumen, they reveal a catholic appreciation that enabled him to admire all good art, the old masters and the modern French painters. When Sargent painted his famous Four Doctors in 1905, Welch talked to him by the hour about painting; later he was able to quote at length erudite comparisons Sargent had made between Reynolds and Gainsborough, Hals and Rembrandt. He was so interested by what the artist told him about the Dutch school that as soon as the sittings were over he made a special trip to the galleries of Holland, following an itinerary Sargent gave him. After his early New York period, however, he seems rarely to have attended art shows in the United States, when he would have had to spare the time from pressing duties.

Welch was, of course, an omnivorous reader. Sitting up in bed till dawn, he enjoyed everything from books on ancient Greece and Rome, from the history and literature of the Middle Ages, to modern novels and detective stories. Factual books were his great delight. Visitors to the University Club are still shown with reverence a battered set of the *Encyclopædia Britannica* which Welch is said to have worn out almost single-handed; he is reputed to have read it through several times. And the members of the Maryland Club, refusing to be outdone, also ascribe their battered *Encyclopædia* to Welch, adding proudly that he also wore out their *Dictionary of National Biography*. Not only did Welch have a set of the latter work in his rooms, but he enjoyed it so much that he sent a copy to his niece. "You must have the books handy and get the National Biography habit," he wrote. "There are no such short biographies anywhere. . . . I have made the greatest use of it for the history of English medicine. It will be easy for you to become erudite in English literature."

That Welch should early have been attracted by the historical side of medicine grew naturally out of his habits of mind. He remembered: "My interest began while I was in pursuit of pathology, as far back as my student days in Breslau." He attended Heinrich Haeser's lectures, which he found "deadly dull."

While Welch was in New York and during his first Baltimore years he was too busy laying the foundations for pathology to give much thought to medical history; when in 1886 he outlined the projected medical school he failed to mention the subject, although Billings had nine years before urged that it be taught at the Hopkins.[5] In 1888, however, Welch made up for this omission, advocating in a speech at Yale "the study of the history of medicine, a subject which notwithstanding its interest and values is much neglected. Nothing is more liberalizing and conducive to medical culture than to follow the evolution of medical knowledge."

Osler and Kelly, both of whom were historical-minded, came to Baltimore in 1889, and a year later Osler took the lead in founding the Johns Hopkins Hospital Historical Club, of which Welch was elected the first president.[6] At the inaugural meeting Welch spoke on the value of historical studies to the physician and year after year he addressed the club, whose meetings, Cole tells us, "exerted a deep and lasting influence on all the students and assistants. They stirred into life a new side of our personalities, the cultivation of which is important, even in those whose chief interest is science, since the scientist requires more than the ability to reason, he needs imagination." Welch continued his interest in the club all during his professorship of pathology; shortly after he resigned to go to the School of Hygiene, the meetings lapsed for a time.[7]

Welch's historical talks at the Hopkins, and the many others which he gave outside the walls of the university, covered a wide range of subjects. He spoke on Greek medicine, on the medicine of the seventeenth century, on English medicine and its influence in America; he traced briefly the evolution of pathology or of the modern laboratory; he delivered appraisals of famous scientists such as Virchow and Koch. Nor were these purely historical addresses his only discussions of the subject; he was likely to take a long view on any matter about which he spoke. Thus in writing up experiments or advocating medical reforms, he almost invariably dealt with what had gone before; his mind continually called on the past to shed its light on the present.

In one of his historical addresses, Welch explained: "My purpose is . . . to point out from readily accessible data some of the more important influences that have determined the development of medical science." Relying on standard works in several languages, many of which he had in his own library, he never attempted to get back to first sources. Indeed, he usually covered so broad a field that detailed research was unnecessary; he would, for instance, discuss the whole history of pathology in an hour. A wide range of biographies and biographical reference books sufficed to give him most of the information he needed, since he usually approached the science of a period through the work of its outstanding representatives; he always placed special emphasis on the medical genealogy of who studied with whom.

Dr. Thomas McCrae, of the Hopkins staff, recalled that Welch spent an entire summer studying English medicine of the early nineteenth century. "He showed me the large number of cards which he had written; there were several hundred of them. He said that he had enjoyed himself much more than he could have on any vacation." The quantity of such notes testifies to Welch's industry, but the complete lack of system with which he filed them away on any chair or bookcase or in any drawer where there was yet room makes us wonder whether, once the notes were made, he was ever able to consult them again. Fortunately he did not need to, since the very act of writing facts down engraved them on his memory, and once his mind was charged with information on a subject he could summon up the information at will. Welch's memory was one of his most amazing characteristics. When he heard a strange disease discussed, he would say something like "There is a description of a similar case in the *Münchener Medizinische Wochenschrift* for 1903, volume thirty-four, page one hundred and seven . . . yes, I think on page one hundred and seven." And he would be right. As Osler said, "In addition to a three-story intellect Welch has an attic on top." This attic was crammed with exactly memorized information.

Welch was able to deliver an accurate historical talk from an outline jotted down shortly before a meeting; or if a scheduled speaker failed to turn up, he could do almost as well from no notes at all. Even when he wrote out a speech, he was likely to do it at the last moment, and often entirely from memory. Thus in 1907 he composed his address as president of the American Association for the Advancement of Science without notes in the Pullman car on the way to the meeting in Chicago; the resulting speech, in which he showed, as he loved to do, that medicine "continued for many centuries to be the shelter for most of the natural sciences," was said by Garrison to be "the best study ever made of the interrelationship of medicine and science." [8]

Welch's contribution as a historical writer did not rest on the discovery of new facts, but rather on his broad culture, which extended far beyond the limits of specialized scientific history and enabled him to create general syntheses which caught the imagination of his hearers. In a typical speech on Vesalius he pointed out that in 1543, "the very year of the publication of Vesalius' great work, the epochal contribution of Copernicus established the theory of the solar system. . . . Toward the end of this century . . . came the discoveries of the great Spanish and Portuguese explorers, opening up a new world. . . . Another great in-

fluence to open men's minds to new knowledge was the revival
of classical learning." Printing and cheap paper had been known
for a hundred years, he continued, and the sixteenth century
was "the age of Raphael, of Titian, of Michael Angelo and of
Leonardo da Vinci, indeed one of the greatest periods in the
world's history of art. . . . The artists themselves were often
anatomists and loved to make anatomical drawings. Leonardo da
Vinci, the most varied genius probably who ever lived . . .
ranks as a great anatomist. . . .

"This was also a marvelous period in literature, both in poetry
and in prose. It is interesting to recall that one of the great names
of French literature, Rabelais, was a medical man and a contemporary of Vesalius." In botany it was the time of the herbal-
ists, most of whom were physicians and who had much influence
on medicine. Gesner, one of the fathers of modern zoology, was
also a contemporary, as were the humanistic physicians, including Linacre, who "were characterized by love of classical learning, and often believed that the salvation of medicine rested on
going back to the original writings of Hippocrates, of Galen, of
Dioscorides and of Celsus."

A deep scholar of pathology and bacteriology, Welch never
forgot that his historical addresses, for all their interest and
charm, were not original contributions; he allowed only a few
of them to be published, eliminating works that a lesser man
might have pointed to with pride. And when at seventy-six he
was appointed professor of the history of medicine, he showed
that all the honours and adulation he had received had failed
to dull his realistic evaluation of himself and his work. His election as president of the American Association of Medical History drew from him the comment: "For a budding historian, I
have a running start." He told his niece that he would have to
go "to school again." [9]

In his capacity as schoolboy, Welch soon had a suitable es-
capade to report. "Mary Garden, who summoned me to her
dressing room after the third act of 'Resurrection,' in which she
is really wonderful, and kissing me on both cheeks (all male
Baltimore wildly jealous), made me promise to visit her at Monte

Carlo, where she has her summer villa, but I do not take this too seriously." He enjoyed having his friends tease him about "the divine Mary."

II

On May 20, 1927, Welch sailed to Europe for another period of study and to buy books on medical history for the library. "Simon Flexner," he wrote, "seems rather distressed at my going over alone, but I rather prefer to be foot-free and to strike my own pace; besides I am feeling very well and fit, and anticipate no trouble. The six months will be all too short for doing all that I should like and have planned."

Welch had already resolved that the chair of history of medicine he filled would have to be expanded if the subject were to be adequately handled. "I want to get launched as soon as possible a genuine Institute of Medical History connected with the professorship and the library—altogether a good-sized job," he wrote on May 15, 1927. As he noted in his diary a few months later, "A mere 'Lehrstuhl' of medical history is like a chair of anatomy, physiology, pathology, etc., without laboratory, assistants, staff, and budget." Welch had never been satisfied with professorships that did not present opportunities to train young men in methods of research. Indeed, the idea of a historical institute must long have been in his mind, for on September 30, 1924, he wrote Arnold C. Klebs, whom he had recently visited at Nyon, Switzerland: "I shall interest myself more than I have done in that institute for the history of science, which if properly located, conducted and supported, should be an important undertaking."

Naturally, Welch hurried to Leipzig, where Karl Sudhoff had founded "the only well developed Institute of Medical History"; since Sudhoff's retirement it had been under the directorship of Henry E. Sigerist. Welch wrote that he had "a most interesting and enjoyable week there with Sudhoff and Sigerist. I am delighted with both, and especially with Sudhoff, who is a truly great man in his own field. We had walks and talks and luncheons and dinners together, and I obtained some idea of what a real Institute for the History of Medicine should be." Welch's visit confirmed his belief that a mere chair of history was not enough.[10]

From Leipzig Welch went to Carlsbad for his usual cure, and then to the International Congress of Medical History at Leiden. "This enabled me to meet the leading medical historians of Europe, who, I must say, welcomed me with open arms to their ranks, although I have no right to claim admission to such a gathering of Fach-historiker." It was, he wrote, "a new crowd for me to get in with." He stayed at an uncomfortable hotel so as to be in the same quarters with the historians, and he found his personal talks with them more interesting than the sessions, at one of which he presided. Welch's formal contribution was limited to taking part in the discussions. "In reply to a remark by Klebs that Wu Lien Teh's monograph on plague, which he praised, has the usual slight and unsatisfactory reference to the history of plague . . . I said that the historians of plague—'Pest-Schriften' investigators—often show lack of knowledge of the important facts now known about plague and mentioned that plague is really an epizootic disease and narrated the story which the Jesuit missionary in Peking in 1921 told about the rodent (marmot-like) in Western China and Tibet harboring plague and taboo against touching the animal on part of Tibetans—whereas Chinese, without these taboos, contracted disease." Writing up the conference for the *Nederlandsch Tijdschrift voor Geneeskunde,* G. van Rijnberk stated that Welch's remarks were the most important made at the congress.

On the spur of the moment, some of the historians made a pilgrimage to Boerhaave's statue, where Tricot-Royer spoke extemporaneously for France and Welch for America. Although Welch noted in his diary that his remarks were not important, Klebs remembers them as the feature of the occasion, and the Swedish medical bibliophile Erik Waller wrote that they made the greatest impression on him of anything said at the congress. To Waller's request for a copy of his speech Welch replied that he could not recall what he had said. In his educational addresses, Welch often referred to Boerhaave. "It would be interesting to trace," he said on one occasion, "the evolution of methods of clinical instruction from their inception, or rather revival, in Padua by Montanus about the middle of the sixteenth century to the present time. We should follow the conveyance of these methods by the elder van Heurne . . . from Padua to Leyden, where in the course of a century they reached the high development attained under the great Boerhaave . . . and whence influences, spreading in the eighteenth century first to Göttingen, Halle, Vienna, and Edinburgh, can be traced continuously down to this very day and to the medical schools of America."

Welch noted that the Leiden conference marked the first time French and German medical historians had met together since the war of 1914. All along in his travels he commented on signs of continuing unrest; at Carlsbad he had remarked that the changing of all street names from German to Czech was "disgustingly puerile"; in Leipzig he wrote: "The Germans I see on the streets and the crowds in cafés and restaurants seem quiet, serious, not much gayety. . . . The general effect is drab, indeed melancholy. . . . Few auto-cars on the streets. The effect is of serious work and determination, and hard times and absence of fun and gayety. . . . His told of the dreadful economic status of the practitioners in Germany due to Kassen (panel) practice —poorly paid—15 pfenning a visit! Overcrowding of profession—best talent now going into industries rather than medicine —difficulty of getting assistants in medical sciences."

Passing through Paris in August, Welch interviewed both President Vincent of the Rockefeller Foundation and Abraham Flexner about getting an endowment of at least $500,000 for his projected Institute of the History of Medicine. To Flexner he wrote: "You thought, I am sure, that you were providing a soft, easy, comfy couch for me to fall into in my declining years, and I have never really told you how appreciative and grateful I am, but I cannot, in view of what I see in this wonderful opportunity, take up the job in that spirit. I was never more interested in any undertaking and would like to throw myself into it energetically and enthusiastically." Both Vincent and Flexner were encouraging; they suggested that his plans, when completed, be laid before the General Education Board.

Having attended the World Population Conference in Geneva, Welch spent a delightful ten days at Nyon with his old friend Arnold Klebs, the medical historian and bibliographer, to whom Welch had written: "No one is so informing and helpful as you in connection with my new job." Indeed, Welch seems to have leaned more on Klebs during this period than he had leaned on any other friend during his entire career; and the letters he wrote to his adviser are couched in terms he never used when he was younger. "You are the best comrade I know, and I cannot begin to tell you what a lot of information and inspiration I got from you. . . . Much love to you and Mrs. Klebs and untold (only too literally untold!) thanks for all your hospitality, kindness, and good comradeship." Welch noted in his diary that he kissed Mrs. Klebs on leaving, as he kissed Lady Osler the next year. He seems to have relaxed some of the reticences he had for so long observed; now many of his letters to friends are signed "love," and once he sent love to all his colleagues at the Hopkins.

In Nyon Welch discussed his tasks with Klebs by the hour, and he spent days in Klebs's historical library, copying down the titles of books and journals, and noting the names of booksellers. The Hopkins had given him $5000 before he sailed to buy books for the new medical library, and this sum was subsequently expanded to $12,500 by two separate grants from the General Education Board. Welch, however, had started out very cautiously; although he discussed bibliography with every medical historian he met and obtained lists from many bookstores, he made no actual purchases until shortly before his visit to Nyon. He was working his way gradually into a new field.[11]

With Klebs, Welch motored to Bad Homburg, where he presided at one session of the Deutsche Gesellschaft für Geschichte der Medizin, but took no very active part in the meetings; again his interest was in personal conversation with the historians there assembled. Then, "throwing off temporarily my disguise as a medical historian and assuming that of a hygienist," he accompanied "an international group of sanitarians under the auspices of the League of Nations through Hungary and Jugo-Slavia." [12]

Having attended the formal openings of the State Hygienic Institute at Budapest and the State Institute and School of Hygiene at Zagreb, Welch wrote of his delight at finding that the leading hygienic positions in Poland, Czechoslovakia, Hungary, and Yugoslavia were held by graduates of the Baltimore School of Hygiene. In each Balkan city the visitors conferred with the local sanitarians on curriculum; Welch commented: "The Rockefeller-aided institutes and schools—Warsaw, Prague, Budapest, Zagreb—make a group, and they propose cooperative work and exchanges on certain themes, as scarlet fever, etc., and question raised of publishing a journal representing them more particularly."

As with his fellow-scientists Welch was whisked from one city to another, for the first time in all the papers that have come down to us he expressed irritation at being dragged through so many scientific institutions. "Trogir," he wrote, "is a romantic city, and I wish we were shown less malaria and more art. . . . I insisted upon being shown the famous cathedral, but it was growing dark when we returned to Trogir and the view of the beauties was tantalizing." In Zagreb he put his foot down and refused to accompany the party to Belgrade and Macedonia; before he joined them some days later at Split, he enjoyed a short respite of sightseeing. He attended "the third performance of an opera by a Croatian composer—of course in Croatian—title something like 'Medvedgradska Kraljica,'—Scene 13th century —the black queen—snake motives. A really fine performance in a beautiful, good-sized opera-house—2 or 3 grand operas weekly and other nights the drama—in addition there is an operetta theatre. What a contrast to American cities of same size (130,000 inhabitants)! Voices and acting good—like a first class metropolis."

Typically, Welch was interested in the political condition of the countries he visited. "Hungarians consider their government a monarchy—no desire for a republic . . . land still in large estates . . . whereas in Jugo-Slavia the government is more democratic—no titles, not even 'excellency' allowed. Estates divided up and given to peasants—I understand without compensation—look up agrarian situation in two countries. Hungarians extremely dissatisfied with Trianon treaty."

At Dubrovnik (formerly Ragusa) on the Adriatic Welch settled down for an indefinite rest. He wrote Weed, the dean of the medical school, that he wished to have his leave of absence extended for the remainder of the academic year; it could be regarded, he pointed out, as a sabbatical, the first he had ever taken in his forty-three years at the Hopkins. He wished "to go on with this work of collecting books," and "to get acquainted with more workers in the field of medical history and to inform myself better about methods and results of study and research, especially in Universities, in this subject." The leave, of course, was granted.

To his niece he wrote: "Ragusa is more than a compensation for missing Biarritz. Here I am in the land of palms, oranges, figs, olives, cigars, pomegranates, cactus, with the most delightful, soft, balmy, warm days, excellent sea bathing, warm sun in the day time, but cool at night; a nice room with a balcony (where I have my breakfast) looking out on the unequalled blue of the broad Adriatic, with old medieval Fort Lorenzo in the foreground and a good view of wonderful city walls, only equalled to-day by those of Carcassone and Aigues-Mortes, and perfectly preserved—a city springing from old Epidamas, with reminiscences of the worship of Aesculapius—fine monasteries, churches, palaces, dating from the 13th, 14th, 15th centuries, a city full of romance and historical interest through Greek, Roman, Venetian days up to the present. Why look further for a place to settle down and read and rest and write and bathe and loaf to my heart's content? Given the opportunity, my capacity to loaf is unlimited."

However, the old war horse could not resist a bugle call. On receiving an invitation from Russell to "accompany him on a tour to the various anti-malarial stations which [L. W.] Hackett has established under the International Health Division of the Rockefeller Foundation in Italy," Welch hurried across the Adriatic to Rome, and took a strenuous ten days' trip that ended up in

Sicily. He noted: "I need only say that the results of the anti-larval use of Paris green (which is the central feature of [L. W.] Hackett's method—Gambusia being used also when practicable) are excellent and have eliminated malaria in Bianconovo and Sermoneta and lessened it elsewhere. Hackett has had to overcome serious obstacles and criticism, due mainly to international jealousies and reactionary opinions. Main reliance of Italians has been curative and prophylactic use of quinine, which is distributed free by the State—antilarval work considered impracticable. The widow of Celli has been among those attacking Hackett's methods. The ambassador from Argentina to Italy—a medical doctor—Ferris?—has led in opposing Anglo-Saxon vs. Latin methods, &c!! and largely through him a 'School of Malariology,' not a part of university, but under Ministry of Public Instruction, and supported by Mussolini—President V. Ascoli (prof. med., Rome) has been established. Perhaps a good thing and not opposed by Hackett, but motives in creating school were antagonistic."

On November 28 Welch settled in Taormina for more than a month of rest while the other members of the party returned to Rome. "This hotel is a beautiful old Dominican Monastery . . . and is fitted up with wonderful preservation of cloisters, church, corridors, and rooms (once the cells of the monks) as a most comfortable, luxurious abode. . . . I am sitting in my room looking out at the sea with its marvelous coloring and down into the lovely garden still ablaze with flowers,—roses, geraniums, marigolds, chrysanthemums, coxcomb, and many of which I do not know the names. The orange and lemon trees are loaded with fruit—figs, olives, almonds growing everywhere. . . . Glorious Aetna dominates it all, wonderful at sunrise (which I have actually seen) and last night indescribably beautiful in the most wonderful sunset which I have ever seen, and now by the full moon standing out at night with a silver white glow of its stupendous cone. I do not see how earth can offer anything more beautiful than Taormina at this time of the year."

From Taormina, Welch wrote the medical historian James J. Walsh, who was writing a book to be called *Laughter and*

Health: "Your idea about the gift of laughter to compensate the handicaps of an erect posture is, I fancy, entirely original." Then characteristically he allowed his mind to play with the novel theme; he discussed William James's theory that emotional sensation is the result rather than the cause of the particular muscular movements of each emotion, "just the opposite of the ordinary, common sense view of the sequence of events." Walsh, he continued, might be led into consideration of what the Germans call *Stimmung,* for which there is no exact English word; mood, temperament, tone are all included under *Stimmung,* he pointed out, adding that Halsted always wanted his patient to be in the right *Stimmung* before he operated.

After a prolonged stay in Naples, Welch reached England on May 10 to attend the Harvey Tercentenary celebrations held by the Royal College of Physicians at London, Oxford, and Cambridge. Again he was singled out among the distinguished delegates for special honours and was asked to speak.[13]

In London he was happily continuing his negotiations with officials of the General Education Board toward securing an endowment of $500,000 for his Institute of the History of Medicine, when he received a series of shocks. The first was Abraham Flexner's retirement from the board. "Have you really resigned . . . ?" Welch asked his friend. "I feel like an orphan bereft of his parental support, if you go." Instantly Welch turned to Dr. Rose, president of the board, writing him, he noted in his diary, "about desire to secure endowment, yielding $25,000 per annum for Institute of Med. History. Asked if after a year he might not consider taking presidency of J.H.U.—that I did not expect him to answer now."

When Rose turned up in London a month later, Welch received another shock; Rose told him that the "General and International Education Boards have used up about all the money set apart for medical education, which will hereafter be under Foundation, and that question of endowment for an institute of med. history I should take up with Vincent and especially Pearce . . . who is now the one charged with all grants through the Foundation for medical education." To Klebs Welch complained: "The various Rockefeller boards are being completely reorganized with such changes in personnel that I shall have to impress others than those I have previously relied upon with the importance of an institute of the history of medicine at J.H.U." Back in Paris in July, Welch saw Vincent, who showed continued interest in his project and urged him to write Richard M. Pearce.

On other matters Vincent was less enthusiastic. "I got the impression that on the whole Vincent is disappointed with outlook so far as enlisting good men either on staff of board, or in general for careers in public health. Thinks our School in Baltimore has turned out very few able men for public health careers, which do not attract best type." Concerning the foreign schools founded by the International Health Board, Vincent "questions certain policies, such as the separation so much insisted on by Rose of public health institutes from universities." Welch himself had questioned this policy in Prague.

Book buying had increasingly become Welch's major activity. At first, as we have seen, he sought advice and purchased little, but by February 1928 he had spent $3000. Seven months later he noted in his diary: "I have no idea what the total of my orders amounts to, but I am willing to pay out of my own pocket any excess over the appropriation of $12,500." Welch had found getting his accounts into shape a "nightmare. . . . Really an army of clerks is needed for this work, which is far more time-consuming and complicated than I had foreseen."

Difficulties crept in from many directions. To begin with, Welch had failed to take with him lists of the books already in the libraries of the medical school and hospital, nor did he write for them until he had been buying for many months. When the lists finally arrived, a hasty survey showed Welch he had bought fourteen books the medical school already owned. "There are doubtless more," he commented sadly, adding that those he had found had cost $143.59, "a goodly sum to have wasted."

Welch was never sure that he himself was not buying several copies of the same book. Since it had not occurred to him to keep his records on cards until it was too late, he relied on unsystematic lists of what he had purchased, which, as they mounted in number, were impossible to correlate with one another. Attempting to extricate himself, he made compilations, but they merely served to increase the sea of paper in which he floundered. Then there were the letters from scores of bookstores quoting prices, which should be compared before purchases were made, and which were all drawn up in different ways. Furthermore, he had many bibliographies of desirable works sent him by his friends, as well as lists in his own hand of books in the libraries he had visited. Soon bills began flooding in, which should be compared with records of purchases that were no longer findable. An unending fall of sheets of every size snowed him under—they fill six large boxes among his papers—and the individual entries must have run close to a hundred thousand.

"Another handicap," Welch wrote, "has been the absurd attempt to write my day's doings in a journal, which I shall never attempt again, as it precludes at the end of the day doing anything else and becomes an incubus, a nightmare, an obsession, a soul-destroying task." Indeed, his journal of this trip was the fullest he had kept so far; written in black ink and annotated in several other colours, it fills six large diaries and covers even the most insignificant event several times.

But the purchasing itself was fun. "I am in correspondence with half a dozen book dealers to whom I have sent lists of desiderata. It is a great game and quite fascinating," Welch wrote from Naples. He enjoyed rummaging through old bookstores; he would spend hours sitting in dark rooms redolent with the smell of old leather and dust while he pored over stock lists, or he would climb up on ladders himself and examine the shelves. When he saw books he wanted, his heart contracted a little, and sometimes he made lucky strikes. After a piece of good fortune in London he noted: "I shall gloat over Arnold Klebs who told me these were impossible to find now." Then, of course, there were the stalls on the quais in Paris, those most romantic of all bookshops; Welch could never pass them by, and often he had to take a taxi to get all his purchases back to the hotel.

Welch searched not for rare books but for useful ones; he was planning a working library for scholars. "This is of course something quite different from a bibliophilic collection like Osler's— I am not going in for that at all, although it would be nice if some one presented the library such treasures." Cole tells us that Welch could not be called a bibliophile. "A bibliophile is generally thought to be one who values a book chiefly because of its age, its rarity and the beauty of its binding and typography. Dr. Welch is a friend and lover of books, but I think his affection is more than 'skin deep.' I cannot imagine his eyes sparkling over the possession of a book simply because it is old and has original wrappers and uncut pages." Welch said to Klebs: "You fellows want first editions and I prefer last editions."

Having too broad a conception of history to believe it could be divided into narrow categories, Welch bought many books that might seem at first glance only remotely relevant to medicine. "My idea is that there should be at least something in the library relating to nearly all branches of history. The various sets of the Cambridge historical series, including modern, ancient and mediaeval history and general literature . . . are a case in point. Then there should be some works treating of such subjects as history of law, education in general, agriculture, social life, institutions, etc. I have got many general bibliographical and biographical dictionaries and other works—rather specialized in biographies. . . .

"I think there is scarcely any subject which, for the study of the history of medicine, does not possess significance; the history of medicine requires information on all the conditions of civilization of the particular period under consideration. How can one grasp its real significance without knowing the state of contemporary knowledge of all departments of science and philosophy? Such a broad background for study and research in medical history necessitates a collection of books embracing all fields of knowledge." To Klebs Welch wrote: "If I leave a monument my year's work on this collection will be a major stone."

III

Welch landed in New York on September 23, 1928. While abroad, he had failed to answer several letters and a cable asking him whom he would recommend for librarian of the Welch library; now he joined in offering the position to Garrison, who, however, hesitated for more than a year before he accepted in January 1930.[14]

Although Dr. Emanuel Libman [15] gave $10,000 to establish the Noguchi Lectureship in the History of Medicine, the organization of the new department proceeded slowly. During the academic years of 1928–29 and 1929–30, the library was occupied, but no formal instruction was attempted. Welch negotiated with the Rockefeller Foundation for the additional endowment of $500,000 so that his chair might be expanded to the institute he desired, but without result.

On Commemoration Day, February 22, 1929, Welch made his first official speech before the university as an incumbent of his new chair. Having credited Osler with initiating the interest in the history of medicine at the Hopkins, he insisted that such an interest was not, as some "Philistines" argued, a decadent fleeing into the past. "That interest in historical matters can be an extremely stimulating influence upon the development of thought is evident when we consider that the Renaissance itself came from the depths, from the wilds of the past. . . . I think there has never been a time when the past has had more wisdom to give in the proper interpretation of history than at present. What we lack is the historical sense . . . some knowledge of the whole development of the thought and culture of mankind through the ages. I venture to say that anyone imbued with this spirit, possessing something of this knowledge, would not make the blunders which we make in our legislative halls, when we do not know what laws are enforceable and what laws are not, and we would not go bluntly against all the teaching of human experience." [16]

Welch proceeded in a few trenchant paragraphs, for which he

stated his obligation to the works of Garrison and Sigerist, to show the vast field open to medical historians. "The study of the relation of the knowledge applicable to medicine and the biological sciences at a given period to culture in general, is one of the most fascinating lines," he continued. "I have indicated that one may have the interest of Osler in biography and bibliography, and again one may be interested in the idea that a summary of the past will have a tremendous effect on the future work in human health, life, and death. However empirical the physician's vision may be, his ideas on the nature and origin and spread of disease influence his practice." And these ideas, Welch implied, often grew out of the non-scientific culture of the period.[17]

Again Welch advocated establishing an institute of the history of medicine to supply "a staff of earnest, serious workers" who, in combination with the library that had already been founded, "would permeate the whole school and create an atmosphere. Then, too, we need a museum." Referring to the Leipzig institute as an example of what was required, and pointing out that "a strong effort is being made to establish a like institution at the University of Berlin," he argued that the growing interest in the subject showed that the time was ripe for its development as an important university discipline.

"And now the benefits. . . . We are so absorbed in tremendous additions to our medical knowledge, in the great discoveries in the biological field, that the cultural aspect, the humanizing aspect, is often lost sight of. We should remember the great advantage to all society, not merely to the individual patient, to be derived from this aspect. All that will be brought to the front, will be cultivated with this kind of cultural interest which I claim for the history of medicine. I think this will permeate the whole study [of medicine]." Every teacher in the medical school should be brought to recognize that "the best line of approach to whatever subject he is teaching is really the historical one, not to formulate the existing line, but rather the way knowledge came to be." Indeed, he continued, the best contributions to medical history came not from professional historians but rather from scientists with a historical interest, who were able to handle the medical aspects with more authority.[18]

On October 17 and 18, 1929, the library and department of the history of medicine were officially dedicated, the principal addresses being delivered by Cushing, Abraham Flexner, and Sudhoff. Although Welch presided on the second day, his main function was, as he told Cushing, to "sit and blush." Uneasy at the amount of credit being given him for forwarding medical history at the Hopkins, Welch in his remarks as chairman again insisted that Osler's contribution was the greatest, and he praised, because of their work in establishing the medical school library, Gilman, Hurd, and particularly Halsted, "who . . . circularized our alumni with the view of securing funds." To emphasize the part Halsted had played, Welch broke into the ceremonies in his own honour by giving a dinner to the memory of his old colleague.

One of the guests at the dinner, John A. Kingsbury, the director of the Milbank Memorial Fund, did a lot of whispering behind Welch's back, securing the support of the other guests for an international celebration of Welch's eightieth birthday, which would centre upon the simultaneous presentation of an etched portrait to forty-five scientific institutions. When Welch went to Atlantic City to recuperate from the dedications, Kingsbury persuaded him to take along an etcher, Alfred Hutty. Kingsbury refused to explain his reasons, merely writing: "If you are real good until your next birthday, you may get a birthday present."

From Atlantic City, Welch confided to Kingsbury that Hutty had been approached in the hotel lobby by "an attractive, beautifully gowned young woman. . . . They walked on the boardwalk. She told him of her unhappy home life with an uncongenial husband, etc., etc. I told him that doubtless snapshots were taken of them together, which will be used for some sinister purpose. After that he wished me to protect him by taking him to the movies." Welch hoped that Kingsbury "would be capable of seeing the possibilities of the thrilling episode in his innocent young life."

Kingsbury in the meantime was rounding up a distinguished

committee and arranging for the events which were described in the first chapter of this book. When the full plans were revealed to Welch, he demurred, agreeing in the end only because the festivities would be most valuable in publicizing the importance of the public health movement. To this attitude he adhered, writing after it was all over: "I feel that it was all a tribute to scientific medicine and public health, for which I appeared at the moment as a kind of symbol—as the most ancient in service." [19]

On May 22, 1930, Welch made perfect his record of realizing all his institutional desires. The General Education Board appropriated $250,000 as endowment for his Institute of the History of Medicine, adding a grant of $12,500 a year for five years "to enable Dr. Welch to arrange the work of the Department in accordance with his ideas of its needs." Instantly Welch wrote Sir D'Arcy Power, the distinguished British surgeon and medical historian, asking him to be the first of a series of visiting lecturers. He also added Dr. John R. Oliver to the permanent staff of the department, which had up till then consisted of Welch and Dr. Stephen d'Irsay, a Hungarian pupil of Sudhoff's and Sigerist's, whom Welch had got to know in Europe and who had begun his work at the Hopkins in the fall of 1929.

Welch had been invited by the trustees of the Huntington Library in San Marino, California, to stay a month there during the summer of 1930, "examining the collection of books, mss., etc., with especial reference to their use and value for historical research in medicine and science, and to advise the trustees about such research." Welch was so interested that he remained three months, spending, as he tells us, almost every day from nine-thirty to four-thirty in the library, "my happy hunting grounds. There is no limit to the joys of browsing over the books. . . . It is a place for scholars—such quiet and peace and delight for the book-lover and historian . . . altogether a paradise. . . . I have only dipped into the treasures—one could spend a lifetime in following the trails."

Dr. Max Farrand, the director of the library, writes: "We were all impressed by his eager curiosity . . . perhaps the expression most frequently heard from him was 'How extraordinary!' . . .

Every note on a manuscript that might refer to illness or an unusual physical condition, with the treatment that had been applied, would attract him . . . and he would make a record of it. . . . Dr. Welch intended to study our English collection, but his attention was called to early, unknown Mexican material, and he was amazed to learn that there was information of that sort, at so early a date, on this continent. That had to be disposed of before he turned to the English books and manuscripts." Welch noted alphabetically in an address book the names and achievements of many Central American doctors, as well as the bibliography of the subject. Since, as Farrand tells us, "Welch's primary interest was in finding something new for the library in Baltimore," he ordered many photostats of material bearing on what he called the "century and more of medical and scientific activity before Jamestown and Plymouth Rock."

Welch was greatly helped in evaluating the contents of the library by the presence of Charles Singer, the distinguished British medical historian, who had just delivered the first Noguchi Lectures in Baltimore. Although Welch never managed to make the formal report which was desired, he wrote Farrand that "the library offers opportunities for certain fascinating studies in the by-paths of medical and scientific history, especially for England, but that the broader highways of such history are represented by only a few works, except in the field of incunabula in which the library is exceptionally strong. . . . With the present resources of the Library I certainly should not advise attempting to make the library a centre for research in world history of medicine and science. . . . I see wonderful possibilities of cooperative effort between the Mt. Wilson Observatory, the California Institute of Technology and the Huntington Library, each a top-notcher in its own field. If the right man could be found, research in the history of science could be developed here through such combined effort with unequalled opportunities in this country."

California amused and interested Welch, who had always liked the carnival side of life. He was delighted by attending a meeting of the Wednesday Breakfast Club in Hollywood at which several hundred men and women gathered to eat ham and eggs as a ritual of friendship. "Songs about ham and eggs," he noted in his diary. "Altogether the affair was worth attending once as a remarkable spectacle and performance, and a characteristic feature of Los Angeles."

To the horror of some of his more conservative friends, Welch visited the Angelus Temple "and witnessed the extraordinary spectacle of Amy MacPherson addressing the huge assembly —several thousand—on her visit to Palestine. Young men and women—perhaps 200 of them—were garbed in what purported to be Palestinian costumes. A string band and saxophone played —all exciting and colorful—much applause. Amy herself wore a native Palestine costume with high head decoration. . . . With her blond or red hair, fair complexion, graceful figure, ease of manner and speech, and rather pleasant, well modulated voice I could understand something of the appeal which she makes— an appeal which is fundamentally sexual.

"My most unique experience was an invitation to tea from Mary Pickford and Douglas Fairbanks. Mary seated me at a table and brought up Dolores del Rio, Mae Murray and a lot of movie stars to sit beside me. Afterward came invitations to luncheon and evidently I could have got deep into the Hollywood life, but I drew out when I saw what was coming. I have been photographed with Mary and Douglas, both still life and in the talkies. I shall be very much embarrassed if my friends see me in the news reels, as I believe has occurred. Mary is really charming—good hearted and generous, and I like Douglas Fairbanks very much."

That fall formal instruction began at the institute. Sir D'Arcy Power came as visiting lecturer; Garrison, Oliver, and d'Irsay gave courses; and Welch delivered weekly lectures, scheduled for January, February, and March, on the history of British surgery and related subjects. The faculty, he wrote Cushing, was "rather overdoing it, I fear," for the institute was not well enough known to attract students and the courses were poorly attended.

It had been clear to Welch that he no longer possessed the energy to initiate successfully one of the most difficult ventures he had ever attempted; early in that academic year, he had insisted that he be allowed to retire. On December 1, 1930, President Ames notified Cushing of his unanimous election as Welch's successor. Two days later Cushing refused, but when he learned in February that the position had been offered to Singer, he expressed willingness to reconsider his refusal. On March 27 Singer declined the offer, which was then again made to Cushing, who asked to be allowed to reserve his decision until his successor at Harvard had been appointed. Thus the matter stood when Welch's retirement became official on July 1.

Welch had already gone abroad to attend several academic celebrations and conferences, and to receive the Harben Medal, awarded triennially by the Royal Institute of Public Health to the individual who had done most to advance that subject. During August, his official duties over, he hid from his friends in London, loafing, visiting bookshops, going to plays and movies. "I have never cared much for the latter," he wrote, "but the movie chairs are so comfortable and they let you smoke anywhere in the theatre, so that I spend many evenings in the picture theatre. Really some of the movies are very amusing and enjoyable." [20]

In Paris he stayed at the same hotel with Cushing, who writes: "At about 6:30 [a.m.] there was a knock on my door and hopping up I opened it to find Popsy standing there in his pajamas. 'There's trouble in store for us,' said he. 'Please come to my room immediately. There's been a murder there.'" Cushing followed Welch to his room, where the old gentleman closed the door and said: "After I had turned in I was aroused by someone opening the French window. I lept from the bed and grappled with him and finally hurled him over the balcony onto the street—not without serious loss of blood. We must get out of Paris before the police learn of this." Whereupon he opened the windows and on the balcony was a gory mass of bath towels and newspapers. Investigation revealed that in the middle of the night Welch had spilled a bottle of red ink.

Although Welch returned to Baltimore in the fall, he adhered to his retirement; the professorship of the history of medicine remained vacant, Garrison temporarily assuming the executive work of the institute. Sigerist was the visiting lecturer that year. His success was instantaneous, and on November 23, 1931, Cushing wrote Welch that he wished to resign as a candidate for the professorship, since he felt Sigerist was the right man. Welch, who had noted in his diary during the summer that Sigerist's visit "will be the greatest stimulus ever given to appreciation of importance of medical history in America," agreed. In December, Sigerist was offered the position. After returning to Germany, he cabled his acceptance on May 1, 1932; he had foreseen Hitlerism and the disastrous effect it would have on the Leipzig institute he headed.

A few months after Sigerist had taken over (in the fall of 1932), Welch wrote that he was "making a great success of the Institute of the History of Medicine, which is an immense satisfaction to me. I think his coming to Johns Hopkins is one of the most important events in the history of the University for years." The department at the Hopkins was well under way.

Welch's activities as a historian had also been effective outside the university. The students of the University and Bellevue Hospital Medical College organized in 1929 the William Welch Society for the study of medical history, and some three years later a group of his pupils and admirers banded together as the Welch Bibliophilic Society "to carry out," as they said, "an idea which belonged to Dr. Welch," namely, the publication of significant but unavailable medical documents; their first volume was a reprint of Welch's speech "The Interdependence of Medicine and Other Sciences of Nature." When in March 1933 the University of Pennsylvania founded a chair of the history of medicine, Abraham Flexner wrote Welch: "Once more you may have the satisfaction of realizing that you have started in Baltimore work which has been influential elsewhere."

CHAPTER XX

Last Adventures

IN October 1931 Welch returned from Europe to test the joys of retirement after more than a half-century of intense activity.[1] But the machine that had been geared high so long refused really to rest; hardly a day passed when Popsy did not sally forth into the world. There were dinners to attend and dinners to give: he sometimes gave as many as three or four a month. There were speeches to listen to and speeches to deliver: although he refused many invitations, he found himself on his feet before many gatherings, and although now his talks rambled a little, the points he had once made so concisely spilling into numerous words, the eyes of his listeners shone with affection and when he sat down the applause was deafening. Still pilgrims found their way to his door seeking advice: college presidents, hospital directors, potentates from foundations, and always the young who were trying to organize their careers. Sometimes these were the grandchildren of the men he had advised fifty years before. He told the youthful members of the William Welch Society at Bellevue College that he had been loath to come there to speak, since he questioned their wisdom "in facing the reality of one whose name may possibly become almost a myth or a legend."

There were deaths of old friends to record on his calendar, deaths, and funerals, and memorial meetings at which he talked enthusiastically of his juniors now departed and invoked again the shadows of great scientists who had passed from life into history. "I suppose I am the only man here," he would say, "who remembers Cohnheim," and then the past would rise like a flood into his mind, and he would talk on and on with his eyes turned inward. But he was not one to stay home with his memories: trains rushed him to New York, to Norfolk, and to Washington, where he spent hours as he had always done in reading at the Surgeon General's Library. No gala occasion at the University Club was complete without Welch as toastmaster, and he met with his friends for intimate joking dinners. What if the "old gang" was a new gang now; the food was still good, the wine still warmed the blood despite that idiocy prohibition, and Shriver was gay as Venable had been. A month before he died, Welch wrote Shriver his appreciation of "the atmosphere of good fellowship which you have cultivated and promoted as a distinctive feature of our Club."

The club remained the centre of his life; here he ate his meals, here he spent long hours in the library sitting in that chair by the bay window in which no one else dared sit, raising his head sometimes to look out the window at the vivid green of Mount Vernon Place. Late, late into the night burned the light beside his chair, while the rumble of Charles Street directly below his window hushed to a whisper and then petered out at last. It was often two or three in the morning before the portly old man closed his book and wandered home. Shriver tells us: "The night before the Norris murder, a member of this Club was held up in front of the home of Mr. Haxall, on St. Paul Street, by Socoloff, one of the four convicted in the Norris murder. A few days afterwards, Dr. Welch was joking with this member about his having been held up, and the member retorted: 'You who are walking around these streets at all hours of the night and early morning had better be more careful or the bandits will get you.' And Dr. Welch rejoined: 'But I never go home until after the bandits have gone to bed.' " He had not lost his faith that the evils of destiny would not strike him.

He disliked anything that suggested he was being put on the shelf. If there was no important business to transact, the secretary of the club did not notify him of meetings of the board of management, but he would appear none the less and preside as usual. In 1932 Dr. Joseph H. Pratt tried to compliment him by saying that he did not seem a day older than when Pratt had been a student thirty-seven years before. Popsy replied: "That does not prove a thing. I may have been senile then."

Welch testified to his vigour in January 1932 by making a

strenuous two weeks' trip to Minneapolis, Rochester, Minn., Madison, and Chicago; he gave five more or less formal lectures, and inspected many medical institutions, being particularly impressed with the Mayo Clinic.

During his later years, one of Welch's major interests was the Milbank Memorial Fund, of whose advisory council he was chairman from May 1922 to March 1932. He was friendly with Kingsbury, the director, and enthusiastic about the activities of the fund in setting up practical demonstrations of public health procedures to work out improved methods which could thereafter be taken over by the state. "The results," he wrote, "are already of great significance. Not the least important of these results is the determination of values to health from expenditures of public money."

To suggestions that he take part in a campaign to rebuild the economics of the medical profession from the ground up, Welch turned a deaf ear and a non-committally benevolent smile. He refused to become a member of the Committee on the Costs of Medical Care, and when its report was published his reaction was typical. "It seems to me that there is altogether too much excitement and bad blood aroused on both sides by the Wilbur Report, and regrettable things are said and done, which prejudice sane discussions and action. After all the interests of the public will decide the controversy, but the whole question should be envisaged in a better temper and with more tolerance for conflicting sentiments and views than appears now to be the case."

In 1932 he said: "I don't believe we could do without health insurance, though I should not like to raise that question." He had previously made it clear, however, that he would deeply regret "the eventual disappearance of the private practitioner as we know him today. . . . There was something so fine about the best type of family doctor in the old days. My father was a country doctor and I know something of the life and what it meant to patients, so that I cannot help feeling that every effort ought to be made to rescue this situation."

Before the presidential election that put Franklin D. Roosevelt into the White House for the first time, Welch was dining quietly at his club when a messenger from Governor Ritchie of Maryland asked him to come at once to the Belvedere Hotel. There he was taken into a smoke-filled room where the Governor sat surrounded by his friends and told that he had been selected to make the speech nominating Governor Ritchie at the Democratic convention about to begin in Chicago. Welch remembered that he had to think fast in giving the reasons why he could not consent; none that he thought of was convincing, apparently, until he pointed out that Hoover, who would certainly be the Republican nominee, had made an address for his eightieth birthday. This succeeded in getting him out of the room without making any commitment, but he was so afraid that further pressure would be put upon him that he fled to New York; he stayed at the University Club, telling his friends with a twinkle in his eye that he was "in hiding." When Roosevelt had been nominated and the campaign got under way, he admitted that his predilection was for Hoover, "influenced to some extent by personal feelings, but I really think that the urgent problems of the moment are so largely fiscal that Hoover and the group of his advisers are better qualified to handle them. . . . Then I did resent so much Roosevelt's stab at the League of Nations."

Welch's "hiding" was rather a public affair; all his friends knew where he was. He was importuned by MacCallum to allow his features, voice, and gestures to be recorded for posterity in a ten-minute talking picture during which he was to review his career. Since he was expected to speak informally, as if reminiscing to his pupils, it was arranged that I was to be present as an audience for him to talk at. Cushing thus summarizes Welch's own account of what happened: "He had arrived promptly at the hour set and found his audience—i.e. Flexner—all gathered about to hear his reminiscences. Moving picture people are not punctual and he was obliged to entertain his audience for half an hour before the movie people came in and adjusted their cameras and lights and another fifteen or twenty minutes before the 'sound' people got their apparatus installed. By this time he had entirely forgotten his memorized speech. What's more, someone suddenly said, 'Are you ready? Let's go!' and he found himself in the glare of lights so powerful that his audience—i.e. Flexner— he was supposed to be addressing in familiar and informal fashion promptly disappeared from view and he never saw them again till it was all over."

Welch heaved a sigh of relief, but soon the telephone rang and the recording company told him that the picture would have to be done again; "there was an underlying rumble or hum from the machine or camera or something," Welch wrote unenthusiastically. When he was shown the negative of the film—"I appear coal black in spotless robes of angelic white"—he insisted the hum was unnoticeable except to an expert, that the film was, in fact, "much better than I had expected." But it was no use; an appointment was made for refilming. He bowed to the inevitable with his usual good grace. "I think that I can do better next time, and am glad to have another try at it," he wrote MacCallum. "I am really very grateful to you and Flexner for arranging the show. It interests me more than I expected, and I should like to make a success of it." But he insisted that he would not need an audience this time, as the audience would again be invisible.

I was there at the refilming, however, and I recorded in my diary: "Dr. Welch was in excellent form and good voice, and the matter was interesting. The material just covered ten minutes. There is no doubt that the film as now made is an improvement over the first effort. . . . Dr. Welch was in excellent spirits after the recording in contrast to what I thought was depression after the first attempt."

Welch found his "hiding" at the University Club so agreeable that, instead of spending a week or so as he had planned, he stayed without interruption from June 6 to October 1. "I have had a rather absurd summer. . . . The ostensible excuse was that I had some writing to do and had told editors and printers that I would not leave until this was in their hands." His principal task was preparing a biographical account of Libman to serve as an introduction to three volumes of contributions by Libman's pupils, but, as he admitted to Libman, he put off composition until his last day in New York and then did it in a rush. "An evidence of senility which you might study is the difficulty of breaking daily routine—newspapers, books, trips to the beaches, etc., reading your papers—and settling down to actual writing."

Welch spent his mornings in the library of the University Club—"a restful and delightful retreat"—and after lunch set out adventuring. Systematically the old gentleman visited every bathing beach accessible from the city, his portly form in his favourite one-piece bathing suit mingling happily with the crowds of the proletariat at places such as Coney Island, where he often spent the night. The children sticky with Eskimo pie or gleeful with little buckets, the sportive adolescents giggling and wrestling in the sand, the harried fathers of families trying to round up their squawking broods, all these amused him and filled him with a sense of life; the medical Brahmin had never enjoyed exclusive watering places. Undoubtedly the side-shows knew him, and who can tell what daring shoot-the-chutes thrilled the wastrel of eighty-two? He took long sunbaths on the beach, getting too sunburned as a matter of course, and he enjoyed bathing most when the surf was highest.

"In truth New York is not such a bad summer resort," he wrote. "I have had plenty of sea and sun bathing, and am able to tell old New Yorkers more than they know about the attractions of bathing-places from Coney Island to Babylon and Fire Island and from Atlantic Highlands to Asbury Park." As a result of his exhaustive survey he announced that of all the bathing places Jones Beach was the best.

It is reported that when bathing was impracticable, he rode to the end of all the street-car lines in the city, and then he would alight and prowl through strange parts of town even the oldest New Yorkers do not know. He went to art galleries and concerts and plays and movies galore.

Shortly after his return to Baltimore he was invited to deliver the Beaumont Lecture at Yale in December; after much urging he reluctantly accepted and announced his subject as "Nathan Smith." Soon he had also agreed to talk before the Twentieth Century Club at Hartford. He commuted for days to Washington investigating Nathan Smith's career, but as the time for the trip approached he became, for the first time in the memory of his friends, worried about his health. "I am off on a lecturing jaunt tomorrow to Hartford and New Haven," he wrote. "Incredible that I let myself be inveigled into this at this time of year."

The trip to Hartford was made on a cold train, and when he arrived he felt so ill that he rushed from the station to Dr. Walter Steiner's office. Steiner sent him to Dr. Charles Y. Bidgood, who was able to bring him relief. Although his doctors managed to persuade him to cut the dinner of the Twentieth Century Club, he insisted on making the speech. "He gave us, as might have been expected, a rare treat," wrote the editor of the *Hartford Courant*. "One would never have suspected that he had been in any discomfort."

At the importuning of his doctors, Welch cancelled the Beaumont Lecture, but after enjoying a good night he wrote: "It seems to me that I might have gone to New Haven." The eighty-two-year-old physician was so unused to being ill that he refused to accept the evidence of his own medical knowledge. Indeed, there is reason to believe that at the end of the previous summer he had already experienced symptoms of his malady, although he told no one, not even his physicians. It had undoubtedly been more than a psychic premonition that had made him dread the trip to Hartford.

When word reached Baltimore that Welch had been taken ill and had actually cancelled a speech, consternation reigned. He was "amazed on arrival here that the most absurd and exaggerated (à la Mark Twain) rumors of my illness had preceded me." Shriver was later to remind the members of the University Club: "You will recall that the newspapers at the time of his return from this trip were filled with sensational accounts of his illness—that he was returning to Baltimore in a private car, in the care of doctors, nurses, and other attendants. Those of you who happened to have been in the Club that evening were awaiting with anxious expectation further news of his condition— one member having reported that he had seen someone who said that he had seen Dr. Welch carried on a stretcher into his St. Paul Street house. About 7:30 o'clock, to the amazement of all present, Dr. Welch appeared in the dining room and ordered a substantial dinner." Undoubtedly Welch enjoyed his dramatic entrance.

Although his malady would not leave him alone, Welch journeyed to Atlantic City and New York, made several speeches, attended committee meetings and at least one funeral. On January 30, 1933, he gave his last dinner party—fourteen covers; it preceded a meeting of the Historical Society at which he presided. Two days later he entered the Johns Hopkins Hospital, leaving the University Club at about 1:30 p.m. "That evening, in the dining room," Shriver remembered, "a number of us were discussing his going to the hospital and his condition, and to the surprise of everyone, Dr. Welch again entered the dining room. Some member, in great surprise and almost instinctively, said: 'How did you escape?' and Dr. Welch replied: 'They told me at the hospital that they would not need me until bed time, so I took a cab and came over here for dinner.' After dinner, he came up into this room [the library] and at the western-most south desk did considerable writing, and from here he made his return directly to the Hopkins Hospital, from which he never came out alive."

When on February 10 it was decided that an immediate operation was necessary, Welch asked to speak to his doctors, Dean Lewis and Warfield T. Longcope. The latter recalls: "It did not seem to occur to him for an instant that both Lewis and I were greatly honored that he should have asked to see us, for he apologized profusely for bringing us to the hospital at such a late hour of the evening, and thanked us repeatedly for coming out on such a bad night. It was snowing hard. He excused what he spoke of as his inconsiderate request by saying that it seemed to him somewhat unconventional and a little irregular to be operated on suddenly in the middle of the night, and thought that he would like to talk the matter over with us. When we told him that we considered the operation absolutely necessary, he very quietly said that it had best be done as soon as possible. It was obvious that he regarded it as serious, but his decision was made almost in an impersonal manner."

During the summer following the operation Welch felt so much better that he played with the idea of going to Norfolk and Atlantic City. The trip had continually to be postponed, but he did not repine. He was happy in the hospital, he insisted. "I tell Young he runs a watering resort superior to Bedford Springs, which would be my alternative at present." According to Longcope, "he praised the food and said that the hospital cook was in some respects better than the chef at the Maryland Club." He encouraged his friends, however, to bring him delicacies.

His mail was prodigious. Although he steeled himself to allowing his stenographer to handle a few of the replies, in most cases this seemed unbearably impersonal to him; he would get his physicians to write answers for him, or occasionally answer a letter himself, but this "tired and worried him." Frequently he read his letters to his doctors; Longcope remembers that "his pleasure at receiving a letter from John D. Rockefeller, Jr., was unbounded. He sent many of his letters from important people to the Welch Library to be preserved. His room was full of flowers and he always drew attention to the beauty of any particular bouquet and remarked upon the kindness of the person who had sent it."

Despite the pleasure that visitors gave him, he refused to let his friends come to Baltimore specially to see him; they had to pretend that they were brought to town by other business. At first, his doctor tells us, "he protested that he could not receive ladies while he was in his bed or sitting up in his dressing gown, but before long he accepted his situation and many of his old friends came in to see him."

To his callers Welch talked about everything except his illness. His mind had turned back to his own past, and he discussed by the hour the events of his life, reminiscing charmingly and in great detail, with very little of the romantic heightening that is usual when the old dream again of their robuster years; such autobiographical errors as he made were slips of his memory or a slurring over of unpleasant things he did not wish to think of now. He talked of his colleagues, some of them dead, and of science, and of the serious books he had read, and of world affairs, and when, as sometimes happened, younger men brought him the problems of the institutions he had once led, they found that his mind was still clear and his advice still pertinent. He continued to keep up to date with medical literature.

"It is astonishing how his wealth of associations persists despite his long illness," Barker wrote. "He always has something of genuine interest to recount when one visits him." Longcope added: "He reads everything and talks in a marvelous way about all manner of things. I must have spent at least an hour with him each day without realizing that I had been there for more than fifteen minutes. . . . On the days when he felt well, a visit to him was a most stimulating and uplifting experience. One day Sigerist and I left the room and as we walked down the corridor we simultaneously remarked that we had been spiritually elevated in much the same way as if we had been deeply moved by some religious experience. Dr. Welch, completely oblivious of his physical body, had carried us soaring to rare heights."

Welch's spiritual elevation was not, however, based on religious faith; indeed, he did not like to be reminded of his ancient beliefs. Mrs. Kellogg records that one of the few times she ever saw him exasperated was when Dennis teased him about the conversion he had experienced as a boy. The history of religion, however, interested him as an aspect of the history of thought—he sometimes studied it with greater eagerness—and he never flaunted his views; indeed, many of his friends commented on his perpetual unwillingness to discuss philosophical subjects. Barker tells us: "Though I think he was an agnostic, he was always careful, especially in mixed company, to avoid the expression of agnostic views, and there has been some correspondence in the Baltimore papers since his death intimating that some of the churchmen here thought him to be a believer."

Once during Welch's last illness Barker induced him to talk on the subject. "I asked Welch if he had any conception of how the universe itself could have begun. He said no, it was beyond him; that many people thought of it only as mind and that in the last analysis nothing but concepts of the human mind were available. Of course, you could refer it to God, but then you got no

further. Dr. Welch said that physicists seem to be more susceptible to religious beliefs than biologists, for instance Millikan
is a firm believer and a church member. He asked if I had
read Needham's book called *The Sceptical Biologist.* . . . He
thought it was well worth reading, and he thinks that biologists
are more skeptical than physicists; he thinks that very few biologists have any conception of a survival of the human psyche after
death."

In the fall of 1933 Welch's condition took a turn for the worse.
By November he was suffering a series of attacks so serious that
after he recovered from each one his doctors commented on the
"astounding recuperative power" of this very old man. In the
periods between them, his cheerfulness also amazed the physicians who had seen so many men go down the road to death. "Dr.
Welch," Longcope wrote, "continues more and more remarkable
for in the last few days he has been mentally just as active and
energetic and apparently just as happy as at any time during his
stay in the hospital. If one could forget temporarily his physical
condition, a visit to him is an inspiration, and when one sees him
daily as I do, the physical state becomes entirely subordinate to
his marvelous spirit."

On December 17 his nephew, Senator Walcott, wrote: "While
he does not discuss symptoms, I think he is beginning to look
upon the immediate future with a good deal of apprehension. I
think it shows in his face. . . . I marvel at his detached point of
view, his utter selflessness, as he discusses with the greatest interest and keenness all kinds of world problems, scientific, economic, and political." Nine days later Longcope added: "As you
probably realize, he has been in excellent spirits and very happy
for some time, but except for that there has been no material
change."

The feverish attacks continued. When on February 25, 1934,
during another lull, I visited Welch, he discussed the affairs of
the Pasteur Institute, and gossiped about Garrison and Klebs as
if nothing were wrong. However, as I wrote in my diary, "Twice
during this full hour's talk Dr. Welch laughed at some passing
amusing incident. His laugh had changed. I was afraid each time

that the laugh might turn into weeping. It did not. Was the effect due to the change in Dr. Welch's features? He is much thinner, or is there some loss in emotional control?"

"As he grew weaker he saw fewer friends," Longcope remembers. "On his [eighty-fourth] birthday the letters, telegrams, flowers, books and presents pleased him immensely, and he even became somewhat emotional on reading some of them. The huge cake with its forest of candles attracted his attention, but he would not have it in his room. For some days, visits and long conversations had tired him considerably and he was greatly fatigued after his birthday. Very soon he started to fail rapidly. Fever developed. He could see no visitors. . . . He was completely unconscious for several hours before his death on April 30th at 5:30 P.M.," from cancer.

Looking back over Welch's fourteen months in the hospital, MacCallum tells us that Welch never once asked anyone about "his prospects of recovery. To have done so would have led to tragic commiseration and this he must have known only too well." Longcope adds that when Welch was sinking, he "must himself have observed the changes that were taking place, but he never made any serious reference to his loss of weight, his failing strength, or his increasing pallor. He occasionally complained of abdominal pain and once when I was examining his abdomen he asked me whether I could feel his liver. . . . Even during the periods when he was at his worst he rarely complained, and when I would ask him at my morning visit how he was he always said, 'Oh, I am all right.' When he was really feeling well, he said this with gusto and with an expression that would lead one to believe that he was in the best of health. When he was not so well, he said it in a slightly dubious, hesitating manner, as though his health was, after all, not worth bothering about very much."

Welch was holding to his lifelong habit of not confiding in anyone, irrespective of who that person was or what he knew. Always he had been surrounded with people, and during most of his life he had moved on a public stage toward public ends, but always he had kept the inner core of his being inviolate. And when the final trial came, he did not change. While his body suffered, his mind struggled to maintain before the world the same placid exterior that had been his banner and his shield. Popsy, the physician who had been so greatly beloved, died as he had lived, keeping his own counsel, essentially alone.

ACKNOWLEDGMENTS

ORGANIZATIONS AND HONOURS

NOTES TO THE TEXT

INDEX

Acknowledgments

The authors wish to acknowledge their special indebtedness to Mrs. Jean Webber Conti for invaluable aid in classifying the material on which this book is based, for work on the appendix notes and in preparing the index. Miss Wilhelmina Broemer, Dr. Welch's secretary, also assisted in the organization of the papers.

Dr. Welch's niece, Mrs. Frederick S. Kellogg, has kindly placed at our disposal her memories of her uncle, and her rich collection of family letters and papers. Other members of the Welch family, notably Frederic C. Walcott, William S. Walcott, and Philip Curtiss, have been of great assistance.

In the preparation of the manuscript itself, the authors have profited by the criticism of Helen Thomas Flexner, Agnes Halsey Flexner, and Marshall A. Best. Dr. William G. MacCallum has kindly read the proof and given us the benefit of his advice.

Many of Dr. Welch's friends and colleagues have loaned us correspondence and discussed with us his career; the institutions with which he was associated have permitted us to consult their files. Particular mention should be made of Alexander C. Abbott, Lewellys F. Barker, Walter Lester Carr, China Medical Board, Henry C. Coe, Rufus Cole, Harvey Cushing, Max Farrand, Allen W. Freeman, General Education Board, George E. Hale, Johns Hopkins University and Medical School, John A. Kingsbury, Arnold C. Klebs, Warfield T. Longcope, John D. Rockefeller, junior, Rockefeller Foundation, Rockefeller Institute for Medical Research, F. F. Russell, Florence R. Sabin, and Francis Carter Wood.

Other individuals and institutions to whom we are grateful for supplying us with documents and information are:
C. G. Abbot, Mrs. Lewis G. Adams, Joseph S. Ames
Helen Bayne, Stanhope Bayne-Jones, Clifford W. Beers, Mrs.

Joseph Colt Bloodgood, Richard A. Bolt, Isaiah Bowman, George E. Brewer, Paul Brockett, Mrs. Elliott Bronson, Thomas R. Brown, Mr. and Mrs. William H. Buckler, Perry Burgess, Walter C. Burket

Walter B. Cannon, Alan M. Chesney, Mrs. Juliana Keyser Clark, Barnett Cohen, Alfred E. Cohn, Frederick Collin, E. C. Cort, Thomas S. Cullen

Mrs. H. D. Dakin, Charles B. Davenport, S. Griffith Davis, William M. Davis, Wilburt C. Davison, George Derby, L. Doljanski, J. A. Doull

Mrs. Leonard Elsmith

Harold Farmer, John H. Finley, Morris Fishbein, Abraham Flexner, Lawrence F. Flick, Homer Folks, William W. Francis, F. R. Fraser, John C. Frer h, R. H. Freyberg, John F. Fulton

Fielding H. Garrison, Mrs. Andrew F. Gates, Frederick P. Gay, Miss Elizabeth Gilman, Mrs. Henry May Gittings, Jerome D. Greene, Alan Gregg, Selskar M. Gunn

Ivan C. Hall, Louis P. Hamburger, E. M. Hanrahan, junior, John A. Hartwell, Ludvig Hektoen, Justin Herold, Guy Hinsdale, Charles McH. Howard, W. T. Howard, William H. Howell, Edward H. Hume

Henry Barton Jacobs, Mrs. Theodore C. Janeway, Mrs. Philip K. Jessup, George T. Johnson, Mrs. J. Hemsley Johnson

Howard T. Karsner, Miss Florence Keen, Mrs. Vernon Kellogg, Howard A. Kelly, Mrs. John C. Kendall, S. Adolphus Knopf, E. B. Krumbhaar

Dwight W. Learned, Emanuel Libman, Sidney Licht, S. D. Ludlum

P. Stewart Macaulay, L. L. Mackall, Archibald Malloch, Theodore Marburg, Thomas McCrae, E. B. McKinley, Milbank Memorial Fund

National Tuberculosis Association, New York Academy of Medicine, New York University Medical College, John R. Nicholson, George H. F. Nuttall

John Rathbone Oliver, Eugene L. Opie

Edwards A. Park, Stewart Paton, Raymond Pearl, Peiping Union Medical College, William Pepper, H. F. Pierce, Henry S. Pritchett

F. V. Rand, Maj. Gen. C. R. Reynolds, R. H. Riley, G. Canby Robinson, Paul B. Roen, Sir Humphry Rolleston, Mrs. Edward W. Root, Peyton Rous

George Sarton, W. A. Sawyer, Henry Sewall, Alfred Jenkins Shriver, Henry E. Sigerist, Wilson G. Smillie, Mrs. Theobald Smith,

Winford Smith, Alfred Stengel, Charles Wardell Stiles, Mrs. Carl Stoeckel, George L. Streeter, Richard P. Strong

Carl Ten Broeck, Miss Lillia M. D. Trask

Henry R. Viets, George E. Vincent

Augustus B. Wadsworth, F. C. Waite, J. J. Walsh, George H. Weaver, Lewis H. Weed, H. G. Weiskotten, George H. Whipple, Huntington Williams, William H. Wilmer, C.-E. A. Winslow, Milton C. Winternitz, R. W. Wood, Sir Almroth Wright

Organizations and Honours

I

ORGANIZATIONS OF WHICH WELCH WAS A MEMBER

As a result of the continually increasing importance of his position, Welch was invited to join a large number of scientific and civic organizations; usually he accepted. Since all the bodies to which he lent his name are too numerous to be included here, we have merely listed those in which he was most active.

American Association for the Advancement of Science: In 1902, made opening address before the newly formed Section of Physiology and Experimental Medicine (*Papers and Addresses, 3,* 280). President, 1906. (Two speeches, *Papers and Addresses, 3,* 83 and 284.)

American Association of Pathologists and Bacteriologists: Charter member. President in 1906. On the death of Harold C. Ernst, became custodian of the gold-headed cane, an institution begun by Dr. Ernst. Succeeded by Theobald Smith.

American Association of the History of Medicine: First President, 1927.

American Foundation for Mental Hygiene: Honorary President, 1928–1934. See Chapter XVI.

American Medical Association: Member of the House of Delegates (1902–1903), Trustee (1903–1909), President (1910–1911).

American Public Health Association: Honorary chairman of the committee to organize a laboratory section in 1899. (Address, *Papers and Addresses, 1,* 615.)

American Red Cross: Chairman of the Health Advisory Committee, 1922; delegate to the conference that organized the League of Red Cross Societies, Cannes, 1919. See Chapter XVII.

American School Hygiene Association: Member of the Council, 1919.

American Social Hygiene Association: President, 1917–1919. President of the All-America Conference on Venereal Diseases, 1920. Member of the Presidents' Committee of Fifty on College Hygiene, 1922, and of the Executive Board of the Committee on Research in Syphilis, 1928.

Association of American Physicians: President, 1901. In his remarks in acceptance of the Kober medal of the Association (*Tr. Assn. Am. Physn.,* 1927, *42,* 11) Welch said of this association: "I was present not only at its birth, but, I think, now as the sole survivor, also at its conception, when, if my memory serves me correctly, in January, 1886, a small group of physicians, which included Osler and Pepper from Philadelphia, Francis Minot and Fitz from Boston, and Draper and Kinnicut from New York, were invited to meet in the office of Francis Delafield in New York to consider the desirability of founding a national association of the character realized six months later and of selecting the first founder members. Only those familiar with the factional troubles, the disturbed professional conditions and the general state of medical education, science and art in this country at that time can realize the full significance of the brief introductory remarks of the first president of the Association, Dr. Delafield, who had in eminent degree the gift of multum-in-parvo speech, when he expressed our purpose to create a society without medical politics and without medical ethics, where no one cared who the officers were and where one would find fellow-workers in medicine and pathology understanding and capable of intelligently discussing the papers presented, and from whom one could learn. I need not tell you at this forty-second annual meeting that the hopes and wishes of the founders have been fulfilled beyond all expectation in the history of this Association, membership in which still remains the high ambition of aspiring young clinicians and pathologists in spite of the later creation of many specialized national societies, not a few of these being offshoots from this parent stem."

Baltimore Alliance: From 1920 to 1925 served on Board of Directors of this organization for budgeting the city's charitable expenditures.

Carnegie Institution of Washington: Member of Board of Trustees, 1906–1934; Chairman of Executive Committee, 1909–1916. See Chapter XIII.

Charter Revision Commission, City of Baltimore: See Chapter XVI.

Commission on Acute Respiratory Diseases: Appointed Chairman, 1904.

Committee of Fifty: A body that conducted a ten-year survey of the liquor problem (1893–1903). Member of Physiological Committee. Welch's paper on "The Pathological Effects of Alcohol," published in *Physiological Aspects of the Liquor Problem,* New York, 1903, 2, 349.

Committee on Public Health Nursing Education: 1919–1923(?).

Hall of Fame, New York University: Original elector. In 1920, when Morton's name was on the ballot and the question of credit for the discovery of anæsthesia was under discussion, Welch supported Morton.

Happy Hills Convalescent Home for Children: President of Board of Trustees, 1922–1934. After Welch's death a bronze plaque in his honour was dedicated at Happy Hills on June 5, 1935.

History of Science Society: Member of Council from 1924; President, 1931.

Hooper (George Williams) Foundation for Medical Research, University of California: Member of the Board of Trustees, 1913–1922.

International Committee for Mental Hygiene: Advisor of the organizing committee in 1923; Vice-President of the First International Congress on Mental Hygiene in 1930. Honorary President of Committee, 1930–1934. See Chapter XVI.

International Health Board: Member, 1913–1927. Original member of Rockefeller Sanitary Commission, 1909–1913. See Chapter XVI.

League of Nations Health Section: See Chapter XVII.

League of Nations Non-Partisan Association, Maryland Branch: President, 1923–1929.

Maryland Peace Society: Vice-President in 1910, when a meeting held in February led to the organization of the American Society for the Judicial Settlement of International Disputes.

Maryland Public Health Association: Charter member, and first President, 1897.

Maryland Social Hygiene Society: Member of Board of Directors, 1919–1934.

Maryland State Board of Health: See Chapter XVI.

Medical and Chirurgical Faculty of the State of Maryland: President, 1891–1892.

Milbank Memorial Fund: Chairman of the Advisory Council, 1922–1932. See Chapter XX.

National Academy of Sciences: President, 1913–1916. During his presidency the National Research Council was organized. See Chapter XVII.

National Association for the Study and Prevention of Tuberculosis (later, name changed to *National Tuberculosis Association*): President, 1911. See Chapter XVI.

Sixth International Congress on Tuberculosis, Washington, 1908: President of Section I, Pathology and Bacteriology. See Chapter XVI.

National Committee on Mental Hygiene: Vice-President, 1909–1923; President, 1923; Honorary President, 1924–1934. See Chapter XVI.

National Institute of Social Sciences: In 1919 the Institute awarded Welch its gold medal "in recognition not only of your life-long service in behalf of medical science, but also in consideration of the assistance you have rendered the Surgeon-General of the Army, during the present war." Welch was in Europe, for the Red Cross Conference at Cannes, when the medal was presented at a dinner on April 25; Theodore Marburg accepted it in his behalf. On his return from Europe Welch accepted the Institute's invitation to membership.

National Organization for Public Health Nursing: Member of the Advisory Council, 1919.

New York Academy of Medicine: Fellow, 1879; Honorary Fellow, 1904.

Peking Union Medical College: Member of the Board of Trustees, 1915–1931. See Chapter XVIII.
Rockefeller Institute for Medical Research: President of the Board of Scientific Directors, 1901–1933; member of the Board of Trustees, 1910–1933. See Chapter XIII.
Society of American Bacteriologists: President in 1901.
Yale Alumni Association of Maryland: President in 1919.

II

SOCIETIES OF WHICH WELCH WAS AN HONORARY MEMBER

Académie de Médecine, Paris
Académie Royale de Médecine de Belgique
American Academy of Arts and Sciences
American Philosophical Society
American Society of Clinical Pathology
American Therapeutic Society
Association of American Veterinarians
Berliner medizinische Gesellschaft
British Association for the Advancement of Science
British Medical Association
College of Physicians of Philadelphia
Comité International d'Histoire des Sciences
Deutsche medizinische Gesellschaft in New York
Deutsche Zentralkomitee zur Erforschung und Bekämpfung der Krebskrankheit
Gesellschaft der Aerzte in Wien
Harveian Society of London
Harvey Society of New York
Hollywood Academy of Medicine
Hufelandische Gesellschaft, Berlin
International Anti-Tuberculosis Association
International Society for Microbiology
Istituto Storico Italiano dell'Arte Sanitaria
Kaiserlich Deutsche Akademie d. Naturforscher zu Halle ("Academia Leopoldina")
Maryland Society of Bacteriologists
Pathological Society of Great Britain and Ireland
Pathological Society of London
Phi Beta Kappa
Physiological Society (British)
Reale Accademia Medica di Roma
Royal College of Physicians, Edinburgh
Royal Medical and Chirurgical Society, London
Royal Sanitary Institute, London
Royal Society of Medicine, London
Schlesische Gesellschaft für Vaterländische Cultur
Sigma Xi
Società Medica Chirurgica di Bologna
Société Royale des Sciences Médicales et Naturelles de Bruxelles
Society of Medical Officers of Health, England

United States Veterinary Medical Association
Washington Medical and Surgical Society
Wiener Gesellschaft für Mikrobiologie

III

HONORARY DEGREES, DECORATIONS, AND MEDALS

1894: LL.D., Western Reserve University
M.D., University of Pennsylvania
1896: LL.D., Yale University
1900: LL.D., Harvard University
1903: LL.D., University of Toronto
1904: LL.D., Columbia University
1907: LL.D., Jefferson Medical College
1910: LL.D., Princeton University
1911: Order of the Royal Crown, second class (Germany)
1915: LL.D., Washington University
Order of the Rising Sun, third class (Japan)
1916: LL.D., University of Chicago
1919: Gold medal awarded by the National Institute of Social Sciences in recognition of valuable services during the World War. Distinguished Service Medal and citation, United States Army
1920: Order of the Cross of Mercy (Kingdom of Serbs, Croats, and Slovenes)
1922: Gold medal of the University of Vienna
1923: M.D., University of Strasbourg
Sc.D., University of Cambridge
Legion of Honour—officer
1925: W. W. Gerhard gold medal awarded by the Pathological Society of Philadelphia
1926: Order of St. Olav, commander of the second class (Norway)
Diploma of the Distinguished Service Medal, United States Army
1927: Kober gold medal, with diploma from Association of American Physicians
1929: D.Sc., Western Reserve University
1930: LL.D., University of Southern California
Gold medal of the American Medical Association
Litt.D., University of Pennsylvania
LL.D., University of the State of New York
1931: Harben gold medal awarded for public health service by the Royal Institute of Public Health
1932: D.Sc., University of Maryland
D.Sc., New York University

APPENDIX C

Notes to the Text

The notes which contain further material than simple source references have been indicated by numbers in the text; they will be found here arranged according to chapters. These notes are followed, under each chapter heading, by the source references, which are indicated by page and paragraph number, the numbers referring to the place where the paragraph begins.

When no collection is specified, the document in question will be found among the Welch papers that are to be deposited in the William H. Welch Medical Library at Baltimore. The abbreviation W.P. means Welch papers. *P. & A.* refers to *Papers and Addresses by William Henry Welch*, edited by W. C. Burket, 3 vols., Baltimore, 1920. The Cushing papers are in the Yale Medical Library, and the Mall papers belong to the Department of Embryology, Carnegie Institution of Washington, Baltimore.

CHAPTER I TEXT NOTES

1. It is not clear whether the London regional station of the British Broadcasting Company succeeded in picking up the Washington broadcast as it was scheduled to do. Describing the meeting held by the London School of Hygiene and Tropical Medicine, John F. Fulton said (to Harvey Cushing, April 9, 1930; Cushing papers, copy W.P.): "President Hoover's speech from Washington consisted chiefly of thunderstorms." This suggests that something was received; but John A. Kingsbury stated that because of atmospheric conditions "the attempt was unsuccessful." (*Summary of Celebrations outside of Washington in Honor of the 80th Birthday of Dr. William Henry Welch*, May 1, 1930, ms.)
2. According to a report published by the Twentieth Century Fund (*American Foundations and Their Fields*, N.Y., 1935), in 1934 fifty-six American charitable foundations gave $9,166,582 specifically for medicine and public health. In addition, $722,133 was given for the physical and biological sciences in general, while other grants classified more specifically under this heading include: $3356 for the study of anatomy: $408,641 for biology; $15,300 for biochemistry; $37,606 for genetics; and $138,390 for physiology. Under social sciences we find that $189,843 was donated for psychology. The basis of classification does not make it clear what percentage of the $4,768,263 spent for social welfare was used to further health, but some must have been, since the agencies supported include camps, homes, and settlements.

CHAPTER I SOURCE REFERENCES

3, ¶1. Full references to the events of Welch's life touched on briefly in this chapter are appended to those later sections of the text where these matters are fully discussed. A description of the ceremonies held on Welch's eightieth birthday, including transcripts of speeches delivered in many places and of many messages of congratulation, may be found in *William Henry Welch at Eighty*, ed. by Victor O. Freeburg, N.Y., 1930.

3, ¶2. Kingsbury, John A., *Summary of Celebrations outside of Washington in Honor of the 80th Birthday of Dr. William Henry Welch*, May 1, 1930. John F. Fulton to Cushing, April 9, 1930, Cushing papers, copy W.P.

7, ¶2. Barker to Welch, April 8, 1920.

7, ¶3–4. Cushing, ms. account of Welch's eightieth birthday, coll. John F. Fulton, copy W.P.

CHAPTER II TEXT NOTE

1. Crissey lists the children of Benjamin and Louisa Guiteau Welch as: Asa Guiteau (1789–1851); Irad (1792–1796); Luna Selina (1795–1873); Benjamin (1798–1873); Louisa Pamela (1801–1865); Alice (1804–1843); James (1807–1886); Phebe Sophia (1810–1822). (Crissey, T. W., *History of Norfolk, Litchfield County, Connecticut, 1744–1900*, Everett, Mass., 1900, p. 468.)

CHAPTER II SOURCE REFERENCES

9, ¶2. *New England Historical and Genealogical Register*, Boston, 1865, *19*, 55; *ibid.*, 1869, *23*, 417. Papers in coll. Philip Curtiss, Norfolk, Conn.

9, ¶3. Flexner, S., notes on a visit to Norfolk, Aug. 9–11, 1937. Crissey, Theron Wilmot, *History of Norfolk, Litchfield County, Connecticut, 1744–1900*, Everett, Mass., 1900, p. 466.

10, ¶1. Crissey, *op. cit.*, p. 467.

10, ¶2. Flexner, J. T., *Doctors on Horseback*, N.Y., 1937. Crissey, *op. cit.*, p. 468. Welch's incomplete memorial to his father enclosed in his letter to his sister, March 23, 1898.

10, ¶3. Crissey, *op. cit.*, p. 470. Welch, *op. cit.* Eldridge, Joseph, *Discourse Delivered . . . at the Funeral of Benjamin Welch, M.D.*, N.Y., 1850.

11, ¶1. Crissey, *op. cit.*, pp. 470, 473, 475. *Catalogue of Berkshire Medical Institute*, 1831.

11, ¶2. Crissey, *op. cit.*, pp. 469, 472.

11, ¶3. Letter to William Wickham signed by S. A. Pettibone, Haven Smith, and Newton Kasson, Oct. 30, 1838. Crissey, *op. cit.*, p. 475.

12, ¶1. *Penn Yan (N. Y.) Chronicle*, April 28, 1932. *Obituary Notice of Henry Clark Collin*, source unknown, coll. Frederick Collin, copy W.P. *Cyclopedia of Biography containing a History of the Family and Descendants of John Collin*, Hudson, 1872, pp. 20–21.

13, ¶3. All Emeline Collin's childhood writings are among the Welch papers.

14, ¶3. William Wickham to Emeline Collin, Sept. 6, 1843.

15, ¶1. *Ibid.*, Oct. 9, 1843.

15, ¶2. Emeline Collin to William Wickham, Nov. 14, 1843.

15, ¶3. William Wickham to Emeline Collin, Dec. 1, 1843.

16, ¶1. Emeline Collin to William Wickham, Dec. 30, 1843.

17, ¶2. *Ibid.*, June 13, 1844.

17, ¶4. William Wickham to Emeline C. Welch, July 24, 1846.

18, ¶1. Emeline C. Welch to William Wickham, July 13, 1846.

18, ¶2. William Wickham to Emeline C. Welch, July 15, 1846.

19, ¶2. For details of Emeline C. Welch's last illness and death, see her correspondence with her husband. Also: William Wickham to Harriette Collin Seward, Oct. 7, 1850. Elizabeth Loveland Welch to Emeline's grandmother, probably written Oct. 1850.

CHAPTER III   TEXT NOTES

1. The children of Dr. John Hopestill Welch were: Elizabeth Bell (Mrs. Ellsworth D. Ives), 1851–1914; Mary Emeline (Mrs. George D. Harrison), 1853–1918; John William, 1853–1927; Olive Collins (Mrs. Philip Everett Curtiss), 1854–1929; Alice Louise (Mrs. Andrew F. Gates), 1860–   . (Philip Curtiss to S. Flexner, Aug. 25, 1939.)

2. Benjamin Welch, jr., was in his own day the best known of the five doctor brothers. He received the fullest education, attending both the Yale Medical Institution and Jefferson Medical College; he collected a library of medical classics which included the works of Morgagni, Baillie, Bichat, Laennec, and Bright. His specialty being surgery, he invented a splint that was mentioned in Samuel David Gross's famous practice of surgery. William Wickham was in the habit of calling him in for consultation on difficult cases; indeed, Crissey tells us that people in Norfolk used to say, "Don't give up hope before having sent for Dr. Benjamin." (Crissey, *History of Norfolk*, Everett, Mass., 1900, p. 474.) After leaving Norfolk, Benjamin made his headquarters first in Litchfield and then in Salisbury.

His Yale address reveals that he was a deeply religious man who considered all life's manifestations, whether in health or disease, as under the influence of laws "founded by the Will of God." Belonging to the school of vitalists, he believed that the origin and phenomena of life are due to a vital principle, as distinguished from a purely chemical or physical force.

In his practice Dr. Benjamin was sound, basing his actions on "anatomy and physiology [which] have been aptly termed the alphabet of the science of medicine." He appreciated the quantitative work of Lavoisier in chemistry and of Liebig in animal nutrition, and he was a follower of Jacob Bigelow who, in 1835, enunciated the doctrine of the self-limitation of infectious diseases which Oliver Wendell Holmes said had done "more than any other work or essay in our own language to rescue the practice of medicine from the slavery to the drugging system which was a part of the inheritance of the profession." (Garrison, F. H., *An Introduction to the History of Medicine*, Phila., 1929, p. 440.) Benjamin himself puts the matter tersely: "The most important duty of the physician is, after all, to watch the tendencies of nature, to aid those which are salutary, to moderate such as are in excess, and to arrest and subdue such as tend to dissolution." (Welch, Benjamin, *Annual Address to the Graduating Class in the Medical Institution of Yale College*, Jan. 27, 1853, New Haven, 1853.)

It is difficult to say how much influence Benjamin Welch had on his brilliant nephew, but the chances are it was not very great since he died before William Henry took up the study of medicine, and the evidences indicate that as a boy William Henry shied away from medical knowledge.

CHAPTER III   SOURCE REFERENCES

20, ¶1. Crissey, Theron Wilmot, *History of Norfolk, Litchfield County, Connecticut, 1744–1900*, Everett, Mass., 1900, pp. 472–73.

20, ¶2. Crissey, *op. cit.*, pp. 472–73. Alice Welch Gates to S. Flexner, June 3, 1939.

21, ¶1. E. W. Kellogg to S. Flexner, Oct. 27, 1936. Philip Curtiss to S. Flexner, Jan. 15, 1940. John W. Welch to Welch, Feb. 9, March 2, 14, 1864.

21, ¶2. Ms. Account of conversation between Nellie Battell Stoeckel and S. Flexner, Norfolk, Feb. 12, 1937, p. 5. Alice Welch Gates to S. Flexner, June 3, 1939.

21, ¶3. Welch to sister, Jan. 17, 31, 1864, April 6, 1861. W. K. Harrison to Welch, May 22, 1865.

22, ¶2. Welch, *Remarks at the Unveiling of a Tablet in Memory of Miss Isabella Eldridge in the Congregational Church*, Norfolk, June 26, 1921, ms.

23, ¶4. Crissey, *op. cit.*, p. 278.

24, ¶2. Alice Eldridge Bridgman to Welch, Feb. 5, 1931.

24, ¶3. Conversation between Philip Curtiss and S. Flexner. S. Flexner's notes on a visit to Norfolk, Aug. 9–11, 1939, p. 4.

24, ¶4. William R. Rice quoted in Crissey, *op. cit.*, p. 280.

25, ¶1. Announcement of Winchester Institute, coll. Mrs. Elliott Bronson, Winchester, Conn., photograph W.P.

25, ¶3. Crissey, *op. cit.*, p. 479. Welch to sister, Jan. 1, 1865.

25, ¶4. Samuel Dennis to Welch, Dec., 1864. Alfred M. Millard to Welch, March 25, 1865.

26, ¶1. Father to Welch, Jan. 18, 1864.

26, ¶2. Welch to Benjamin Walcott, June, 1864. Diary of Dennis, Jan. 21, 1865, coll. N. Y. Acad. Med.

26, ¶3. W. K. Harrison to Welch, May 22, 1865.

27, ¶1. Charles W. Peck to Welch, May 24, 1865. Diary of Dennis, *op. cit.*, March 20, April 13, 1864.

27, ¶2. Welch to sister, Feb. 7, 1864.

27, ¶3. Emeline C. Welch to William Wickham, undated.

28, ¶1. Sister to Welch, March 1, 1864. Welch to sister, March 6, 1864.

28, ¶2. Sister to Welch, March 9, 1864.

28, ¶3. Welch to sister, March 13, 1864.

28, ¶4. Welch to sister, May 23, March 27, 1865.

29, ¶1. Alice Welch Gates to S. Flexner, Jan. 23, 1939.

29, ¶2. Cushing, ms. account of conversation with Welch, Jan. 23, 1908, Cushing papers, copy W.P.

30, ¶1. Ms. account of conversation between George T. Johnson and S. Flexner, Norfolk, Feb. 12, 1937. Barber, W. L., Address before Litchfield County Med. Soc., undated clipping.

30, ¶2–31, ¶1. Walcott, W. S., jr., ms. account of Welch and William Wickham.

31, ¶2. Philip Curtiss to S. Flexner, Sept. 16, 1937. Conversation between Nellie Battell Stoeckel and S. Flexner, *op. cit.*

31, ¶3. Conversation between Mrs. Stoeckel and S. Flexner, *op. cit.*

31, ¶4. *Ibid.* Walcott, W. S., jr., *op. cit.*

32, ¶1. Eddy, Rev. Hiram, Remarks at funeral of William Wickham Welch, Norfolk, Conn., *Litchfield County Leader*, Aug. 5, 1892. Barber, *op. cit.*

32, ¶3. Welch, W. W., *Annual Address to the Candidates for the Degree of Doctor in Medicine in the Medical Institution of Yale College*, Jan. 15, 1857, New Haven, 1857. Welch, Benjamin, *Annual Address to the Graduating Class in the Medical Institution of Yale College*, Jan. 27, 1853, New Haven, 1853. Virchow, Rudolf, "Cellular-Pathologie," *Arch. path. Anat.*, 1855, *8*, 3.

33, ¶1. William Wickham's ledger. Walcott, W. S., jr., *op. cit.* MacCallum, W. G., "William Wickham Welch," in *Dictionary of American Biography*, N.Y., 1936, *19*, 624.

34, ¶1. Conversation between George T. Johnson and S. Flexner, *op. cit.* Conversation between Philip Curtiss and S. Flexner.

34, ¶2. MacCallum, *op. cit.*

34, ¶3. Barber, *op. cit.*

34, ¶4. Crissey, *op. cit.,* p. 475.

34, ¶5. Crissey, *op. cit.,* pp. 242, 238, 240, 251, 249–254, 343–353.

35, ¶1. Minnie Welch to Welch, Nov. 25, 1865. Welch to sister, May 23, 1864.

35, ¶2. Grandmother, undated note. Father to Welch, Jan. 28, Feb. 25, 1865.

36, ¶1. Kellogg, E. W., ms. account of Emily Sedgwick Welch, Jan. 1937. Welch, Emily S., *John Sedgwick, Major-General,* N.Y., 1899.

36, ¶2. Welch to sister, Feb. 4, 1866.

37, ¶1. Sister to Welch, Feb. 28, 1866.

37, ¶2. Welch to sister, March 7, 1866.

37, ¶3. *Ibid.,* March 23, 1866.

37, ¶4. Sister to Welch, May 9, 1866.

38, ¶1. Welch to sister, May 12, 1866.

38, ¶2. Kellogg, E. W., *op. cit.*

39, ¶1. Father to Welch, May 13, 1865.

39, ¶2. Welch to sister, March 7, 1866.

40, ¶1. Welch to sister, June 13, 1865. Diary of Dennis, 1865, *op. cit.*

40, ¶2. Welch to sister, Aug. 2, 1866.

CHAPTER IV   SOURCE REFERENCES

41, ¶1. Sister to Welch, Sept. 17, 1866.

41, ¶2. Welch to sister, Nov. 24, 1866.

41, ¶3. Welch to Dennis, Dec. 1, 1866, coll. N. Y. Acad. of Med., copy W.P.

42, ¶2. Dennis to Welch, Oct. 28, 1866. Alfred M. Millard to Welch, Oct. 13, 1866. Bagg, Lyman H., *Four Years at Yale,* New Haven, 1871. Welch to Dennis, Sept. 22, 1867, coll. N. Y. Acad. of Med., copy W.P.

42, ¶3. Frederick Collin to S. Flexner, May 29, 1939.

43, ¶1. Welch to sister, Jan. 23, 1867.

43, ¶2. Sister to Welch, Feb. 17, 1867.

43, ¶3. Sister to Welch, Feb. 28, 1867.

44, ¶1. Welch to sister, Nov. 24, 1866.

44, ¶2. Welch to father, June 27, 1869.

45, ¶1. Welch to brother-in-law, Feb. 27, 1890.

45, ¶2. Welch to father, June 27, 1869. *The Nation,* 1883, *37,* 413, 431, 447, 469, 470. *The Independent,* 1871, *23,* No. 1157, p. 4. Dwight W. Learned to Welch, Feb. 20, April 21, 1871.

45, ¶3. Learned to Welch, March 4, 1871.

45, ¶4. J. G. K. McClure to Welch, Jan. 31, 1871.

46, ¶1. *The Nation,* 1870, *10,* 70.

46, ¶2. *Catalogue of the Officers and Students in Yale College, 1865–74.*

46, ¶3. Edward S. Dana to Welch, Nov. 5, 1933.

47, ¶1. *The Nation,* 1870, *10,* 70; 1870, *11,* 69, 70, 91, 137, 173, 235, 350, 384, 385, 402; 1871, *12,* 355, 379, 417; 1871, *13,* 42, 258; 1872, *15,* 59.

47, ¶2. Welch, *The Decay of Faith*, 1870, ms.

49, ¶2. Welch, *The Realm of Law*, 1870, ms.

50, ¶2. Lauriston L. Scaife to Welch, July 22, 1920.

50, ¶3. Scaife to Welch, Aug. 10, 1870.

51, ¶2. Welch to E. W. Kellogg, Jan. 3, 1907.

51, ¶3. *Biographical Record of the Class of 1870*, compiled by Lewis W. Hicks, Boston, 1911. Scaife to Welch, Feb. 4, 1871. McClure to Welch, Jan. 31, 1871.

51, ¶4. Learned to Welch, Aug. 20, 1870. William Hutchison to Welch, Sept. 17, 1870. H. A. Newton to Welch, Sept. 14, 1870. Isaac S. Newton to Welch, Sept. 20, 1870 (2 letters).

52, ¶1. Welch to Dennis, May 14, 1871, coll. N. Y. Acad. of Med., copy W.P.

53, ¶1. Learned to Welch, Oct. 26, Nov. 12, Dec. 2, 10, 1870, Jan. 6, 21, Feb. 6, 20, March 4, 14, 27, April 11, 21, May 3, 10, 17, 31, June 13, 21, July 5, 21, Aug. 1, 1871. Welch to sister, June 25, 1871.

53, ¶2. Welch to sister, June 25, 1871.

53, ¶3. Learned to Welch, Jan. 21, 1871.

54, ¶1. Learned to Welch, March 27, 1871.

54, ¶2. Learned to Welch, April 11, 1871.

CHAPTER V   TEXT NOTES

1. Welch spoke of his having gone to the Sheffield Scientific School during 1871 in his speech before the Alumni Association of the College of Physicians and Surgeons, New York, March 19, 1926 (ms.), from which the extract in the text is quoted; he also told S. Flexner and others the same story. However, on p. 207 of the *Biographical Record of the Class of Seventy, Yale University, 1870–1904*, Boston, n. d., we read: "During the year after graduation Welch taught school in Norwich, New York. The following autumn and winter he studied medicine at home." Many documents among the Welch papers show that he was in Norfolk during the period in question. Letters from Learned, addressed to him there, are postmarked Sept. 20, Oct. 6 and 21, Nov. 18, 1871, and Jan. 16, 1872. His letters to his sister of Oct. 9, 1871, and Jan. 25, 1872, are written from Norfolk, and his letter to her from New Haven on Feb. 18, 1872, much of which is quoted in the text, makes the matter clear.
2. On March 22, 1878, Welch wrote his sister from New York: "It is so much more interesting to have something to write people than to discourse on the weather, that I have been waiting to have things come to a focus, before pouring out my soul to you."
3. Dr. Lafayette B. Mendel tells us that Allen had studied abroad and was "reputed to have been an inspiring teacher and especially an expert analyst who conducted researches on some of the compounds of alkali metals. He was forceful and thorough. As an illustration of this, . . . he took up the study of Russian, Swedish and other foreign languages in order that he might read scientific literature in the original. He was interested in natural history and became an expert amateur botanist describing many new species about New Haven. . . . Allen is said to have been interested in his *good* students. . . . He had red hair, a birthmark on his face, and was indifferent about clothes, [which] made him seem like an uncouth person, though despite his disregard of social conventionalities, he had a fine mind. About 1887, having suffered from bad health, he went west, settled in a cabin near Mt. Rainier, and made a living by collecting and selling botanical specimens." Welch referred to him as a remarkable professor in his address before the Alumni Association of the College of Physicians and Surgeons in 1926.
   Although there is no mention of George Frederick Barker in Welch's letters

while he was at Sheffield, he often spoke in his later years of having sat in on Barker's lectures. Barker, a graduate of the Sheffield Scientific School, was professor of physiological chemistry and toxicology in the Yale Medical School, 1867–1873. He was a member of the National Academy of Sciences and finally became professor of physics at the University of Pennsylvania. (Lafayette B. Mendel to S. Flexner, March 5, 21, 1920. Memo. of conversation between S. Flexner and Welch, March 16, 1920.)

4. There is no evidence to show that William Wickham ever lacked funds for necessities and such simple luxuries as he desired; quite the contrary. However, a continual sense of strain on the pocket-book is typical of men of the physician's temperament.

5. Huxley's address "On the Physical Basis of Life" was delivered at Edinburgh on Nov. 8, 1868; see: Huxley, Thomas H., *Methods and Results*, N.Y., 1896, p. 130.

6. On Jan. 11, 1873, Welch wrote to his father: "One of our best clinics this year is that on nervous diseases by Dr. Seguin. He is a young doctor . . . and has studied in Paris for some time and with Dr. Brown-Séquard, by whom he is highly recommended. His is the only really systematic clinic we have. He takes up each time some disease and treats it exhaustively, illustrating the symptoms by patients. He is now giving two interesting lectures on locomotor ataxia, a disease for the first time described about ten years ago." That Welch was much impressed by Seguin is shown by the fact that he preserved his notes on this course for the rest of his life.

CHAPTER V   SOURCE REFERENCES

55, ¶1. Welch, Address before Alumni Assn. of College of Physicians and Surgeons, N.Y., March 19, 1926, ms.

55, ¶2. Welch to sister, Oct. 9, 1871. Learned to Welch, Sept. 20, Oct. 6, 21, Nov. 18, 1871, Jan. 16, 1872.

56, ¶1. Learned to Welch, Jan. 15, 1872.

56, ¶2. Welch to sister, Feb. 18, 1872.

57, ¶2. Welch to sister, March 30, 1872.

57, ¶4. Gilman, D. C., "The Sheffield Scientific School of Yale University," in *University Problems in the United States*, N.Y., 1898, p. 109. *Biographical Sketches and Letters of T. Mitchell Prudden*, ed. by Lillian E. Prudden, New Haven, 1927, p. 13.

58, ¶2. Welch to sister, June 15, 1901.

58, ¶3–4. Welch to sister, Oct. 27, 1872.

59, ¶1. Welch to sister, Jan. 25, 1874.

59, ¶2. Welch to sister, Oct. 27, 1872, April 13, 1873.

59, ¶3. Welch to father, Jan. 11, June 9, 1873, Nov. 5, 1874, Nov. 9, 1875.

60, ¶2–5. Welch to sister, June 8, 1873.

60, ¶6. Welch to father, June 14, 1873. Franklin B. Dexter to Welch, June 11, 1873.

61, ¶1. Welch, "Some of the Conditions Which Have Influenced the Development of American Medicine, Especially during the Last Century," *Bull. Johns Hopkins Hosp.*, 1908, *19*, 33, *P. & A.*, *3*, 288.

61, ¶2. Welch, Address before Alumni Assn., P. & S., *op. cit.*, p. 8. Welch to father, June 15, 1873. Welch to sister, March 7, 1875.

62, ¶1. Welch, Address before Alumni Assn., P. & S., *op. cit.*, pp. 8–9. Flexner, A., *Medical Education in the United States and Canada*, Bull. No. 4, Carnegie Foundation for the Advancement of Teaching, N.Y., 1910, p. 268.

62, ¶2. Welch, Address before Alumni Assn., P. & S., *op. cit.*, p. 11.

62, ¶3. *Ibid.* James, Henry, *Charles W. Eliot*, Boston, 1930, *1*, 279.

63, ¶1. Welch, Address before Alumni Assn., P. & S., *op. cit.*, p. 14. Biography of Alonzo Clark (1807–1887): Kelly, H. A., and Burrage, W. L., *American Medical Biographies*, Balto., 1920, p. 222.

63, ¶2. Welch, Address before Alumni Assn., P. & S., *op. cit.*, p. 12. Welch to father, Oct. 3, 1873. Biography of Edward Curtis (1838–1912): Kelly and Burrage, *op. cit.*, p. 268.

63, ¶3. Welch to father, May 14, 1875.

63, ¶4. Welch, Address before Alumni Assn., P. & S., *op. cit.*, p. 16. Biography of Edward C. Seguin (1843–1898): Kelly and Burrage, *op. cit.*, p. 1029.

64, ¶1. Welch to father, March 3, 1874.

64, ¶2. Welch to father, June 9, 1873.

64, ¶3. John B. Isham to Welch, July 13, 1873. Welch, Address before Alumni Assn., P. & S., *op. cit.*, p. 15.

65, ¶1. Cushing, ms. account of conversation with Welch, Jan. 23, 1908, Cushing papers, copy W.P. Welch, Address before Alumni Assn., P. & S., *op. cit.*, pp. 15–16.

65, ¶2. Welch to father, Nov. 2, 1873. Welch, Address before Alumni Assn., P. & S., *op. cit.*, pp. 15–16. Welch to father, Jan. 18, 1874.

66, ¶1–2. Welch, Address before Alumni Assn., P. & S., *op. cit.*, pp. 17–18.

66, ¶3. Welch to sister, March 7, 1875. Welch to father, April 9, 22, May 5, 1875, March 31, 1874. Welch, Address before the William Welch Soc. of the Univ. & Bellevue Hosp. Med. Coll., N.Y., Feb. 25, 1930, *Bellevue Violet*, 1930, *6*, 192.

67, ¶1. Welch to sister, March 7, 1875.

67, ¶2. Welch to sister, Feb. 14, 1875.

68, ¶1. Welch to father, Feb. 22, 1875. Welch to sister, March 7, 1875.

68, ¶2. Welch, Address before Alumni Assn., P. & S., *op. cit.*, p. 17. Ms. account of conversation between S. Flexner and Welch, March 16, 1920.

68, ¶3. Welch to father, Nov. 5, 1874, May 14, 1875.

69, ¶1. *Ibid.*, July 22, 1875.

69, ¶2. Welch to sister, May 6, 1875.

69, ¶3. Welch, "Remarks in Acceptance of a Medallion," Balto., April 2, 1910, in *In Honour of William H. Welch*, Balto., 1910, 40, also, somewhat edited, *P. & A.*, *3*, 360.

70, ¶1. Jacobi, Abraham, "Remarks at a Dinner in Honour of Welch," April 2, 1910, in *In Honour of William H. Welch*, p. 20.

70, ¶2. Francis Carter Wood to S. Flexner, June 10, 1937. Wood, *Francis Delafield, His Life and Achievements*, 1926, ms., coll. F. C. Wood, N.Y. Biography of Francis Delafield (1841–1915): Kelly and Burrage, *op. cit.*, p. 302.

70, ¶3. Conversation between S. Flexner and Welch, March 16, 1920, *op. cit.* Welch to father, June 9, 1875.

71, ¶2–72, ¶3. Welch to father, Jan. 3, 1876.

73, ¶1. Welch to father, Feb. 23, 1876.

73, ¶2. Welch to father, April 9, 1875.

73, ¶3. Welch to father, Feb. 23, 1876.

74, ¶1. Welch to father, March 9, 1876.

74, ¶3. Welch to father, March 21, 1876.

75, ¶3. Welch to sister, March 19, 1876.

CHAPTER VI   TEXT NOTES

1. In a letter to John C. Kendall (Sept. 11, 1876, copy W.P.) Welch thus described his itinerary: "We left Strassburg one morning about eight o'clock and rode by rail until noon into the heart of the Black Forest, whence we walked to Schaff-hausen on the Rhine (26 miles). From there we went by rail to Zurich, sailed on the Zurich lake to Horgen, thence to Zug on foot, sailed on the lake of Zug to Arth, whence we ascended the Rigi and were rewarded by a glorious sunrise; after this our journey included the lake of Luzerne, the St. Gothard Pass, into Italy, the lakes of Maggiore and Como, a couple of days in Milan, the Engadine valley, Albula Pass, and return by the lake of Constance and Munich, through Bavaria to Leipsic—a dry enough enumeration for you."

2. There is an element of mystery about Welch's statement that he went to Leip-zig primarily to study with Heubner, for in his letters home Heubner is not mentioned. He selected Leipzig, he wrote from Strasbourg, because "I am told that Vienna and Berlin are poor places to study pathology, so that as far as I can learn Leipzig offers the most attractions." (Welch to father, July 3, 1876.) It seems very strange that Welch, whose father felt that he was wasting his time studying abstract matters, should have neglected to mention that he had taken a major step for what his father would have considered so practical a reason.

3. Welch went to Europe provided with $1,000. He said in his letter of Dec. 18, 1876, to his father that when his first letter of credit expired in the coming April he would probably have drawn on it about $600, so that it would be cancelled with $400 remaining. We have little evidence as to the source of this thousand dollars. According to his letter of March 9, 1876, to his father, Welch had $300 saved from his year's teaching in Norwich which he intended to use for his European studies. On March 21, 1876, he wrote his father that Stuart had offered to lend him $500 for the purpose, but that he would be guided by his father in the acceptance of it. If he did accept this loan, there is still $200 to be accounted for, presumably supplied by his father. When he asked his father for a second letter of credit he spoke of making the amount again $1,000 by adding $600 to the remaining $400. In this letter (Dec. 18, 1876) he spoke of his gratitude "to you and mother," which might mean that Stuart's money was not a part of the first amount. The new letter of credit received in April was for £100, so that the amount sent him was $500, not $600. He expressed gratitude to his father, speaking of the sacrifices which he knew were required, with no mention of Stuart; nor is there any word about money supplied by Stuart in any letters to his sister at this time. Welch himself was in doubt about when he incurred the debt to Stuart, for when he returned the $500 to his brother-in-law he wrote him: "I could not learn defi-nitely from father or mother when it was that you sent me the $500, but I think that it was when I received the second letter of credit abroad." (Jan. 5, 1881.) On Feb. 13, 1886, he sent his step-mother $500 which he said was "in partial payment of the money which you so generously advanced to me during my studies in Europe ten years ago."

4. Welch reviewed his research on pulmonary œdema at the request of S. J. Meltzer twenty-five years after the first publication. In this interval his theory had been the subject of criticism and repetition. In his critical review Welch maintained his original position. He admitted another factor, however, which could not have been apparent before the days of Koch's bacteriology. Welch said: "In one respect I am in agreement with Sahli; namely, that a larger number of cases of pul-monary œdema are referable to inflammatory changes in the vascular walls than is generally supposed. My opinion is based upon the results of the systematic bacteriological examinations which are made at all autopsies at the Johns Hop-kins Hospital. Not only in irregular and localized œdemas, but also in not a few extensive and even general pulmonary œdemas, plate cultures from the

lungs show numerous colonies of bacteria, most frequently streptococci and lanceolate micrococci [pneumococci], so numerous that they must have been in active growth in the lungs." (Welch, "Theory of Pulmonary Œdema," in Meltzer, S. J., "Edema," *Am. Med.*, 1904, *8*, 195, *P. & A.*, *1*, 36.)

5. The myth has grown up that Robert Koch was the country doctor almost miraculously transformed into the great scientist. Nothing could be farther from the truth. Koch was the pupil of Jacob Henle the anatomist and George Meissner the physiologist, at Göttingen, where as a student he won the prize for his discovery of ganglionic nerve cells in the uterus, and he carried out successfully a research on the formation of succinic acid in the human organism. An academic career was open to him but he chose instead practical medicine. (Heymann, Bruno, *Robert Koch*, Leipzig, 1932, pp. 39–41. Welch, "History of Pathology," address to the Med. Dept. of the Univ. of Pittsburgh, Dec. 5, 1913, *Bull. Inst. Hist. Med.*, 1935, *3*, 1.)

6. Welch kept all his lecture notes in German. In a small notebook which he used in Breslau he listed the lectures he attended:

Haidenhain
Pbl.	Thierische Wärme—Montag, 4–5
Pbl.	Gescheidlen—Chemie d. Harns—Montag, 5–6
Magnus	Augenspielcursus 2 mal wöchentlich.
	(Stunde von Hewer [illegible word])
	[illegible name] Str. 17, oder 176—1 Trippe
Cohn	Augenspielcursus & Klinik
	Dientag u. Freitag 5–6
	Neue [illegible name] Str. 5.
Berger	Krankh. d. Nerv. syst. Pv.
	Sonnabend 3–5 Begins Mai 5.
	Krankh. d. Gehirns Pbl. unbestimt

Voltolini
Cohn	Ausgew. Kap. d. Allg. Botanik
	Montag, 5-6.

7. Charles Scott Roy of Cambridge, who had followed Welch as a student with Cohnheim, decided on his return to England to translate Cohnheim's book, *Vorlesungen über allgemeine Pathologie*, Berlin, 1877–1880. He wrote Welch for his consent and Welch gave it with alacrity. However, Roy never completed the translation, which was afterwards done by several persons and brought out in the Sydenham Society series. (Ms. account of conversation between Welch and S. Flexner, Nov. 16, 1920.)

CHAPTER VI   SOURCE REFERENCES

77, ¶1. Welch to father, April 27, 1876.

77, ¶2–3. Welch to stepmother, May 8, 1876.

78, ¶1. *Ibid.* Welch to sister, May 15, 1876.

78, ¶2. Welch to sister, *ibid.*

78, ¶3–79, ¶2. Welch to John C. Kendall, Sept. 11, 1876, copy W.P. Welch to father, May 22, July 3, 1876.

79, ¶3. Welch to sister, June 18, 1876.

80, ¶1. Welch to sister, May 15, 1876.

80, ¶2. Welch to father, July 3, 1876. Welch to sister, June 18, 1876. Welch to father, May 22, 1876. Welch to sister, July 8, 1876.

80, ¶3. Welch to sister, May 29, 1876.

81, ¶1. Welch to stepmother, June 6, 1876.

81, ¶2. Welch to stepmother, July 23, 1876.

82, ¶2–3. Welch to Kendall, Sept. 11, 1876, copy W.P. Welch to sister, Aug. 30, 1876, with enclosure.

82, ¶4. Welch to stepmother, Sept. 16, 1876. Welch to father, Dec. 18, 1876.

83, ¶1–2. Welch to father, Oct. 18, Dec. 18, 1876, Feb. 25, April 15, 1877. Welch to sister, April 26, 1877.

84, ¶1. Ms. account of conversation between Welch and S. Flexner, March 16, 1920.

84, ¶2. Welch to father, Oct. 18, 1876.

84, ¶3–85, ¶1. Welch to sister, Nov. 18, 1876.

85, ¶2–86, ¶1. Welch to father, Feb. 25, 1877.

86, ¶3. Welch to father, Oct. 18, 1876.

87, ¶1. Welch to sister, Oct. 22, 1876.

88, ¶1. Welch to sister, Oct. 1, 1877.

88, ¶2. Welch to stepmother, Jan. 29, 1877.

88, ¶3. Welch to stepmother, Sept. 16, 1876.

88, ¶4. Welch to stepmother, Jan. 29, 1877.

88, ¶5. Welch to stepmother, Sept. 16, 1876. Welch to father, June 10, 1877.

89, ¶1. Welch to Kendall, Sept. 11, 1876, copy W.P.

89, ¶2. Welch to sister, Nov. 18, 1876, March 12, 1877.

90, ¶1. Welch to sister, Jan. 1, 1877. Welch to stepmother, Dec. 31, 1876.

90, ¶2. Welch to father, Feb. 25, 1877, Oct. 18, 1876.

91, ¶1. Welch to stepmother, Jan. 29, 1877.

91, ¶2. Welch to father, Dec. 18, 1876. Welch to stepmother, March 26, 1877.

91, ¶3. Welch to Kendall, Sept. 11, 1876, copy W.P. Welch to father, April 15, 1877.

92, ¶1. Welch to sister, Sept. 21, 1876.

92, ¶2–93, ¶2. Welch to stepmother, Nov. 8, 1876. Garrison, F. H., *John Shaw Billings: a Memoir*, N.Y., 1915, p. 207.

93, ¶3. Welch to father, Dec. 18, 1876.

94, ¶1. Welch to father, Feb. 25, 1877.

94, ¶2. Welch to stepmother, March 26, 1877. Welch to father, April 15, 1877.

94, ¶3. Flexner, S., "William Henry Welch," *Science*, 1920, *52*, 417, *P. & A.*, *1*, xi.

94, ¶4–98, ¶1. Welch to father, Sept. 23, 1877.

98, ¶2. Cohnheim, Julius, *Vorlesungen über allgemeine Pathologie*, Berlin, 1882, *1*, pp. 501–7.

98, ¶3. Welch, "Zur Pathologie des Lungenödems," *Arch. f. path. Anat. u. Physiol. u. f. klin. Med.*, 1878, *72*, 375, *P. & A.*, *1*, 3. Welch to stepmother, Oct. 22, 1877. Welch to father, Dec. 26, 1877.

99, ¶1. Welch to Dennis, May 31, 1877, coll. N. Y. Acad. of Med., copy W.P. Salomonsen, Carl, "Lebenserinnerungen aus dem Breslauer Sommersemester 1877," *Berlin klin. Woch.*, 1914, *51*, 485.

100, ¶1. Heymann, Bruno, *Robert Koch*, Leipzig, 1932, p. 151.

100, ¶3. *Ibid.*, p. 211. Welch, Address before Alumni Assn., P. & S., N.Y., March 19, 1926, ms., p. 5.

101, ¶1. Welch, *The Influence of Koch and His Students*, before Laennec Society,

March 27, 1911, ms., p. 4. Welch to stepmother, Oct. 22, 1877. Heymann, *op. cit.*, p. 213. Welch to father, Dec. 26, 1877.

101, ¶2. Welch to stepmother, Aug. 17, 1877. Flexner, S., "William Henry Welch," . *op. cit.* Conversation between Welch and Florence R. Sabin, Dec. 1, 1933.

102, ¶1. Welch to sister, Feb. 9, 1877. Welch to stepmother, July 20, 1877. Welch to Dennis, Aug. 27, 1876, coll. N. Y. Acad. of Med., copy W.P.

102, ¶2. Welch to Dennis, May 31, 1877, coll. N. Y. Acad. of Med., copy W.P.

102, ¶3. Welch to Dennis, Sept. 10, 1877, coll. N. Y. Acad. of Med., copy W.P.

102, ¶4. Welch to father, June 10, 1877.

103, ¶1. Welch to stepmother, July 20, June 18, 1877.

103, ¶2. Welch to sister, June 24, 1877.

104, ¶1. Welch to sister, Aug. 3, 1877. Welch to Dennis, June 10, 1877, coll. N. Y. Acad. of Med., copy W.P.

105, ¶1. Welch to Dennis, June 10, May 12, Dec. 24, 1877, coll. N. Y. Acad. of Med., copies W.P.

105, ¶2. Welch to Dennis, Sept. 21, 1877, coll. N. Y. Acad. of Med., copy W.P.

105, ¶3. Welch to Dennis, Dec. 5, 1877, coll. N. Y. Acad. of Med., copy W.P.

106, ¶1. Welch to Dennis, June 29, 1877, coll. N. Y. Acad. of Med., copy W.P. Cohnheim, Julius, *Vorlesungen über allgemeine Pathologie*, Berlin, 1877–1880.

106, ¶2. Welch to Dennis, Dec. 24, 1877, coll. N. Y. Acad. of Med., copy W.P. Welch to father, Dec. 26, 1877. Welch to sister, Dec. 31, 1877.

106, ¶3. Welch to sister, Oct. 29, 1877. Welch to father, Nov. 25, 1877. Flexner, "William Henry Welch," *op. cit.*

107, ¶1. Flexner, *ibid.* Welch to Dennis, Dec. 5, 1877, coll. N. Y. Acad. of Med., copy W.P.

107, ¶2. Welch to sister, Nov. 19, 1877.

107, ¶3. Welch to sister, Dec. 16, 1877.

108, ¶1. Flexner, *ibid.* Welch to father, Dec. 26, 1877.

108, ¶2. Flexner, *ibid.*

109, ¶1. Welch to stepmother, Jan. 19, 1878. Welch to sister, Jan. 27, 1878.

109, ¶2. Welch to stepmother, Jan. 19, 1878. Welch to Dennis, Jan. 21, 1878, coll. N. Y. Acad. of Med., copy W.P.

109, ¶3. Welch to sister, Jan. 27, 1878.

CHAPTER VII   TEXT NOTES

1. In 1910 Welch said: "That period in New York is one which I delight to recall. . . . *It was in the beginning of pathological anatomy in this country.* The seeds had been sown in New York and had been developed by Dr. Fitz in Boston, but it was first possible at Bellevue to appreciate pathological anatomy as an important subject in the medical curriculum. Those with whom I was associated there, such men as Dennis, my dear friend, Edward Janeway, and above all Austin Flint—were men from whom I received great assistance." (Welch, "Remarks at a Testimonial Dinner," Balto., April 2, 1910, in *In Honour of William H. Welch*, Baltimore, 1910, 40, also, somewhat edited, *P. & A., 3*, 360.)
2. Welch's charming manner and obvious competence secured him privileges from the Babies' Hospital, and from the coroner, with whom Welch stipulated he was

not to testify in court. Furthermore, he worked in the dead house of the New York State Women's Hospital, in 1880 becoming clinical registrar there, an arduous job which, however, paid him $250 a year. (Welch to sister, Feb. 23, 1879, March 1, 1880. Flexner, S., "William Henry Welch," *Science*, 1920, *52*, 417, *P. & A.*, *1*, xi.)

3. Flint's offer to Welch cannot be exactly dated, since it was not mentioned in the correspondence of the period.

4. Cohnheim wrote Gilman (Feb. 4, 1884, coll. Hopkins Library, copy W.P.): "*Dies veranlasst mich nun, . . . dass ich am geeignesten für grade dies Fach der Allgemeinen Pathologie Mr. Welch aus New York halte. Mr. Welch ist mir seit Jahren bekannt, hat längere Zeit bei mir gearbeitet und ich halte ihn für einen ebenso scharfsinnigen als gedankenreichen Arbeiter.*"

5. In 1932 Welch wrote to MacCallum (Nov. 13, coll. MacCallum, abstract W.P.): "So far as I know the designation of the chair at Johns Hopkins as simply 'professorship of Pathology' without epithet was unprecedented. When I chose this title I expected to be attacked for this appropriation to a single chair of the whole science or study of disease, but for some reason there was no criticism, and now the designation is so familiar that no one realizes its significance. My choice of the title was deliberate. One reason was to avoid the cumbersome 'pathological anatomy and general pathology' still in use in Germany. Another and more important reason was to stake out the claim that the chair really should cover, even if it did not actually cultivate, the whole broad field of the origin and nature of disease."

6. The articles for Pepper's *System* follow conventional lines, but with full use of the European literature. Welch assisted in the preparation of two editions of Flint's *Practice of Medicine*, the fifth edition, which was published in 1881, and the sixth, published in 1886. In the former Welch brought the pathology into line with the German point of view, but the bacteriology is not especially notable. On the other hand, the sixth edition, in the revision of which Welch was given a free hand and for which he was paid $600 (undated memorandum of agreement signed by Flint and Welch, coll. N. Y. Acad. Med., copy W.P.), is a modern text in all respects. Indeed, so full are the sections on pathology and bacteriology that they may be regarded as the first complete treatise on these two subjects to reach the rank and file of the medical profession.

CHAPTER VII   SOURCE REFERENCES

111, ¶1. Welch to sister, April 2, 1878.

111, ¶2. Flexner, S., "William Henry Welch," *Science*, 1920, *52*, 417; *P. & A.*, *1*, xi. Welch, Address before William Welch Soc., Univ. & Bellevue Hosp. Med. Coll., Feb. 25, 1930, *Bellevue Violet*, 1930, *6*, 192. Sabin, Florence R., ms. account of interview with Welch, Dec. 1, 1933, p. 4. MacCallum, W. G., ms. account of conversation with Welch, May 15, 1927, p. 4.

111, ¶3. Flexner, *op. cit.* Welch, *op. cit.* Sabin, *op. cit.* MacCallum, *op. cit.* Welch to father, March 22, 1878. Welch to sister, March 22, 1878.

112, ¶1-3. MacCallum, *op. cit.*, p. 4. Welch to sister, April 21, 1878.

113, ¶1. Welch, "Remarks upon Receiving the Kober Medal," May 4, 1927, *Tr. Assn. Am. Physn.*, 1927, *42*, 11.

113, ¶2. Welch to father, May 16, 1878. Welch to sister, April 2, 1878, June 22, 1879.

113, ¶3. Welch to sister, Dec. 8, 1878.

114, ¶2. Welch to father, March 22, July 21, 1878. Welch to sister, March 22, June 7, Sept. 15, Dec. 8, 1878, Sept. 29, 1879. Welch, Address before William Welch Soc., *op. cit.* MacCallum, *op. cit.*, p. 6.

114, ¶3. Welch to father, May 22, 1878. Biography of Austin Flint, sr. (1812-1886):

Carpenter, W. M., "In Memoriam," *Tr. Med. Soc. of N. Y.*, Syracuse, 1887, p. 556; *Dictionary of American Biography*, N.Y., 1931, *6*, 471.

115, ¶1. Welch to father, May 16, 1878.

115, ¶2–116, ¶1. Welch to father, May 22, 1878.

116, ¶2–3. Welch to sister, June 7, Oct. 13, 1878. Flexner, *op. cit.*, containing Welch to Prudden, Oct. 9, 1878. MacCallum, *op. cit.*, p. 5. Sabin, *op. cit.*, pp. 4–5. *Biographical Sketches and Letters of T. Mitchell Prudden*, ed. by Lillian E. Prudden, New Haven, 1927, p. 34.

117, ¶2. Hugh T. Patrick to Arnold C. Klebs, Nov., 1932, Cushing papers, copy W.P.

117, ¶3. Coe, Henry C., *Reminiscences of William H. Welch*, ms.

117, ¶4–118, ¶1. Conversation between Walter Lester Carr and J. T. Flexner. Carr, Address before William Welch Soc., Univ. and Bellevue Hosp. Med. College, Oct. 17, 1930, ms.

118, ¶2. Carr, *op. cit.* Welch, Address before William Welch Soc., *op. cit.*

118, ¶3. Winslow, C.-E. A., *The Life of Hermann M. Biggs*, Phila., 1929, p. 267. Carr, *op. cit.* Welch, *op. cit.*

119, ¶1. Winslow, *op. cit.*, p. 268.

119, ¶2. Conversation between Carr and J. T. Flexner.

119, ¶3. Welch to sister, Dec. 22, 1878. Cushing, *The Life of Sir William Osler*, Oxford, 1925, *1*, 297, f.n. Welch, Address before P. & S. Alumni Assn., March 19, 1926, ms., p. 11.

120, ¶1. Welch to sister, June 18, 1881.

120, ¶2. Welch and Meltzer, S. J., "Zur Histiophysik der roten Blutkörperchen," *Centralbl. f. d. med. Wissensch.*, 1884, *22*, 721. Welch and Meltzer, "The Behaviour of the Red Blood-Corpuscles When Shaken with Indifferent Substances," *J. Physiol.* (London), 1884–1885, *5*, 255; *P. & A.*, *1*, 42.

120, ¶3. Welch to sister, Sept. 15, 1878. *Catalogue of the Faculty and Alumni of the Bellevue Hospital Medical College, 1861 to 1881*, N.Y., 1884, p. 13. Patrick to Klebs, *op. cit.*

121, ¶1. Patrick to Klebs, *op. cit.*

121, ¶2. Welch, Address before William Welch Soc., *op. cit.* Welch to sister, April 7, 1881.

122, ¶1. Welch's lecture notes for Sept. 22, 1882.

122, ¶2. *Ibid.*, Oct. 27, 1883.

122, ¶3. Coe, *op. cit.*, p. 4.

122, ¶4. Ms. account of conversation between Welch and S. Flexner, Nov. 16, 1920.

123, ¶1. Flint, Austin, *A Treatise on the Principles and Practice of Medicine*, Phila., 1881, *1*, iii. Welch to sister, Nov. 2, 1879, Feb. 4, July 12, Aug. 5, Nov. 15, 1880. Welch to brother-in-law, Jan. 5, 1881. Welch to father, April 4, 1881. Flexner, S., "William H. Welch," *op. cit.*

123, ¶2. MacCallum, Interview with Welch, May 15, 1927, *op. cit.*, p. 4.

123, ¶3. Welch to sister, Sept. 15, June 7, 1878, June 10, Oct. 27, 1883.

124, ¶1. Welch told this story both to S. Flexner in 1920 and to Joseph H. Pratt, who repeated it in the *New Eng. J. of Med.*, 1934, *210*, 1038.

124, ¶2. Welch to sister, April 30, 1881, Jan. 14, 1884, Dec. 26, 1881. Kellogg, E. W., ms. account of Welch.

125, ¶1. Welch to sister, Dec. 22, 1878. S. Flexner's recollections.

125, ¶2. Welch to sister, Feb. 4, 1880.

125, ¶3. Welch to sister, Sept. 20, 1882, March 14, 1883.

126, ¶1. Kellogg, E. W., *op. cit.*

126, ¶2. Welch, "In Memoriam—William Stewart Halsted," *Bull. Johns Hopkins Hosp.*, 1925, *36*, 34.

126, ¶3. Welch to stepmother, Oct. 25, 1879.

127, ¶1. Coe, *op. cit.*, p. 5.

127, ¶2. Billings to Gilman, March 1, 1884, coll. Hopkins Library, copy W.P. Mac-Callum, *op. cit.*, p. 6. Sabin, *op. cit.*, p. 6.

128, ¶1. Billings to Gilman, March 1, 1884, coll. Hopkins Library, copy W.P.

128, ¶2. Billings to Gilman, March 9, 1884, coll. Hopkins Library, copy W.P.

128, ¶3. Welch to father, March 11, 1884. MacCallum, *op. cit.*, pp. 6–7.

128, ¶4. Alice Welch Gates to S. Flexner, Feb. 2, 1939.

129, ¶1–2. Welch to father, March 11, 1884.

129, ¶3. Welch to stepmother, June 21, 1885. Gilman, *Ninth Annual Report of the President to the Trustees of the Johns Hopkins University*, 1884, p. 10. Barker, ms. account of talk with Welch in Hopkins Hosp., July 14, 1933, copy W.P.

130, ¶1–3. Welch to father, March 11, 1884.

130, ¶4. Welch to sister, March 11, 1884.

131, ¶2. Welch to sister, March 23, 1884. Dennis to Stuart Walcott, March 25, 1884. Andrew Carnegie's memorandum to his bankers, April 24, 1884, coll. N. Y. Acad. of Med., copy W.P.

131, ¶3. William Wickham to Stuart and Emma Walcott, March 14, 1884. Dennis to Stuart Walcott, March 14, 1884.

132, ¶1. H. M. Alexander to Welch, March 15, 1884, coll. N. Y. Acad. of Med., copy W.P.

132, ¶2. Welch to sister, March 23, 1884.

133, ¶2. Alexander to Welch, March 28, 1884, coll. N. Y. Acad. of Med., copy W.P.

133, ¶3. George H. Williams to Welch, March 25, 1884.

134, ¶1. MacCallum, *op. cit.*, p. 7. Shriver, A. J., Address at unveiling of Welch plaque at Happy Hills Home, June 5, 1935.

134, ¶2–3. Welch to father, March 31, 1884.

135, ¶1–3. Welch to stepmother, April 3, 1884.

135, ¶4. Welch to father, April 9, 1884.

136, ¶1. Welch to Dennis, Sept. 27, 1884, coll. N. Y. Acad. of Med., copy W.P.

137, ¶1. Welch to father, April 9, Aug. 20, Sept. 11, 1884. Welch to sister, Sept. 15, 1884. Welch to Gilman, May 29, 1884, coll. Hopkins Library, copy W.P. Welch, "Simple Ulcer of the Stomach," in Pepper, Wm., *Syst. Pract. Med.*, Philadelphia, 1885, *2*, 480. "Cancer of the Stomach," *ibid.*, 530. "Hemorrhage from the Stomach," *ibid.*, 580. "Dilatation of the Stomach," *ibid.*, 586. "Minor Organic Affections of the Stomach," *ibid.*, 611.

CHAPTER VIII   TEXT NOTES

1. Welch wrote the Board of Trustees of the Hopkins on April 1, 1886 (coll. Hopkins Library, copy W.P.) that while in Europe he had spent $1,207.77 for ap-

paratus and $291 for books. In addition he left orders at the Cambridge Scientific Company totalling $577.46, and for four microscopes ($335) and a kymographion "which was to cost in the neighborhood of $200." This meant that, including custom house fees, freightage, etc., he spent $842.31 more than his appropriation of $2,000. The apparatus, he wrote, "includes that necessary for post mortem examinations, and for bacteriological, experimental and microscopical work. The books are such as are required for constant reference in a pathological laboratory and embrace several sets of journals. They were obtained in considerable part at very reasonable rates at the sale of Prof. Cohnheim's library."

2. Speaking at his eightieth birthday celebration at the New York Academy of Medicine (*William H. Welch at Eighty*, ed. by Victor O. Freeburg, N.Y., 1930, p. 64), Welch said: "During the year I spent abroad, chiefly in Germany, working with Flügge and Koch in bacteriology, before entering upon my duties in 1885 at Johns Hopkins, I visited Pasteur's laboratory. I shall never forget the circumstances of my visit when he put aside his test-tubes and showed me around his laboratory." This story is almost certainly apocryphal, since it contradicts the evidence of the letters he wrote home at the time. Furthermore, although such an incident would have been of great interest to his pupils and colleagues, he never spoke of it until the very end of his life.

3. According to Prudden's account of this incident, noted by S. Flexner on March 3, 1920, he and Welch discussed the matter of destroying the cholera cultures and set out together to drop their test tubes in the Spree. This may well be the correct version, as Welch was not averse to making a good story better.

CHAPTER VIII   SOURCE REFERENCES

138, ¶1. Welch to Gilman, April 18, 1885, coll. Hopkins Library, copy W.P.

138, ¶2. Welch to father, Nov. 8, 1884.

138, ¶3. *Ibid*. Welch to Gilman, Dec. 18, 1884, coll. Hopkins Library, copy W.P.

139, ¶1. Welch, *The Influence of Koch and His Students*, before Laennec Society, March 27, 1911, ms., p. 9.

139, ¶2. Welch to Gilman, Dec. 18, 1884, coll. Hopkins Library, copy W.P. Flexner, S., "William Henry Welch," *Science*, 1920, *52*, 417, *P. & A.*, *1*, xi. Hume, E. E., *Max von Pettenkofer*, N.Y., 1927.

139, ¶3. Welch to stepmother, Dec. 1, 1884.

140, ¶1. Welch to Gilman, April 18, 1885, Dec. 18, 1884, coll. Hopkins Library, copies W.P.

140, ¶2. Welch to father, Jan. 7, 1885.

140, ¶3. Conversation between Welch and S. Flexner.

141, ¶1. Welch to stepmother, Jan. 18, 1885. Welch to Gilman, April 15, 1885. Welch to Trustees, Hopkins Univ., April 1, 1886, coll. Hopkins Library, copies W.P.

141, ¶2. Welch to Gilman, Dec. 18, 1884, April 18, 1885, coll. Hopkins Library, copies W.P.

142, ¶1. Carl Ludwig to Welch, Aug. 5, 1885.

142, ¶2. Alfred L. Loomis to Welch, Dec. 30, 1884.

142, ¶3. Welch to father, Jan. 25, 1885.

142, ¶4. Welch to stepmother, May 23, 1885.

143, ¶2. Welch to stepmother, Dec. 11, 15, 1884. Welch to father, Jan. 7, 1885. Welch to stepmother, Jan. 18, 1885. Welch to father, Jan. 25, April 17, 1885.

143, ¶3. Welch to Gilman, April 18, 1885; F. T. Frelinghuysen to J. A. Kasson, Jan.

22, 1885, coll. Hopkins Library, copies W.P. Welch, *The Influence of Koch and His Students, op. cit.*, p. 9.

144, ¶1. Welch, *Influence of Koch*, p. 9. Welch to sister, April 8, 1885.

144, ¶2. Welch to stepmother, June 21, 1885.

145, ¶1. Welch to S. Flexner, July 20, 1920, coll. S. Flexner, abstract W.P.

145, ¶2. Welch to stepmother, June 21, 1885.

145, ¶3. Welch to stepmother, May 23, 1885.

146, ¶1. Welch to Mall, Sept. 9, 1890, Mall papers, copy W.P.

146, ¶2. Welch, *The Influence of Koch*, pp. 1, 2, 6.

146, ¶3. Welch to stepmother, June 21, 1885. Welch to Gilman, June 22, Aug. 4, 1885, coll. Hopkins Library, copy W.P.

147, ¶1. Welch to Gilman, Aug. 4, 1885, *op. cit.*

147, ¶2. Welch, *Influence of Koch*, pp. 10–11.

147, ¶3. *Ibid.*, p. 8.

148, ¶1–2. *Ibid.*, p. 8. Conversation between Welch and S. Flexner, 1920.

149, ¶1. Welch to sister, Aug. 4, 1885.

CHAPTER IX   TEXT NOTES

1. The so-called "Pathological" was at first a small, two-story structure. An amphitheatre for autopsies ran the full height, supplying in railed-off tiers standing room for some thirty men. Beside it on the ground floor was the bacteriological laboratory, a long, narrow room along one side of which a shelf or counter ran under small glass cupboards in which the students kept their cultures; the width of the cupboard showed the students how much of the counter each might use. A small separate room on the same floor was assigned to Welch's assistant, Alexander C. Abbott, for the professor himself preferred to work at the communal table. On the second floor, above the bacteriological laboratory, was the almost identical pathological laboratory.

   After his return to Baltimore, Welch spent $146.30 for alcohol, $124.37 for a janitor and running expenses, and $393.45 for glassware and chemicals. In April he desired an additional appropriation of $410, $100 being for running expenses, $26 for a refrigerator, $200 for glass jars to preserve specimens, and $84 to pay a janitor $4 a week. (Welch to Trustees, Hopkins Univ., April 1, 1886, coll. Hopkins Library, copy. W.P.)

2. Welch listed the subjects to be considered as follows: (1) the history of our knowledge concerning the relations of micro-organisms to fermentation and putrefaction and to disease; (2) the classification and biology of bacteria in general; (3) the methods of demonstration and cultivation of bacteria; (4) general characters of infectious diseases; what is necessary in order to prove the causation of a given disease by a specific organism? (5) modes of infection; bacteria in air, ground, water, and food; (6) bacteria in healthy human beings; (7) micro-organisms in special diseases, such as tuberculosis, splenic fever, cholera, typhoid fever, leprosy, relapsing fever, erysipelas, pneumonia, suppurations, malaria, etc.; (8) diagnosis of diseases by recognition of micro-organisms; (9) theories as to action of bacteria in disease; ptomaines; (10) doctrine of immunity; attenuation of virus; preventive inoculation; (11) disinfectants; bearings of the germ-doctrine of disease on sanitation and on the prophylaxis and treatment of disease. (*Johns Hopkins Univ. Cir.*, 1886, No. 46, p. 54.)

3. Sir Thomas Lauder Brunton (1844–1916): M.D., Edinburgh, 1868; asst. phys. (1875–1897) and full phys. (1897–1904) to St. Bartholomew's Hospital; pupil of Brücke, Kühne, and Ludwig; became a master in the application of the physiological findings of pharmacology to internal medicine, his special field being the

action of drugs on the heart. A warm personal friend of Billings's, he made princely donations to the Surgeon General's Library. (Garrison, F. H., *An Introduction to the History of Medicine*, Phila., 1929, p. 654.)

4. Thomas was undoubtedly referring to the schism in the American medical profession that had come about during the negotiations for the 9th International Medical Congress of 1887 in Washington, the first such Congress held in this country. From the beginning of these negotiations in 1885, the southern and western doctors had shown increasing resentment and distrust of what they called the eastern clique, which seemed to them to have excessive representation in the original organization. The committees originally appointed by Billings, who was violently attacked, were entirely reorganized; many of the eastern doctors withdrew completely and even stayed away from the Congress, with the result that many foreign visitors expressed disappointment at the Congress itself, since they did not meet there the American medical men with whose work they had become familiar. One of the outgrowths of the rift was the organization of the Association of American Physicians (see Delafield, Francis, "Opening Remarks at First Meeting," *Tr. Assn. Am. Physn.*, 1886, *1*, 1) in 1885. It seems natural that Thomas should fear that the factional quarrel, if allowed to influence the organization of the school and hospital, might work to the detriment of so new an undertaking in Baltimore, on the borderline between North and South, East and West. (See: *J. Am. Med. Assn.*, *Med. News*, *Med. Rec.*, *Canada Med. & Surg. J.*, etc., 1885–1887.)

5. Hurd, who had taken his A.B., M.D., and A.M. degrees at the University of Michigan, had been superintendent of the Eastern Michigan Asylum at Pontiac from 1878 until his appointment to the superintendency of the Johns Hopkins Hospital in June 1889. He served as professor of psychiatry from 1889 to 1906 and in 1911, retiring from his hospital post, he became secretary of the Board of Trustees. During his twenty-two years as superintendent he became the personal friend of every worker in the hospital. When the medical school was started Hurd's was a powerful influence in establishing close and harmonious relations between the school and the hospital. He died in 1927. (Hurd, H. M., *The First Quarter-Century of the Johns Hopkins Hospital, 1889–1914*, ed. and extended by L. F. Barker, ms., coll. Hopkins Hosp., excerpts W.P.)

6. Welch continued to examine pathological specimens for the New York profession until he retired in 1917; then he handed them over to his successor, MacCallum, writing: "I have been in the habit of charging five or ten dollars for such examinations, provided the patient pays the fee; otherwise I have not charged anything. I never attempted to develop this sort of work as a paying undertaking." (Welch to MacCallum, Oct. 3, 1915, coll. MacCallum, copy W.P.)

7. References to the published studies mentioned in this section will be given fully in the notes for the following chapter.

CHAPTER IX   SOURCE REFERENCES

150, ¶1–2. Welch to stepmother, Oct. 2, 1885. *Johns Hopkins Univ. Cir.*, 1885, No. 44, p. 28.

151, ¶1. Welch to father, Oct. 11, 1885.

151, ¶3. *Ibid.* Welch to sister, Jan. 18, 1886.

152, ¶1. Welch to stepmother, Feb. 13, 1886.

152, ¶2. Welch to Gilman, June 8, 1886, coll. Hopkins Library, copy W.P.

153, ¶1. W. S. Walcott, jr., to his mother, Aug. 9, 1886. Welch to sister, Aug. 9, 29, 1886.

153, ¶2. Welch to Trustees, Hopkins Univ., May 14, 1887, coll. Hopkins Library, copy W.P. MacCallum, *William Stewart Halsted, Surgeon*, Balto., 1930, p. 60. Sabin, Florence R., *Franklin Paine Mall*, Balto., 1934, p. 76.

153, ¶3. Welch to sister, Feb. 12, 1889, April 4, 1892.

154, ¶1. Ms. account of conversation between Mrs. J. Hemsley Johnson and S. Flexner, Dec. 11, 1935.

155, ¶1. Welch to stepmother, Oct. 2, 1885. In the fall of 1886, 20 Cathedral Street became 506 Cathedral Street through a change in numbering. Welch to sister, Oct. 15, 1886. Notes on conversation between S. Bayne-Jones and S. Flexner.

155, ¶2. Welch to father, Feb. 4, 1889. Welch to brother-in-law, Jan. 24, 1889.

156, ¶1. Welch, Remarks at dinner for William T. Councilman, *P. & A.*, *3*, 423.

156, ¶2. Welch to stepmother, Feb. 13, 1886, May 2, 1891.

156, ¶3. Barker, ms. account of talk with Welch at Hopkins Hosp., July 14, 1933, copy W.P. Welch to sister, Oct. 23, 1888.

157, ¶1. Barker, *op. cit.*

157, ¶2. Thomas, James Carey, memo. of talk with Welch, Aug. 31, 1886. M. Carey Thomas papers, Bryn Mawr College, copy W.P.

158, ¶3. Welch, "John Shaw Billings," remarks at memorial meeting, May 26, 1913, *Bull. Johns Hopkins Hosp.*, 1914, *25*, 251, *P. & A.*, *3*, 400. Barker, *op. cit.*

158, ¶4. Welch to father, Feb. 4, 1889. Welch to Mall, Aug. 17, 1889, Mall papers, copy W.P.

159, ¶1. Welch to sister, June 25, 1886. Hurd, Henry M., *The First Quarter-Century of the Johns Hopkins Hospital, 1889–1914*, ms., coll. Hopkins Hosp., abstract W.P.

159, ¶2. Welch to father, Aug. 12, 1890.

163, ¶4. Welch, "Remarks on Receiving the Kober Medal," May 4, 1927, *Tr. Assn. Am. Physn.*, 1927, *42*, 11. Welch to Mall, June 29, 1898, Mall papers, copy W.P.

164, ¶1. Barker, ms. account of Henry Barton Jacobs's dinner, Feb. 27, 1929, copy W.P. MacCallum, "Dr. Welch," *Bull. Johns Hopkins Hosp.*, 1934, *54*, 383.

166, ¶4. G. H. Whipple to S. Flexner, March 17, 1937.

167, ¶1. MacCallum, "William Henry Welch," *Arch. Path.*, 1934, *17*, 829.

168, ¶2. Welch to sister, June 9, 1891. Welch to E. W. Kellogg, June 10, 1914.

169, ¶1. Welch to S. Flexner, Dec. 8, 1905, coll. S. Flexner, abstract W.P. See also: Welch to MacCallum, May 30, 1908, coll. MacCallum, copy W.P.

169, ¶2. Zinsser, Hans, *Theobald Smith, 1859–1934*, Nat. Acad. Sciences biographical memoir, 1936, *17*, No. 12, p. 288.

170, ¶3. Freeman, A. W., *Memorandum . . . on My Personal Memories of Dr. Welch*, April 22, 1936, p. 29. Welch to sister, July 8, 1898.

171, ¶1. Welch to Mall, June 5, 1889, Mall papers, copy W.P.

171, ¶2. Welch to S. Flexner, March 17, 1899, coll. S. Flexner, abstract W.P.

171, ¶3. The young man in this story was S. Flexner.

171, ¶4. *The Sun*, Balto., July 11, 1910, p. 9.

173, ¶1. R. W. Wood to S. Flexner, May 29, 1934.

173, ¶3. Welch to Dennis, Dec. 9, 1890, May 26, 1899, March 8, 1910, coll. N. Y. Acad. of Med., copies W.P. Welch, "General Bacteriology of Surgical Infections," in Dennis, *System of Surgery*, Phila., 1895, *1*, 249, *P. & A.*, *2*, 436.

174, ¶1. Welch to sister, Jan. 29, 1890.

174, ¶2. *Ibid.* Welch to brother-in-law, Feb. 27, 1890.

175, ¶1. Welch to sister, July 1, 1890.

175, ¶2. Welch to sister, April 9, 1891.

175, ¶3. Welch to sister, March 28, 1891. Welch to stepmother, Feb. 20, 1886.

175, ¶4. "William Wickham Welch," *Dictionary of American Biography*, N.Y., 1936, *19*, 624. Welch to G. H. F. Nuttall, Aug. 19, 1892, Nuttall papers, copy W.P. Welch to sister, April 29, 1893.

176, ¶1. Welch to sister, June 17, 27, July 1, 1895. Welch to stepmother, July 1, Dec. 31, 1895. Welch to Gilman, June 28, 1895, coll. Hopkins Library, copy W.P.

176, ¶2. Welch to stepmother, Nov. 2, 1892. Welch to sister, March 23, 1898.

178, ¶2. This story has been told in a number of published accounts of Welch; it is here told as remembered by S. Flexner.

179, ¶3. Welch and Nuttall, "A Gas-Producing Bacillus (*Bacillus Aerogenes Capsulatus*, Nov. Spec.) Capable of Rapid Development in the Body after Death," *Bull. Johns Hopkins Hosp.*, 1892, *3*, 81, *P. & A.*, *2*, 539.

CHAPTER X   TEXT NOTES

1. In all of Welch's papers he reviews the literature on the subject. The original papers are to be consulted for his comments.
2. For present views on fibrin formation, see Howell, W. H., *A Text-Book of Physiology*, Phila., 1936, p. 481.
3. Among Welch's papers there are two small notebooks containing his notes, in German, on Heidenhain's lectures in Breslau, one on *Haemodynamik* and the other on animal heat (*Thierische Wärme*).
4. For present knowledge of the neurogenic origin of fever, see Howell, *op. cit.*, p. 1055.
5. This point of view is supported by contemporary knowledge, and the curative action of fever (hyperpyrexia) in certain pathological conditions caused by infectious micro-organisms—paresis, for instance—has been established by clinical observations. See MacCallum, W. G., *A Text-Book of Pathology*, Phila., 1940, p. 169.
6. Welch employed two names to designate the pneumococcus: *Diplococcus pneumoniae* and *Micrococcus lanceolatus*. At that time the nomenclature of the micro-organisms was in a confused state. Welch discussed the confusion in the opening paragraph of his paper, "*Micrococcus lanceolatus*, with Especial Reference to the Etiology of Acute Lobar Pneumonia," *Bull. Johns Hopkins Hosp.*, 1892, *3*, 125, *P. & A.*, *2*, 146.
7. "*Micrococcus lanceolatus* was discovered by Sternberg in September 1880, by inoculation of rabbits with his own saliva. It was next found by Pasteur in December 1880, by inoculating rabbits with the saliva of a child dead of hydrophobia. Pasteur's observations were the first to be made public, being announced at the meeting of the Académie de Médecine in Paris on January 18, 1881. They gave rise to no less than six communications to the same Academy in January, February, and March 1881. Sternberg's first publication on this subject appeared on April 30, 1881." (Welch, "*Micrococcus lanceolatus*," *loc. cit.*)
8. This bacillus, first erroneously described as a micrococcus and now called *Bacillus mucosus capsulatus*, was discovered in 1882. Friedländer, C., "Über die Schizomyceten bei der acuten fibrinösen Pneumonie," *Arch. f. path. Anat. u. Phys.*, 1882, *87*, 319; "Die Mikrokokken der Pneumonie," *Fortschr. d. Med.*, 1883, *1*, 715; "Weitere Bemerkungen über Pneumonie," *ibid.*, 1884, *2*, 333.
9. In the light of later chemical studies, Welch's attention to the capsules carrying the active chemical substances (polysaccharides) on which the specific properties of the pneumococcus depend, is worth emphasizing. See Avery, O. T., "The Role of Specific Carbohydrates in Pneumococcus Infection and Immunity," *Ann. Int. Med.*, 1933, *6*, p. 1.
10. It is usual to designate the diphtheria bacillus the Klebs-Loeffler bacillus, because Klebs, although he did not cultivate it, described it in 1883.
11. Fraenkel called the bacillus isolated by him *Bacillus phlegmones emphysematosae* (see Fraenkel, E., *Über Gasphlegmonen*, Hamburg, 1893). In Migula's clas-

sification, the designation *Bacillus welchii* is used. Today the bacillus is classified under the genus *Clostridium* as *C. welchii*.

On June 17, 1895, Welch wrote Fraenkel as follows: "I thank you very much for the cultures of your b. phlegmones emphysematosae. . . . I have already examined the cultures and have no doubt of the identity of your bacillus with mine, and am much pleased that you have come to the same conclusion.

"I have also found this bacillus repeatedly both at autopsies and in living human beings and, like you, I am convinced that it is a wide spread organism. . . . We have found it twice in perforative peritonitis with large development of gas in the peritoneal cavity, in one case it was the predominant organism, so that it must be an inhabitant at times of the intestinal canal. I have had several cases of rapid development of gas post-mortem, similar to the one which I first described. I have also found it in emphysematous phlegmons. . . .

"The method which I first described of injecting directly into the ear vein of a rabbit a culture of the bacillus and then killing the rabbit after five minutes and keeping the body in a warm place for ten or twelve hours or less is a convenient one for demonstrating and separating the bacillus. 'Schaumleber' and 'Schaum-milz' and gas in the blood and elsewhere are produced regularly.

"We have also confirmed your observations as to the pathogenic properties of the bacillus and have found bacilli even more pathogenic than those first described by you. I am delighted that our results are in such harmony.

"As regards nomenclature, would it be presumptuous if I suggest that you adopt the name first given to this organism by Nuttall and myself in an article published in July–August 1892. Your first publication was I believe in Jan. 1893. (Centralbl. f. Bakt. 1893, XIII, 1.) It is, I believe, in accordance with scientific usage to adopt the name first given to a new species, unless this is objectionable. As the bacillus is wide spread and concerned in other conditions and processes besides gaseous phlegmons, it seems to me that the less restricted name b. aerogenes capsulatus is more appropriate than b. phlegmones emphysematosae which commits the organism to a single pathological process."

A point of difference between Welch's observations on his bacillus and Fraenkel's on his related to spore formation. The discrepancy was cleared up by S. K. Dunham (*Bull. Johns Hopkins Hosp.*, 1897, *8*, 68), who found that the Welch micro-organisms also produced spores on particular culture media.

In a letter to Ivan C. Hall of May 13, 1927 (coll. Hall, copy W.P.), Welch wrote: "There is, of course, an enormous literature on gas bacillus infection during the war, together with the discovery of other gas-producing and non-gas-producing anaerobic bacilli in wound infections."

12. A second paper that was to have followed in the *Journal* was never published; the manuscript was found among Welch's papers.

13. The case illustrating the condition found in biliary infection was supplied by Dr. W. T. Howard, jr., of Cleveland, Ohio.

CHAPTER X　　　SOURCE REFERENCES

181, ¶2. Welch, "An Experimental Study of Glomerulonephritis," *Tr. Assn. Am. Physn.*, 1886, *1*, 171, *P. & A.*, *1*, 293.

183, ¶3. MacCallum, W. G., "Glomerular Changes in Nephritis," *Bull. Johns Hopkins Hosp.*, 1934, *55*, 416. MacCallum, *A Text-Book of Pathology*, Phila., 1940.

184, ¶1. Welch, "The Structure of White Thrombi," *Tr. Path. Soc. Phila.*, 1885–1887, *13*, 281, *P. & A.*, *1*, 47.

184, ¶2. Schimmelbusch, C., "Die Blutplättchen und die Blutgerinnung." *Arch. f. path. Anat.*, 1885, *101*, 201. Eberth, J. C., and Schimmelbusch, "Experimentelle Untersuchungen über Thrombose," *ibid.*, 1886, *103*, 39, 1886, *105*, 331.

186, ¶3. Welch, "Thrombosis and Embolism," in *Syst. Med.* (Allbutt), London, 1899, *7*, 155, *Syst. Med.* (Allbutt and Rolleston), London, 1909, *6*, 691, *P. & A.*, *1*, 110, 193.

186, ¶4. Welch to father, Sept. 23, 1877. Cohnheim, Julius, *Untersuchungen über die embolischen Processe*, Berlin, 1872.

187, ¶3. Welch, "Haemorrhagic Infarction," address delivered before the Association of American Physicians, Washington, June 2, 1887, *Tr. Assn. Am. Physn.*, 1887, *2*, 121, *P. & A.*, *1*, 66. Welch and Mall, "Experimental Study of Haemorrhagic Infarction of the Small Intestine in the Dog," *P. & A.*, *1*, 77.

189, ¶4. Welch, "On the General Pathology of Fever," *Boston Med. & Surg. J.*, 1888, *118*, 333, 361, 413, *P. & A.*, *1*, 302. Dalton, J. C., *History of the College of Physicians and Surgeons*, N.Y., 1888, p. 112.

190, ¶1. Welch to sister, March 22, 1888.

195, ¶1. Welch, "Preliminary Report of Investigations Concerning the Causation of Hog Cholera," *Bull. Johns Hopkins Hosp.*, 1889–1890, *1*, 9, *P. & A.*, *2*, 79. Welch and Clement, A. W., *Remarks on Hog Cholera and Swine Plague*, delivered at Chicago, Oct. 20, 1893, Phila., 1894, *P. & A.*, *2*, 86.

198, ¶1. DeSchweinitz, E. A., and Dorset, M., *Bureau of Animal Industry Reports*, 1903, *20*, 157. Dorset, Bolton, B. M., and McBryde, C. N., *Bureau of Animal Industry Reports*, 1904, *21*, 138.

198, ¶3. I am indebted to Dr. Carl Ten Broeck for the information upon which the paragraph on the virus pathology of hog cholera is based.

199, ¶1. Welch, "Remarks on *Diplococcus Pneumoniae*," before Johns Hopkins Hosp. Med. Soc., Feb. 17, 1890, *Bull. Johns Hopkins Hosp.*, 1889–1890, *1*, 73, *P. & A.*, *2*, 120. "The Etiology of Acute Lobar Pneumonia," president's address before Medical and Chirurgical Faculty, Balto., April 26, 1892, *Tr. Med. & Chir. Fac. Maryland*, 1892, *1*, *P. & A.*, *2*, 124. "*Micrococcus lanceolatus*, with Especial Reference to the Etiology of Acute Lobar Pneumonia," *Bull. Johns Hopkins Hosp.*, 1892, *3*, 125, *P. & A.*, *2*, 146. Blachstein, A. G., "Intravenous Inoculation of Rabbits with the *Bacillus Coli Communis* and the *Bacillus Typhi Abdominalis*," *Bull. Johns Hopkins Hosp.*, 1891, *2*, 96. Welch, "Additional Note Concerning the Intravenous Inoculation of *Bacillus Typhi Abdominalis*," *ibid.*, p. 121, *P. & A.*, *2*, 332. Welch, "Experimental Production of Typhoid-Bacillus Carriers," before Johns Hopkins Hosp. Med. Soc., Nov. 2, 1914, *Bull. Johns Hopkins Hosp.*, 1915, *26*, 32, *P. & A.*, *2*, 335.

201, ¶3. Avery, O. T., Chickering, H. T., Cole, Rufus, Dochez, A. R., *Acute Lobar Pneumonia, Prevention and Serum Treatment*, Rock. Inst. for Med. Res. Monographs, No. 7, 1917.

203, ¶1–2. Prudden, T. M., "On the Etiology of Diphtheria," *Am. J. Med. Sc.*, 1889, *97*, 329, 450. Welch and Abbott, "The Etiology of Diphtheria," reported to Johns Hopkins Hosp. Med. Soc., June 2, 1890, and Jan. 9, 1891, *Bull. Johns Hopkins Hosp.*, 1891, *2*, 25, *P. & A.*, *2*, 181. Prudden, T. M., "Studies on the Etiology of Diphtheria," *Med. Record*, 1891, *39*, 445.

203, ¶3. Welch, "The Causation of Diphtheria," *Tr. Med. & Chir. Fac. Maryland*, 1891, 242, *P. & A.*, *2*, 197.

205, ¶1. Welch and Flexner, S., "The Histological Changes in Experimental Diphtheria," before Johns Hopkins Hosp. Med. Soc., May 1891, *Bull. Johns Hopkins Hosp.*, 1891, *2*, 107, *P. & A.*, *2*, 218. Welch and Flexner, "The Histological Lesions Produced by the Toxalbumen of Diphtheria," *Bull. Johns Hopkins Hosp.*, 1892, *3*, 17, *P. & A.*, *2*, 225.

206, ¶1. Welch, "Bacteriological Investigations of Diphtheria in the United States," *Am. J. Med. Sc.*, 1894, *108*, 427, *P. & A.*, *2*, 229.

206, ¶2. Welch, "The Treatment of Diphtheria by Antitoxin," *Tr. Assn. Am. Physn.*, 1895, *10*, 312, *P. & A.*, *2*, 265. Two years later Welch spoke again on diphtheria before a conference of health officers in Baltimore: "Clinical and Bacteriological Diagnosis of Diphtheria," *Maryland Med. J.*, 1896–1897, *36*, 392, *P. & A.*, *2*, 322.

207, ¶3. Welch and Nuttall, "A Gas-Producing Bacillus (*Bacillus Aerogenes Capsulatus*, Nov. Spec.), Capable of Rapid Development in the Blood-Vessels after Death," *Bull. Johns Hopkins Hosp.*, 1892, *3*, 81, *P. & A.*, *2*, 539. See also: Welch, "Aneurism with Demonstration of Bacillus Causing Air in the Tissues," before Johns Hopkins Hosp. Med. Soc., Nov. 2, 1891, *Bull. Johns Hopkins Hosp.*, 1892, *3*, 31.

209, ¶1. Graham, J. C., Steward, S. H., and Baldwin, J. F., "*Bacillus Aerogenes Capsulatus;* Case; Diagnosis; Autopsy; Bacteriological Study," *Columbus Med. J.*, 1893–1894, *12*, 55.

209, ¶2. Welch and Flexner, S., "Observations Concerning *Bacillus Aerogenes Capsulatus*," *J. Exp. Med.*, 1896, *1*, 5, *P. & A.*, *2*, 564. Welch, "Morbid Conditions Caused by *Bacillus Aerogenes Capsulatus*," Shattuck Lecture, before Mass. Med. Soc., Boston, June 12, 1900, *Boston Med. & Surg. J.*, 1900, *143*, 73, *P. & A.*, *2*, 599. Welch, "Distribution of *Bacillus Aerogenes Capsulatus*," Am. Soc. of Bacteriologists, Balto., Dec., 1900, *J. Boston Soc. Med. Sc.*, 1900–1901, *5*, 369, *P. & A.*, *2*, 637.

209, ¶3. Bull, C. G., and Pritchett, Ida W., "Toxin and Antitoxin of and Protective Inoculation against *Bacillus Welchii*," *J. Exp. Med.*, 1917, *26*, 119. Bull, "The Prophylactic and Therapeutic Properties of the Antitoxin for *Bacillus Welchii*," *ibid.*, 1917, *26*, 603. "Gas Gangrene," *Brit. Med. J.*, 1940, *2*, 421. "The Chemotherapy of War Wounds," *J. Am. Med. Assn.*, 1940, *115*, 2194.

210, ¶1. Welch, "Conditions Underlying the Infection of Wounds," before Congress of Amer. Physn. and Surg., Washington, Sept. 22, 1891, *Tr. Cong. Am. Physn. & Surg.*, 1892, *2*, 1, *P. & A.*, *2*, 392. Welch, "Some Considerations Concerning Antiseptic Surgery," before Clinical Soc. of Maryland, Oct. 16, 1891, *Maryland Med. J.*, 1891–1892, *26*, 45, *P. & A.*, *2*, 419. Abbott, A. C., "Corrosive Sublimate as a Disinfectant against the *Staphylococcus Pyogenes Aureus*," *Bull. Johns Hopkins Hosp.*, 1891, *2*, 50.

210, ¶2. The reference to Halsted's subcutaneous sutures may be found in *P. & A.*, *2*, 411 and 435.

CHAPTER XI   TEXT NOTES

1. Welch's statement of the aims of the Medical School ("On Some of the Humane Aspects of Medical Science," *Johns Hopkins Univ. Circ.*, 1886, *5*, 101, *P. & A.*, *3*, 3) was, of course, not the first. We must not forget Gilman's inaugural address, delivered in 1876 ("The Johns Hopkins University in Its Beginnings," in Gilman, *University Problems in the United States*, N.Y., 1898, 1), which so inspired Welch while yet an interne. Giving a course of lectures at the university in 1877–1878, Billings argued that the future medical school should demand a B.A. degree for entrance; that practical instruction should be given in the laboratories and the hospital; that the classes should not exceed twenty-five in number; that research should be stressed as well as teaching; and that the curriculum should be widened to include such subjects as comparative pathology, medical history and bibliography, state medicine and public hygiene, sanitary engineering, forensic medicine, and special courses for the army and navy. This was a visionary scheme which the Johns Hopkins Medical School has not even yet completely realized. (Chesney, A. M., "Two Papers by John Shaw Billings on Medical Education," *Bull. Institute of History of Med.*, 1938, *6*, 285.)

2. In 1888 Thomas had presented a similar suggestion to Gilman in the belief that the fees would offset the extra expense of teaching and that the university would issue the diplomas and thus control the teaching. He wrote (Feb. 10, 1888, coll. Hopkins Library, copy W.P.): "Might it not be well to add that the outlay necessary to provide instruction by the appointees of the Hospital (who would have to be paid for their services to the Hospital) need not be so enormous as to absorb any large proportion of the income of the Hospital—that it would in no sense be the founding of a medical school by the Hospital but simply utilizing the necessary equipment (in men and arrangements) for the teaching purposes

of the University who would be responsible for the Diploma—and that the fees of students might go some way in reimbursing the outlay."

3. The meeting at which the Women's Fund Committee was organized was held at the home of Miss King, daughter of Francis T. King; Mrs. Henry Winter Davis was elected president, and Miss Mary Garrett, secretary. Those present were: Mrs. W. Reed, Mrs. George W. Brown, Mrs. Charles Green, Miss Hall, Miss McLane, Mrs. H. Newell Martin, Miss Gwinn, Miss Morris, Miss M. Carey Thomas, Mrs. Henry M. Hurd, Miss Isabel Hampton, Mrs. Manson Smith, Miss Molly Eaton, Mrs. Barton Brune. (*Baltimore American*, May 4, 1890.)

4. On April 27, 1891, Miss Garrett wrote George W. Dobbin, President of the Trustees (coll. Hopkins Library, copy W.P.), that on May 1 the Women's Fund would pay to the university $109,000. She offered to add another $100,000 on Oct. 1, 1892, "provided that on or before February 1, 1892, there shall be in the hands of the Trustees . . . the remaining sum necessary to constitute an endowment for such school of five hundred thousand dollars, and provided also that the Trustees . . . open the Medical School . . . in October 1892, and will give public notice in February 1892, of its intended opening."

The Trustees accepted Miss Garrett's conditional gift on April 30, 1891, according to *The Nation* (May 7, 1891), "and have pledged themselves to raise the remaining amount needed." Whether they worked hard at it or not is not known, but certainly they did not succeed in raising anything. As a result, Miss Garrett's offer lapsed.

5. The document mentioned in Welch's letter to Cushing (Aug. 8, 1922, Cushing papers, copy W.P.) has disappeared, but among the Welch papers we find the following memorandum, dated 1891, which practically outlines the entrance requirements on which Miss Garrett insisted:

REGARDING MEDICAL INSTRUCTION IN THE JOHNS HOPKINS UNIVERSITY

by William H. Welch

March 18, 1891

A. Plan of Instruction

1. Requirements for *preliminary education:* Such knowledge of *Latin* and of *Mathematics* as is acquired in undergraduate courses in which the chief attention is directed to the natural sciences.

   Especial emphasis should be laid upon good laboratory training in *Physics, Inorganic* and *Organic Chemistry* (excluding Physiological Chemistry), and *General Biology* (Zoology, comparative Anatomy, Botany, general Morphology, general Physiology). Such a reading knowledge of *French* and of *German* should be required as will permit free use of works in these languages by the medical student. It is desirable that the preliminary education should be completed by the twentieth or the twenty-first year of age, at which period medical instruction should begin.

2. The *Medical Course* should be four years in duration.

   a. Studies of the *first* year:—Human Anatomy, Normal Histology, Embryology, Animal Physiology, Physiological Chemistry.

   b. Studies of the *second* year:—Human Anatomy (continued), Pharmacology and Experimental Therapeutics, Pathological Anatomy, Pathological Histology, General Pathology, Bacteriology, Recitations in Theory and Practice of Medicine, and in Theory and Practice of Surgery.

   c. Studies of the *third* year:—Theory and Practice of Medicine, Theory and Practice of Surgery (clinical instruction chiefly), Obstetrics, Gynecology, Instruction in Clinical Laboratory, Hygiene, Legal Medicine, History of Medicine.

   d. Studies of the *fourth* year:—Practical work in the hospital wards and in the dispensary, Attendance upon cases of labor, Practice in Vaccination, Special Subjects—Ophthalmology, Otology, Dermatology, Neurology, Laryngology, Genito-urinary Diseases, etc. During this year the student will be expected to undertake some special work under the supervision of one of the teachers with reference to the preparation of a graduating thesis, involving some original investigation.

B. *Additional Buildings required:*
1. Enlargement of the present Pathological Laboratory so as to furnish a large class room for laboratory instruction, a lecture room and rooms for the director and assistants, and a museum.
2. An anatomical building—to include a dissecting room, a lecture room, laboratories for Normal Histology and for Embryology, a museum and director's room.
3. Provision may be found, at least temporarily, in existing buildings and laboratories for teaching physiological chemistry, experimental therapeutics, human physiology, and for general lectures and recitations. Eventually, it will be desirable to add a building or buildings for pharmacology and experimental therapeutics, for hygiene, for lectures and recitations and the general purpose of medical instruction not provided for in existing buildings. The anatomical building might be planned with reference to addition for these purposes.

C. *Additional Professors:*

The present staff of the hospital and of the university provides instructors in Physiology, Chemistry, Pathology, Medicine, Surgery, Gynecology, Obstetrics, Ophthalmology, Otology, Dermatology, Neurology, Laryngology, Genito-urinary Diseases. Probably some additions to the corps of instructors in the physiological and the chemical departments will be necessary to provide for the teaching of medical students.

Organized medical instruction leading to the degree of doctor of medicine might begin, if a professor of anatomy and a professor of pharmacology and therapeutics were added to the existing staff and a building constructed for anatomical instruction.

In my opinion the anatomical professorship should be filled not by a practitioner of medicine or of surgery, but by a scientific anatomist capable of conducting laboratory instruction in normal histology and embryology, and familiar with the best modern methods of teaching human anatomy. The anatomical department should be made one of the important scientific departments of the University, co-ordinate with those of physiology, pathology, etc.

The professor of pharmacology and experimental therapeutics should also be a trained scientific man and should be supplied with laboratory facilities. He might be selected with reference to the teaching of physiological chemistry.

Eventually, provision should be made for a hygienic laboratory and a professor of hygiene, but this is not essential for the beginning of the course of organized medical instruction.

6. Before the Hopkins Medical School was organized, the medical department of the University of Michigan was probably the most advanced in this country in selecting highly trained investigators to fill its preclinical chairs. It is not an accident that the first three preclinical professors at the Hopkins had all been connected with Michigan. Howell and Abel had both been professors there, while Mall had received his M.D. degree from Michigan and when he went to Chicago had refused an offer to return as professor of anatomy.
7. Welch wrote to his brother-in-law on May 5, 1893 that the three new professors were "the best men in the country in their respective departments. We have got a strong faculty, none stronger anywhere, if I do say it."
8. The second appointment to the medical faculty was that of Matthew Hay of Aberdeen. Welch was informed of this appointment while he was in Germany in 1884–1885, and wrote Gilman on Aug. 4, 1885 (coll. Hopkins Library, copy W.P.): "I am sorry I did not know of Dr. Hay's appointment while I was in England. . . . I received a few days ago a postal card from him and at about the same time your letter referring to his wish to meet me. . . . I look forward with pleasure to our association in the Medical Faculty of the Johns Hopkins."

Hay was assistant in therapeutics to Sir Thomas Fraser at the University of Edinburgh, where he had been graduated in medicine in 1878, after which he spent a short period of study in Strasbourg, Berlin, and Munich. He did not, however, take up residence in Baltimore, being at about the same time elected to the chair of forensic medicine and public health at Aberdeen. Hay's interest proved to be more in administration than in his laboratory. Many years later (Oct. 28, 1929), in connexion with the opening of the Welch Medical Library, Hay wrote Welch recalling "the honor done me in 1884 in the invitation sent me through President Gilman to undertake the duties of the proposed Pharmacological Chair. I am now sorry I didn't go to Baltimore."

9. The woman on the Hopkins faculty referred to was Dr. Florence R. Sabin.

10. The advisory board of the Medical School faculty, created in 1893, became the actual governing body of the school. All appointments were made by it and merely confirmed by the Trustees, as required by charter. (See J. Whitridge Williams to Welch, Nov. 22, 1922. Current announcement of Hopkins Med. Sch.)

11. At the beginning of the Medical School, physiology was taught in Martin's laboratory at the University on Howard Street across town and twenty minutes by horse car from the Hospital site. This was a wasteful arrangement, but inevitable under the circumstances of the small university resources. The Physiological Building, next to the Women's Fund Memorial Building and adjacent to the Hospital, provided also for pharmacology and physiological chemistry, thus releasing much-needed space in the Anatomical Building.

CHAPTER XI   SOURCE REFERENCES

211, ¶1. Francis T. King to Gilman, June 26, 1889, coll. Hopkins Library, copy W.P.

212, ¶2. Gilman, *The Launching of a University*, N.Y., 1906, p. 29. Gilman, 13th Commemoration Day address, *Johns Hopkins Univ. Circ.*, 1888–1889, *8*, 48. George W. Dobbin to Gilman, Feb. 9, 1890, coll. Hopkins Library, copy W.P. Cushing, *The Life of Sir William Osler*, Oxford, 1925, *1*, 372–4. Thomas, H. M., "Some Memories of the Development of the Medical School," *Bull. Johns Hopkins Hosp.*, 1919, *30*, 185.

213, ¶1–214, ¶4. Gilman to Francis T. King, Oct. 11, 1889, with accompanying memo. written May 1905; George W. Dobbin to Gilman, Feb. 9, 1890, coll. Hopkins Library, copies W.P.

215, ¶1. Ira Remsen to Gilman, March 5, 1890. George W. Brown to Gilman, March 10, 1890, coll. Hopkins Library, copies W.P.

215, ¶2. Thomas to Gilman, July 26, 1889, coll. Hopkins Library, copy W.P.

216, ¶1. Dobbin to Gilman, April 7, 1890, coll. Hopkins Library, copy W.P.

216, ¶2. Nancy Morris Davis to Hopkins Univ. Trustees, Oct. 29, 1890, *Bull. Johns Hopkins Hosp.*, 1890, *1*, 103.

216, ¶3. M. Carey Thomas to S. Flexner, June 23, 1934, coll. S. Flexner, copy W.P. Minute adopted by Hopkins Univ. Trustees, Oct. 29, 1890, *Bull. Johns Hopkins Hosp.*, 1890, *1*, 103.

217, ¶1. Gilman to Nancy Morris Davis, *Bull. Johns Hopkins Hosp.*, 1890, *1*, 103.

217, ¶2. *Bull. Johns Hopkins Hosp.*, 1890, *1*, 103. Welch to sister, Nov. 11, 1890.

213, ¶1. *The Century*, 1891, *41* (n.s. *19*), 632.

218, ¶2. Welch to Mall, Nov. 7, 1891, Mall papers, copy W.P.

218, ¶3–219, ¶1. H. M. Hurd to Gilman, Aug. 15, 1890, coll. Hopkins Library, copy W.P. Cushing, *Life of Osler*, *1*, 351. Welch to sister, April 4, 1892. Councilman, W. T., "Osler in the Early Days of the Johns Hopkins Hospital," *Boston Med. & Surg. J.*, 1920, *182*, 341.

219, ¶2. *Bull. Johns Hopkins Hosp.*, 1892, *3*, 139. Gilman, *Report to the Trustees of the Johns Hopkins University*, Dec. 2, 1878, copy W.P.

220, ¶1. Welch to Cushing, Aug. 8, 1922, Cushing papers, copy W.P.

220, ¶2. M. Carey Thomas to S. Flexner, June 23, 1934, coll. S. Flexner, copy W.P. Welch, "Twenty-Fifth Anniversary of the Johns Hopkins Hospital, 1889–1914," *Bull. Johns Hopkins Hosp.*, 1914, *25*, 363, *P. & A.*, *3*, 20.

220, ¶3. Welch, Address at memorial meeting for Mary E. Garrett, May 9, 1915, ms.

221, ¶1–2. Mary Garrett to President and Trustees of Hopkins Univ., Dec. 22, 1892, *Bull. Johns Hopkins Hosp.*, 1892, *3*, 139.

221, ¶3. Gilman, Commemoration Day address, *Johns Hopkins Univ. Cir.*, 1893, *12*, 58.

221, f.n. Welch, "Medical Education in the United States," before Harvey Society, N.Y., April 20, 1916, *Harvey Lectures*, Phila., 1916, 366, *P. & A.*, *3*, 119. Welch, "The Advancement of Medical Education," before Harvard Medical School Assoc., June, 1892, *Bull. Harv. Med. Sch. Assn.*, 1892, p. 55, *P. & A.*, *3*, 41. Pepper, W., Address at Harvard Med. Sch. Assn., June, 1892, *ibid.*, p. 47. James, Henry, *Charles W. Eliot*, Boston, 1930, *2*, 71. Seth Low to James R. Chadwick, *Bull. Harv. Med. Sch. Assn.*, 1892, p. 23. Vaughan, V. C., *A Doctor's Memories*, Indianapolis, 1926. Cannon, W. C., "President Eliot's Relations to Medicine," *New Eng. J. of Med.*, 1934, *210*, 730.

222, ¶3. Welch, *The Johns Hopkins Medical School* Commencement address, June 13, 1893, Balto., 1893, *P. & A.*, *3*, 9.

223, f.n. Welch, Harvard Med. Sch. Assn. address, *op. cit.* Chadwick, address on same occasion, *op. cit.* Vaughan, *op. cit.*

224, ¶2. Howell to S. Flexner, July 19, 1938.

224, ¶4. Welch to Mall, Jan. 12, 1893, Mall papers, copy W.P.

225, ¶1–2. Mall to Welch, Jan. 15, 1893, Mall papers, copy W.P.

225, ¶3. Welch to Mall, Feb. 1, March 4, 1893, Mall papers, copies W.P.

226, ¶1. Welch to Mall, March 10, 1893, Mall papers, copy W.P.

226, ¶2. Mall to Welch, April 4, 1893, Mall papers, copy W.P.

226, ¶3. Biography of Abel: *Science*, 1938, *87*, 566.

226, ¶5. Barker, ms. account of talk with Welch in Johns Hopkins Hosp., July 14, 1933, copy W.P.

227, ¶1. Welch, "Twenty-Fifth Anniversary of the Johns Hopkins Hospital, 1889–1914," *Bull. Johns Hopkins Hosp.*, 1914, *25*, 363, *P. & A.*, *3*, 20.

227, ¶2. Welch to stepmother, Nov. 27, 1893. Welch to brother-in-law, Oct. 1, 1893.

228, ¶2. *The Nation*, 1894, *59*, 288. Welch to brother-in-law, March 7, 1894. Welch to sister, March 13, 1894.

228, ¶3. *Announcement of the Medical School, Johns Hopkins Univ.*, 1893, p. 8. *Ibid.*, 1896, p. 15. Welch to sister, March 13, 1894. Welch to Opie, Oct. 10, 1894, coll. Opie, copy W.P. Welch to Cole, July 1, Aug. 3, 29, 1896, coll. Cole, copies W.P.

229, ¶2. Welch to Gilman, June 27, 1894, coll. Hopkins Library, copy W.P.

230, ¶2. Barker, ms. account of a dinner given by Henry Barton Jacobs, Feb. 27, 1929, copy W.P.

230, ¶3. Welch to Mall, June 11, 1894, Mall papers, copy W.P. Welch to Gilman, July 6, 1897, coll. Hopkins Library, copy W.P.

230, ¶4. Welch, "Remarks at Memorial Meeting for Elizabeth and Emily Blackwell," Jan. 25, 1911, in *In Memory of Dr. Elizabeth Blackwell and Dr. Emily Blackwell*, N.Y., 1911, p. 49.

231, ¶1. Welch to sister, Jan. 25, Feb. 10, 1906.

231, ¶2. Conversation between Welch and S. Flexner.

231, ¶3. Welch to Gilman, April 18, 1895, coll. Hopkins Library, copy W.P. Welch to sister, Sept. 1, 1898.

232, ¶1–3. Howell to S. Flexner, Sept. 15, 1937.

233, ¶1. Welch to stepmother, Oct. 28, 1897.

233, ¶2. Welch, "Remarks at the Presentation of the Candidates for the Degree of Doctor of Medicine at the Commencement of Johns Hopkins University, 1898," *Bull. Johns Hopkins Hosp.*, 1898, *9*, 151, *P. & A.*, *3*, 14. Welch to Gilman, Oct. 3, 1897, coll. Hopkins Library, copy W.P.

CHAPTER XII   TEXT NOTES

1. During Welch's last illness, the Welch Bibliophilic Society reprinted his address, as retiring president of the American Association for the Advancement of Science, on *The Interdependence of Medicine with Other Sciences of Nature* (Balto., 1934). Welch expressed regret to S. Flexner that the address on adaptation had not been chosen instead. The "Adaptation" address was published after his death, as Volume III of the *Fourth Series of Bibliotheca Americana* by the Inst. of the Hist. of Med., Hopkins Univ., 1937.
2. The journals published by Hopkins University were: *American Journal of Mathematics, American Chemical Journal, American Journal of Philology.*
3. Also to be present at the conference were Remsen, Hurd, and Murray, of the Johns Hopkins Press. Welch added to Gilman: "Kelly, Halsted, Abel, and Mall have been consulted and are anxious to co-operate."
4. The associate editors were: For physiology: H. P. Bowditch, Boston; R. H. Chittenden, New Haven; W. H. Howell, Baltimore; for pharmacology: John J. Abel, Baltimore; Arthur R. Cushny, Ann Arbor; H. C. Wood, Philadelphia; for pathology: J. George Adami, Montreal; W. T. Councilman, Boston; T. Mitchell Prudden, New York; for medicine: R. H. Fitz, Boston; William Osler, Baltimore; William Pepper, Philadelphia.

   Among the collaborators were persons both actively and remotely connected with experimental medicine. On the whole, the number of laboratory workers assembled was large, but Welch was careful to include prominent administrators and teachers as well, doubtless to avoid injuring sensitive feelings and to promote the interests and circulation of the *Journal.*
5. The scientific medical journals in the United States were, in the order of their appearance:

		Founder or editor
Journal of Morphology	1887	Charles O. Whitman
Journal of Experimental Medicine	1896	William H. Welch
Journal of the Boston Society of Medical Sciences	1896	Harold C. Ernst
(in 1901 this became the *Journal of Medical Research,* organ of the American Association of Pathologists and Bacteriologists, and, in 1925, the *American Journal of Pathology* under the editorship of Frank B. Mallory)		
American Journal of Physiology	1898	H. P. Bowditch
American Journal of Anatomy	1901	
Journal of Infectious Diseases	1904	Ludvig Hektoen
Journal of Experimental Zoology	1904	Ross G. Harrison
Journal of Biological Chemistry	1905	Christian A. Herter
Journal of Experimental Pharmacology and Therapeutics	1909	John J. Abel
Bio-Chemical Bulletin	1912	

   (See *Reference Handbook of the Medical Sciences*, N.Y., 1915, *5*, 711.)
6. The last number of the *Journal of Experimental Medicine* actually edited by Welch appeared in March 1902 (Vol. 6, No. 3). After the Rockefeller Institute had taken over the *Journal*, the editors, Flexner and Opie, completed Volume 6 by publishing in February 1905, one large issue which bore Welch's name as editor,

and which contained the most important of the manuscripts rescued from Welch's study.

7. The completed puzzle reads: "Orthodox Oxford dons know good old port from logwood."

8. George H. Whipple recalls that during his term as Welch's assistant, 1905–1914, Welch "gradually gave fewer lectures and came over to the Department of Pathology less frequently. During the last few years, it seemed that Monday noon was about the only time we could count on him being in the laboratory, and he often gave his quiz on that day." (Whipple to S. Flexner, May 24, 1941.)

9. The contributors to the volume included S. J. Meltzer and H. G. Beyer, who had worked with Welch in New York, and the following Baltimore pupils: Franklin P. Mall, C. A. Herter, Joseph M. Flint, Henry J. Berkley, Robert L. Randolph, Joseph H. Pratt, George Blumer, Herbert U. Williams, George H. Weaver, John B. MacCallum, George E. Brewer, Harry Friedenwald, James H. Wright, Charles R. Bardeen, Thomas S. Cullen, T. Caspar Gilchrist, J. Whitridge Williams, W. T. Howard, jr., W. G. McCallum, Casper O. Miller, Dorothy M. Reed, Harvey Cushing, Louis E. Livingood, John G. Clark, Hugh H. Young, Stewart Paton, Simon Flexner, John C. Hemmeter, Wm. Royal Stokes, William H. Hudson, E. Bates Block, Eugene L. Opie, Claribel Cone, Arthur Blachstein, Mabel F. Austin, Lewellys F. Barker, Florence R. Sabin, W. S. Halsted.

10. Having succeeded Prudden as professor of pathology at the College of Physicians and Surgeons in New York, MacCallum returned to Baltimore to fill Welch's chair when Welch retired. Opie's excursion was larger: from the Rockefeller Institute to the professorships of pathology successively at Washington University in St. Louis, the University of Pennsylvania, and Cornell Medical School. Winternitz became professor of pathology and dean at the reorganized Yale Medical School. First director of the George Williams Hooper Foundation for Medical Research at the University of California, and then dean of the newly modernized Medical School of the University of Rochester, Whipple won the Nobel Prize in conjunction with George R. Minot and William P. Murphy for his work leading up to the liver treatment for pernicious anæmia, formerly a highly fatal disease.

CHAPTER XII   SOURCE REFERENCES

234, ¶1. Welch, "On Some of the Humane Aspects of Medical Science," *Johns Hopkins Univ. Circ.*, 1886, *5*, 101, *P. & A.*, *3*, 3.

234, ¶2. Welch, "Modes of Infection," annual address, Med. & Chir. Fac., April 27, 1887, *Tr. Med. & Chir. Fac. Maryland*, 1887, 67, *P. & A.*, *1*, 549. Welch to sister, Nov. 2, 1879. Welch to brother-in-law, June 2, 1888. Welch, "Some of the Advantages of the Union of Medical School and University," Yale Commencement address, June 26, 1888, *New Eng. & Yale Rev.*, 1888, *13*, 145, *P. & A.*, *3*, 26. Welch, "Considerations Concerning Some External Sources of Infection in Their Bearing on Preventive Medicine," address on state med., A. M. A., Newport, R. I., June 28, 1889, *Med. News*, 1889, *55*, 29, *P. & A.*, *1*, 567. Welch, "State Medicine," before A. M. A., Indianapolis, 1903, *Indiana Med. J.*, 1903, *21*, 510 (abstr.), ms.

236, ¶3. Welch, "A Consideration of the Introduction of Surgical Anæsthesia," at Mass. Gen. Hosp. on Ether Day, Oct. 16, 1908, *Boston Med. & Surg. J.*, 1908, *159*, 599, *P. & A.*, *3*, 221. Cushing, Note on Welch to Cushing, Oct. 9, 1908, Cushing papers, copy W.P.

237, ¶1. Welch, "The Causation of Diphtheria," annual address, Med. & Chir. Fac., April 29, 1891, *Tr. Med. & Chir. Fac. Maryland*, 1891, 242, *P. & A.*, *2*, 197.

237, ¶2. Welch, "Higher Medical Education and the Need of Its Endowment," address at 50th anniv. of Med. Dept., Western Reserve Univ., Feb. 28, 1894, *Med. News*, 1894, *65*, 63, *P. & A.*, *3*, 46.

237, ¶3. Welch, "The Johns Hopkins Medical School," Commencement address, June 13, 1893, Balto., 1893, *P. & A.*, *3*, 9. Welch, "Medicine and the University," address at Univ. of Chicago convocation, Dec. 17, 1907, *J. Am. Med. Assn.*, 1908, *50*, 1, *P. & A., 3*, 89.

238, ¶1. Welch, "Medicine and the University," *op. cit.*

238, ¶2. Welch, "Laboratory Methods of Teaching," remarks before Amer. Surgical Assn., Balto., May 8, 1901, *Tr. Am. Surg. Assn.*, 1901, *19*, 219, *P. & A., 3*, 71.

238, ¶3. Welch, "Higher Medical Education and the Need of Its Endowment," *op. cit.*

239, ¶1. Welch, "Position of Natural Science in Education," address as presiding officer, Am. Assn. for Adv. of Sc., N.Y., Dec. 27, 1906, *Proc. Am. Assn. Adv. Sc.*, 1906–1907, *56–57*, 617, *P. & A., 3*, 83.

239, ¶2. Welch, "Biology and Medicine," at dedication of Hull Biol. Labs., Univ. of Chicago, July 2, 1897, *Am. Naturalist*, 1897, *31*, 755, *P. & A., 3*, 234. Welch, "Pathology in Its Relations to General Biology," opening of biol. lab., Univ. of Toronto, Dec. 20, 1889, *Bull. Johns Hopkins Hosp.*, 1889–1890, *1*, 25, *P. & A., 3*, 191.

239, ¶3. Welch, "Adaptation in Pathological Processes," president's address, Cong. of Am. Physn. and Surg., Wash., May 5, 1897, *Tr. Cong. Am. Physn. & Surg.*, 1897, *4*, 284, *P. & A., 1*, 370.

242, ¶2. Gilman, *The Launching of a University*, N.Y., 1906, p. 115. Welch to C. A. Herter, May 23, 1888, coll. Mrs. H. D. Dakin, copy W.P.

243, ¶2. Welch to Mall, June 5, Aug. 17, 1889, May 16, 1890, June 26, 1891, Mall papers, copies W.P.

243, ¶3. Welch to Gilman, Oct. 29, 1893, coll. Hopkins Library, copy W.P.

243, ¶4. Welch to Mall, June 2, 1895, Mall papers, copy W.P.

243, ¶5. Welch to sister, Dec. 7, 12, 1895.

244, ¶1. Sabin, Florence R., ms. account of interview with Welch, Dec. 1, 1933, p. 12. Welch to Abbott, Nov. 24, 1895, Abbott papers, copy W.P.

244, ¶2. Welch to S. Flexner, n.d., coll. S. Flexner, abstract W.P. Welch and Thayer, W. S., "Malaria," in *Syst. Pract. Med.* (Loomis), N.Y. & Phila., 1897, *1*, 17, *P. & A., 1*, 463. Welch to sister, Dec. 21, 1895. The article for a new edition of a book of Flint's cannot be traced. The 7th and last edition of Flint's *Practice* came out in 1894.

245, ¶2. Welch to Herter, Feb. 9, 1897, coll. Mrs. Dakin, copy W.P.

245, ¶3. Welch to T. S. Cullen, Nov. 14, 1896, coll. Cullen, copy W.P.

245, ¶4. Welch to Abbott, July 2, 1896, Abbott papers, copy W.P. Welch to S. Flexner, Oct. 25, 1901, coll. S. Flexner, abstract W.P.

246, ¶1. Welch to Mall, July 7, 1896, Mall papers, copy W.P. Welch to Abbott, March 30, 1897, Abbott papers, copy W.P. Welch to Herter, April 19, 1897, coll. Mrs. Dakin, copy W.P.

246, ¶2. Welch to Nuttall, Sept. 6, 1896, Nuttall papers, copy W.P.

247, ¶1. Welch to William T. Porter, July 22, 1897, coll. W. H. Howell, copy W.P.

247, ¶3. Welch to S. Flexner, May 20, 1901, coll. S. Flexner, abstract W.P.

248, ¶1. Howell to S. Flexner, Sept. 15, 1937.

248, ¶2. Welch to Herter, Sept. 6, 1902, coll. Mrs. Dakin, copy W.P.

249, ¶1. Ira Remsen to Welch, June 27, 1903.

249, ¶2. L. Emmett Holt to Welch, Dec. 24, 1903.

250, ¶1. Welch to sister, July 3, 1901.

251, ¶1. Welch to sister, July 26, 1902.

251,¶2. Ames, Joseph S., ms. account of Welch.

252, ¶1. Freeman, A. W., *Memorandum . . . on My Personal Memories of Dr. Welch,* April 22, 1936, p. 30.

253, ¶2. Welch to sister, Sept. 12, 1895.

253, ¶3. Welch to sister, June 8, 1896.

253, ¶4. Welch to sister, May 26, 1905. Cushing, Intro. to Vol. I, *Welch Memorabilia,* Cushing papers, copy W.P.

254, ¶1. Welch to sister, Sept. 28, 1894.

254, ¶3. Welch to S. Flexner, June 18, 1894, coll. S. Flexner, abstract W.P.

254, ¶6. Welch,"Fields of Usefulness of the American Medical Association," president's address, A. M. A., St. Louis, June 7, 1910, *J. Am. Med. Assn.,* 1910, *54,* 2011, *P. & A., 3,* 334.

255, ¶2. Great Britain, *Report of Royal Commission on Vivisection,* London, 1876.

256, ¶2. Welch to Gilman, May 8, 1896, coll. Hopkins Library, copy W.P.

257, ¶1. "Memorial to Congress Protesting Against the Passage of the Antivivisection Bill (S-1552)," *Tr. Assn. Am. Physn.,* 1896, *11,* xxiii. Welch to Cushing, July 27, 1922, Cushing papers, copy W.P.

257, ¶3. Welch to Abbott, Feb. 7, 1898, Abbott papers, copy W.P.

258, ¶1. Welch, "Objections to the Antivivisection Bill Now Before the Senate of the United States," *J. Am. Med. Assn.,* 1898, *30,* 285, *P. & A., 3,* 455. Welch, "Argument against Senate Bill 34, . . ." *J. Am. Med. Assn.,* 1900, *34,* 1242, 1322, *P. & A., 3,* 469.

258, ¶2. Welch to Cushing, July 27, 1922, Cushing papers, copy W.P.

258, ¶3. Extract from letter of Senator James McMillan to his son, n.d., copy W.P. Senator Gallinger to F. A. Stillings, May 9, 1898.

258, ¶4–259, ¶1. Welch, "Argument against Senate Bill 34," *op. cit.*

259, ¶2. Welch to W. W. Keen, Jan. 10, 1917, coll. Florence Keen, copy W.P.

259, ¶3. *Prohibiting Vivisection of Dogs,* hearings before the Subcommittee of the Committee on the Judiciary, U. S. Senate, 66th Congress, first session, on S. 1258, Wash., 1919, 49–56.

260, ¶1.Welch to Cushing, Dec. 5, 1910, Cushing papers, copy W.P.

260, ¶2. Welch to Mrs. Charles Dankmeyer, June 22, 1921, copy W.P.

261, ¶1. Welch to S. Adolphus Knopf, Nov. 7, 1922, Knopf papers, copy W.P. Welch to George E. Vincent, Oct. 29, 1926, Rock. Found. files, copy W.P.

262, ¶1. Welch to W. W. Keen, Nov. 10, 1926, coll. Florence Keen, copy: W.P.

262, ¶2. Welch to Wallace Buttrick, Feb. 25, 1910, China Medical Board files, copy W.P. Welch to G. H. Whipple, April 5, May 10, 18 (1910?), coll. Whipple, copies W.P.

262, ¶3. Welch to F. C. Walcott, Feb. 14, 1907.

263, ¶2. Welch to Mall, May 27, [1897], Mall papers, copy W.P.

263, ¶3. Ray Lyman Wilbur to Welch, April 14, 1911.

265, ¶1. Mall, circular letter, Nov., 1899.

265, ¶2. Welch to S. Flexner, Aug. 9, 1898, coll. S. Flexner, abstract W.P. Mall, printed circular, April 20, 1900. *Contributions to the Science of Medicine Dedicated by His Pupils to William Henry Welch,* Balto., 1900.

265, ¶3. Welch to Herter, May 13, 1900, coll. Mrs. Dakin, copy W.P.

266, ¶1. Councilman, W. T., Presentation address, *Bull. Johns Hopkins Hosp.*, 1900, *9*, 135. Welch to S. Flexner, May 8, 1900, coll. S. Flexner, abstract W.P.

266, ¶2–3. Welch, In acceptance of a volume of contributions to medical science, *Bull. Johns Hopkins Hosp.*, 1900, *9*, 136, *P. & A.*, *3*, 351.

CHAPTER XIII   TEXT NOTES

1. At this point Gates stated that since Rockefeller had founded the University of Chicago in 1889, "it was in his mind, as it was in mine, that the institution of research should be associated . . . with that young and flourishing institution." The affiliation of the Rush Medical College with the university prevented this realization. During the course of the negotiations between the two institutions Gates had written Thomas W. Goodspeed, the secretary of the university, intimating that Rockefeller might at some time endow an institution "simply scientific in its investigations into medical science," and Rockefeller had seen and approved the letter, indicating that the idea had actually taken root in his mind. In a second letter to Goodspeed dated Jan. 19, 1898, Gates wrote: "The whole effect and tendency of this movement [the affiliation] will be to make Rush ultimately the medical department of the University of Chicago, as against that far higher and better conception, which has been one of the dreams of my own mind at least, of a medical college in this country conducted by the University of Chicago, magnificently endowed, devoted primarily to investigation making practice itself an incident of investigation and taking as its students only the choicest spirits quite irrespective of the question of funds. Against that ideal and possibility, a tremendous if not fatal current has been turned. I believed the ideal to be practicable and I hoped to live to see it realized."

2. Formal notification that Rockefeller, sr., was willing to give twenty thousand dollars a year for ten years was made by Rockefeller, jr., in a letter to Holt, April 29, 1901, Rock. Inst. files, copy W.P.

3. For confirmation of this statement see Rufus Cole's address at the dinner given in his honour on the occasion of his retirement as director of the hospital, N.Y., April 30, 1938, Rock. Inst. files.

4. Today the *Studies from the Rockefeller Institute* number 118 volumes. In 1913 the form was entirely changed and, in place of being merely a set of reprints bound annually, they became regular, serially paged volumes, the number issued in any one year being determined by the material available.

5. France had the Pasteur Institute, Germany the Institute for Infectious Diseases (Koch), Russia the Institute for Experimental Medicine, England the Lister Institute.

6. A note in Welch's handwriting attached to Holt to Welch, April 26, 1902, reads: "The Directors are of the opinion that the usefulness of the Institute would be greatly increased if, in addition to the establishment of its own laboratories, a sum of money equal to that now at its annual disposal ($20,000) were available for appropriations to support investigation elsewhere in a manner similar to that now in operation."

7. The charter of the Institute was amended in 1908 to provide for the creation of a Board of Trustees; the organization of the two boards was accomplished in 1910. Welch was one of the two Scientific Directors chosen to serve also as Trustees. To Holt he said: "I think that Mr. Rockefeller, Jr., Mr. Gates and Mr. Murphy understand that I should prefer that some other member of our Board should be Trustee in my place, but I am willing to leave the determination of this matter to them and the other Directors." (Welch to Holt, May 20, 1910, Rock. Inst. files, copy W.P.) This was a characteristic attitude of Welch's, often displayed. He never sought such positions but he was almost never relieved of the choice.

The "Corporation," also formed in 1910, consisted of the Boards of Trustees and of Scientific Directors; the original members were: Frederick T. Gates, John D. Rockefeller, jr., Starr J. Murphy, Hermann M. Biggs, Simon Flexner, C. A.

Herter, L. Emmett Holt, T. Mitchell Prudden, Theobald Smith, and William H. Welch.

8. In 1891, John P. Lotsy came to the Hopkins from Holland to take a Ph.D. in plant pathology. Welch, who was of course not a plant pathologist, read up on the subject so effectively that he was able to direct and follow Lotsy's work and give him his final oral examination in public. We all heard at the time of the competency of the examination; and ever afterward Welch had a broad knowledge of plant pathology and of the men working in the subject.

9. On Nov. 20, 1921, a testimonial dinner was given to Smith on the occasion of the formal opening of the Theobald Smith House in Princeton. Addresses were made by Rockefeller, jr., Welch, and Smith. (Mss. in Rock. Inst. files.) The house in which Smith and his family had lived for eleven years had been turned into a staff house as a permanent memorial to Smith.

CHAPTER XIII   SOURCE REFERENCES

269, ¶2. Gates to Murphy, Dec. 31, 1915, copy W.P.

272, ¶1. Holt, memo. dated March 9, 1921, Rock. Inst. files.

272, ¶2. Herter to Welch, March 15, 1901, coll. Rockefeller, jr., copy W.P.

273, ¶1. Welch to Herter, March 31, 1901, coll. Mrs. Dakin, copy W.P.

273, ¶3. Welch to Theobald Smith, May 5, 1901, T. Smith papers, copy W.P.

274, ¶3. Welch to brother-in-law, May 9, 1901.

274, ¶4. Welch to sister, June 15, 1901.

275, ¶1. Welch to S. Flexner, May 15, 1901, coll. S. Flexner, abstract W.P.

276, ¶3. Memo. in Welch's handwriting, 1901. Holt to Welch, June 16, 1902, with list of 1902 appropriations attached. Instructions to those receiving appropriations from the Rockefeller Institute for Medical Research (printed circular), n.d.

276, ¶4. Vaughan to Welch, July 25, 1901. Ernst to Welch, May 20, 1901. Hektoen to Welch, Oct. 2, 1901. Conn to Welch, July 2, 1901. Adami to Welch, May 21, 1901.

277, ¶2. Welch to Abbott, June 10, 1902, Abbott papers, copy W.P.

277, ¶3. Instructions to those receiving appropriations, *op. cit.*

278, ¶1. Welch to Herter, Feb. 4, 1903, coll. Mrs. Dakin, copy W.P.

278, ¶2. Barker to Welch, June 20, 1903.

278, ¶3. Welch to Rockefeller, jr., Jan. 13, 1902, coll. Rockefeller, jr., copy W.P.

279, ¶2. Rockefeller, jr., to Welch, Jan. 17, 1902, copy W.P.

280, ¶1. Smith to Welch, Feb. 11, 1902, Rock. Inst. files, copy W.P.

280, ¶3. Welch to Prudden, March 5, 1902, Rock. Inst. files, copy W.P.

280, ¶4. S. Flexner to Welch, April 8, 1902, Rock. Inst. files, copy W.P.

281, ¶1. Holt to Welch, April 26, 1902, enclosing first draft of Prudden's memo. *Report and Recommendations of the Directors of the Rockefeller Institute for the Year 1901–02* (incorporating revisions made by Welch).

282, ¶4. Holt to Welch, June 20, 1902, enclosing copies of Rockefeller, jr.'s, telegram to his father, June 13, and his father's reply, June 14.

283, ¶1. Rockefeller, jr., to Welch, June 20, 1902, copy W.P.

283, ¶2. Welch to Holt, Feb. 1, 1903, Rock. Inst. files, abstract W.P. Holt, "A Sketch of the Development of the Rockefeller Institute for Medical Research," *Studies from the Rock. Inst. for Med. Research,* 1907, *6,* 17.

284, ¶2. *Studies from the Rock. Inst. for Med. Research,* 1907, *6,* 1–44. Speakers:

Holt, Welch, Nicholas Murray Butler, Charles W. Eliot. Welch's address also in *P. & A., 3,* 74.

285, ¶1. Business Manager's Reports, 1912–13; Welch to Holt, Nov. 26, Dec. 25, 1906, Rock. Inst. files, excerpts W.P.

286, ¶1. Gates to Holt, May 28, 1907, Rock. Inst. files, abstract W.P.

286, ¶2. Welch to Gates, n.d., 1907 (handwritten draft).

291, ¶2. Welch, "Some of the Advantages of the Union of Medical School and University," *New Eng. & Yale Rev.,* 1888, *13,* 145, *P. & A., 3,* 26. Von Harnack, Adolf, "Gedanken über die Notwendigkeit einer neuen Organisation zur Förderung der Wissenschaft in Deutschland," delivered in 1910, in: *Gesammelte Abhand. zur Kenntniss der Kohle,* Berlin, 1917, vol. 1. Glum, Friedrich, "Die Kaiser Wilhelm-Gesellschafft zur Förderung der Wissenschaften, . . ." in: Brauer, L., *Forschungsinstitut, op. cit., 1,* 359.

291, ¶3–292, ¶2. Welch to S. Flexner, May 24, 1905, Dec. 10, 1908, coll. S. Flexner, abstract W.P.

294, ¶3–295, ¶2. Minutes of Rock. Inst. Exec. Com. meetings of Oct. 22, Nov. 12, 1913, Feb. 5, March 11, April 9, 1914; Minutes of Scientific Directors meetings of Jan. 10, April 18, 1914. Theobald Smith to Henry James, April 16, 1914, Rock. Inst. files, copies and abstracts, W.P.

295, ¶3. Ivanovski, D. A., "Über die Mosaikkrankheit der Tabakspflanze," *Bull. Acad. Imp. Sci.* (St. Petersburg), 1892, *35,* 67. Minutes of Scientific Directors meetings of Oct. 30, 1926, and Jan. 17, 1931.

CHAPTER XIV   TEXT NOTES

1. Welch had already referred to the superiority of laboratory over clinical teaching two years before in practically the same words. (See: Welch, "The Material Needs of Medical Education," at opening of new building of the Coll. of Physn. and Surg., Balto., Dec. 21, 1899, *J. Alum. Assn. Coll. Physn. & Surg.* (Balto.), 1900, *2,* 97, *P. & A., 3,* 63.)
2. That year Harvey Cushing was called from the Hopkins to the chair of surgery, and David L. Edsall from Washington University to the chair of clinical medicine. (See: Cannon, W. B., "President Eliot's Relations to Medicine," *New Eng. J. Med.,* 1934, *210,* 730.)
3. Louis wrote to Dr. James Jackson, sr.: "It did not require much time for me to appreciate fully the sagacity and talent, which your son possesses, in the observation of nature. . . . Soon afterwards, learning that he would ere long return to Boston, I pointed out to him the advantage it would be for science and for himself, if he would devote several years exclusively to the observation of diseases. I now retain the same opinion and am strengthened in it; for the more I become acquainted with him, and the more I notice him applying himself to observation, the more am I persuaded that he is fitted to render real service to science,—to promote its progress." (Jackson, James, *A Memoir of James Jackson, Jr., M.D.,* Boston, 1835, p. 20.)
4. By 1892 a similar laboratory for students and staff was introduced in Leipzig by Curschmann and in 1902 von Müller succeeded to the chair at Munich and still further developed the laboratories in the clinic. The William Pepper Laboratory of Clinical Medicine at the University of Pennsylvania, dedicated in 1895, was a lineal descendant of these clinical laboratories. (Welch, "The Evolution of Modern Scientific Laboratories," address delivered at opening of the Pepper Laboratory, Dec. 4, 1895, *Bull. Johns Hopkins Hosp.,* 1896, *7,* 19, *P. & A., 3,* 200.) So was Barker's laboratory at the Johns Hopkins Hospital, subdivided and provided with heads in biology, physiology, and biochemistry, a development accomplished between 1905 and 1907. (Barker, "The Organization of the Laboratories

in the Medical Clinic of the Johns Hopkins Hospital," *Bull. Johns Hopkins Hosp.*, 1907, *18*, 193.)

5. Welch said that he doubted if Ludwig "had ever had a student to whom he was more attached and who made a more profound impression on him than Mall. It was really remarkable. I remember Ludwig speaking to me more than once of his remarkable intellectual qualities. He used the expression 'intellectual.'" (Welch, "Franklin Paine Mall," *Bull. Johns Hopkins Hosp.*, 1918, *29*, iii.)

6. When Welch, during his last illness, asked Barker how much of his address was Mall's, and how much his own, Barker could not say, after the lapse of thirty years. (Barker, ms. account of talks with Welch, Dec. 13, 1933, copy W.P.)

7. This was just twenty years after Welch, in his 1888 address, had made his first effort to bring university medical education to life at Yale.

8. Welch wrote of Abraham Flexner's report: "I consider it to be one of the most remarkable and influential publications in educational literature. It has had not only a large influence upon professional opinion, but especially a large influence on universities and upon public opinion." (Welch, "Medical Education in the United States," *Harvey Lectures*, Phila., 1915–1916, 366, *P. & A.*, *3*, 119.)

9. In a note written toward the end of his last illness, Welch said: "While the improvements in organization and conduct of the major clinics and in clinical teaching by the opening of the Johns Hopkins Medical School represented a less radical reform in medical education than was accomplished in the preclinical medical sciences, the advance in clinical teaching was a very considerable [one]. In his farewell address to the American medical profession before leaving for Oxford in 1905, Osler said his ambition had been to establish at Johns Hopkins a medical clinic combining the best features of the German clinic and of English clinical training, and in these efforts he achieved a large measure of success." (Osler's exact words were: "My second ambition has been to build up a great clinic on Teutonic lines here . . . lines . . . which have placed the scientific medicine of Germany in the forefront of the world." Osler, *Æquanimitas*, London, 1925, p. 472.) Osler, Welch continued, "introduced three great reforms, (1) the creation of an upper resident staff, corresponding to assistants in a laboratory, of carefully chosen young men who had already served a hospital internship and whose tenure of office was indefinite, lasting often for several years, (2) the introduction of the British system of clinical clerks and surgical dressers, a system far superior to that of *Praktikanten* in German clinics, and (3) the establishment of laboratories as an integral part of the clinic where students were taught laboratory methods of diagnosis, and of examinations of excreta, secretions, blood. . . ." (The note is incomplete.)

10. In a later speech, Welch said that the triumphs of medical research had so impressed laymen and doctors alike that "hospitals are often more eager to contribute to scientific medicine than to participate in the work of medical education." He deplored this tendency to separate hospitals from their teaching function, pointing out that "scientific investigation is the fruit of a tree which has its roots in the educational system, and if the roots are unhealthy and neglected, there will be no fruit." (Welch, "The Hospital in Relation to Medical Science," at opening of Section on Hospitals, A.M.A., Atlantic City, June, 1912, *J. Am. Med. Assn.*, 1912, *59*, 1667, *P. & A.*, *3*, 142; and "Medicine and the University," at Univ. of Chicago, Dec. 17, 1907, *J. Am. Med. Assn.*, 1908, *50*, 1, *P. & A.*, *3*, 89.)

11. Welch had already discussed the importance of social medicine in 1906 in his address at the dedication of the new building of the Harvard Medical School. Hospitals, he insisted, should contribute to the general betterment of the communities they serve. (Welch, "The Unity of the Medical Sciences," *Boston Med. & Surg. J.*, 1906, *155*, 367, *P. & A.*, *3*, 305.)

12. Buckler writes: "After finally convincing the Trustees that he [Welch] would in no circumstances accept the Presidency, he tried to persuade them to offer it to me. When I heard of this (. . . I was at Sardis in Asia Minor), I demurred by letter on the ground that I was inexperienced . . . and Welch wrote that he would see me when he was in Europe that summer. He ultimately spent a day with us . . . when I was able to explain why I deprecated his choice. The post

was never offered by the Trustees . . . but I always have felt it a great honour that Welch should have made that choice and have taken the trouble to urge it as he did." (Buckler to S. Flexner, Nov. 27, 1937.)

13. It is of interest to note that among the officers of the General Education Board at the time of this grant were: Frederick T. Gates, chairman; Wallace Buttrick, secretary; Abraham Flexner, assistant secretary; and among the Board members were: John D. Rockefeller, jr., Walter Hines Page, Starr J. Murphy, Charles W. Eliot, Andrew Carnegie, Edwin A. Alderman, Henry Pratt Judson, and Wickliffe Rose.

14. In his Harvey Lecture on medical education delivered in 1916, Welch said: "The Council on Medical Education of the American Medical Association and the Association of American Medical Colleges entered the field later [after the creation of state licensing boards] and have done a great deal in improving conditions, especially in leading professional opinion on the subject and inciting to a very considerable degree a moral pressure." (Welch, "Medical Education in the United States," *Harvey Lectures*, Phila., 1915–1916, 366, *P. & A., 3,* 119.)

15. The members of the committee of clinicians were: Victor C. Vaughan, University of Michigan, chairman; George E. Armstrong, McGill University; Frank Billings, Rush Medical College; John G. Clark, University of Pennsylvania; Harvey Cushing, Harvard University; George Dock, Washington University; John M. T. Finney, Johns Hopkins University; Samuel W. Lambert, College of Physicians and Surgeons, Columbia University; William J. Mayo; George E. de Schweinitz, University of Pennsylvania. ("Report of the Council on Medical Education," *J. Am. Med. Assn.,* 1914, *63,* 86.)

16. As late as 1928, the Council on Medical Education, of which Arthur D. Bevan had been chairman from its organization until 1918, was still debating the full-time system. Bevan wrote: "The medical educator who sees the future of medical education as a purely university affair, with its clinical teaching conducted in a university-owned hospital . . . officered by full-time salaried men, with the hospital with its patients and the laboratory with its frogs and guinea-pigs, conducted along the same scientific university ideal lines without any contact with the medical profession and the community, surely has no vision and no place in the future development of medical education in this country." (Bevan, "Cooperation in Medical Education and Medical Service," *J. Am. Med. Assn.,* 1928, *90,* 1173. See also: Bevan, "Supplementary Report of Council on Medical Education and Hospitals," *ibid.,* 1928, *90,* 1953.)

17. In 1911, the Royal Commission on University Education in London concluded that it could not accept the point of view that "the University should be satisfied with a different standard and conception of the conditions necessary for the education of its students in the subjects involving clinical instruction from that which it adopts and insists on in the case of all other subjects of university study." (*Royal Commission on University Education in London, Appendix to Third Report,* London, 1911, pp. 1, 305, 342; *Final Report,* 1913, pp. 107, 109, 117. Flexner, A., *Medical education in Europe,* Bull. No. 6, Carnegie Found. for Advance. of Teaching, N.Y., 1912.)

The immediate effect was to bring out in England, as corresponding discussions had done in America, discontent with existing methods of clinical teaching. (See: von Müller, F., "Medical Education and the Universities," *Brit. Med. J.,* 1911, *2,* 1421. Osler, W., "The Hospital Unit in University Work," *Lancet,* 1911, *1,* 211. Osler, "The Medical Clinic," *Brit. Med. J.,* 1914, *1,* 10. Duckworth, Sir D., "Address on Some Requirements for Modern Clinical Teaching," *Lancet,* 1913, *2,* 1448. MacKenzie, J., "On the Teaching of Clinical Medicine," *Brit. Med. J.,* 1914, *1,* 17. Rolleston, H. D., "Universities and Medical Education," *Lancet,* 1912, *2,* 927. Wilson, C. M., "Clinical Units: Their Purpose and Achievement," *Lancet,* 1921, *2,* 33. Allbutt, Sir C., "Some Comments on Clinical Units," *Lancet,* 1921, *2,* 937.)

Beginning in 1919, full-time units in medicine and surgery were set up with funds from various sources: the Rockefeller Foundation, the hospitals themselves, etc. In 1938 London University had five units in medicine, three in surgery, and two in obstetrics. (F. R. Fraser to S. Flexner, Jan. 4, 1938, coll. S. Flexner, copy W.P.) Although in a few cases the heads of the units were made almost independent of teaching and the routine care of the sick, the majority were preoccupied by teaching duties, even if their assistants had time for research. The full-time units were in the nature of supplements to the original organization of the hospital schools, where clinical instruction was also given by the regular staff of professional consultants and their assistants.

Welch commented that the British "think that they have adopted the American plan, but they have not. In their system the older consultants remain in the chief clinical positions, while in America it is the 'big man' who is on full-time, and that makes all the difference." (Sabin, Florence R., Notes on talk with Welch, Dec. 9, 1933.) Welch was interested when Sir Thomas Lewis, who was in charge of a purely research unit alongside a teaching unit at the University College Hospital, London, said that "the prosecution of research in medicine tends in general to unfit for practice, and the more whole-heartedly and continuously research is undertaken and the deeper the research goes, the less fitted the worker becomes for the care of unselected patients." (Lewis, "Observations on Research in Medicine: Its Position and Its Needs," *Brit. Med. J.*, 1930, *1*, 479.) Welch believed that Lewis's opinion arose from the fact that he was not fully acquainted with a really good university medical clinic, since the British hospital units were not the equivalent of a genuine university medical clinic. (Welch, "The Development of the Modern Medical Clinic," address at Univ. of Pennsylvania, Oct. 10, 1930, ms. See also: Lewis, Sir T., "The Huxley Lecture on Clinical Science within the University," *Brit. Med. J.*, 1935, *1*, 631.)

18. Avowedly modelled on a type of fellowship familiar in England, the Welch Fellowships will run for three years with a possibility of renewal, and will vary in amount depending on circumstances, the maximum allowance being set at $6,000 annually with an additional $1,000 for equipment and technical help. Fellows will be free to work in the clinics of their choice.

A statement of the Foundation's reads in part: "From eight to ten years hence the present professors of medicine in eleven out of thirteen most valuable medical schools will begin to retire on account of age. . . . The means to train future professors of medicine, which should be available now, are generally lacking, and, if present and predictable limitations in all schools continue for another ten years, convenience rather than quality will determine the choice of selection of the most important posts in American medicine. . . .

"With the purpose of preparing men of special ability for professorial positions, fellowships must be long in tenure and generous enough to hold men who otherwise have the alternative of certain success in practice. . . . The proposed fellowships are designed to counteract the most serious risk to which our best departments of medicine are now exposed." (Minutes of April, 1941, meeting of the Rock. Found., copy W.P.)

CHAPTER XIV   SOURCE REFERENCES

297, ¶1. Welch, Remarks of president before Assn. of Amer. Physn., *Tr. Assn. Am. Physn.*, 1901, *16*, xvi, *P. & A., 3*, 273.

297, ¶2. Welch, Introduction to *The Medical Sciences in the German Universities*, translated from the German of Theodor Billroth, N.Y., 1925, v–x.

299, ¶2. Von Ziemssen, H. W., *Deutsch. Arch. klin. Med.*, 1874, *13*, 1. *Ibid.*, 1879, *23*, 1. Rieder, H., *Berl. klin. Woch.*, 1902, p. 176.

299, ¶3. Kronecker, H., *Berl. klin. Woch.*, 1895, *32*, 466.

300, ¶1. Sabin, Florence R., *Franklin Paine Mall*, Balto., 1934.

300, ¶2. Flexner, A., *The History of Full-Time Clinical Teaching*, ms.

301, ¶4. Barker, "Medicine and the Universities," *Am. Med.*, 1902, *4*, 143, also in *Medical Research and Education*, ed. by J. McKeen Cattell, N.Y., 1913, p. 223.

302, ¶2. *J. Am. Med. Assn.*, 1902, *39*, 989. Dodson, J. M., "The Modern University

School—Its Purposes and Methods," *J. Am. Med. Assn.*, 1902, *39*, 521. Billings, Frank, "Medical Education in the United States," *ibid.*, 1903, *40*, 1271.

303, ¶1. Bevan, A. D., "Medical Education in the United States; the Need of a Uniform Standard," *J. Am. Med. Assn.*, 1908, *51*, 566. Flexner, A., *op. cit.*

303, ¶2. Howell, W. H., "The Medical School as Part of the University," *Science*, 1909, *30*, 129.

303, ¶3. Welch, "The Unity of the Medical Sciences," at dedication of new buildings of Harvard Medical School, Sept. 26, 1906, *Boston Med. & Surg. J.*, 1906, *155*, 367, *P. & A.*, *3*, 305.

303–304 f.n. Welch, *Medical Research and Practice*, address at Vanderbilt Univ., Oct. 15, 1925, ms.

304, ¶1. Dover Wilson, J., *The Essential Shakespeare*, Cambridge, 1932, p. 20.

304, ¶3. Welch, "Medicine and the University," address at convocation, Univ. of Chicago, Dec. 17, 1907, *J. Am. Med. Assn.*, 1908, *50*, 1, *P. & A.*, *3*, 89.

305, ¶1. Welch to S. Flexner, Nov. 22, 1910, coll. S. Flexner, abstract W.P.

305, ¶2. Gates to Welch, Jan. 6, 1911.

306, ¶1. Welch to Gates, Jan. 8, 1911, Gates papers, copy W.P.

306, ¶2. Gates to Welch, Jan. 10, 1911.

306, ¶3. Gates to Welch, Jan. 30, 1911.

306, ¶4. Welch, "Medical Education in the United States," *Harvey Lectures*, Phila., 1915–1916, 366, *P. & A.*, *3*, 119.

307, ¶1. Welch to sister, Feb. 27, 1903.

307, ¶2. "The Council on Medical Education," *J. Am. Med. Assn.*, 1904, *43*, 468. Flexner, A., *Medical Education in the United States and Canada*, Bull. No. 4, The Carnegie Found. for Advance. of Teaching, N.Y., 1910.

308, ¶1. Rockefeller, John D., *Random Reminiscences of Men and Events*, N.Y., 1909.

308, ¶2. Flexner, A., *I Remember*, N.Y., 1940, 177–9.

308, ¶3. Flexner, A., *Report on the Johns Hopkins Medical School*, confidential pamphlet, 1911.

309, ¶1. Welch to Gates, May 10, 1911, coll. Rockefeller, jr., copy W.P.

309, ¶2. Welch, *Report on the Endowment of University Medical Education*, enclosed with letter to Gates, June 11, 1911, coll. Rockefeller, jr., copy W.P.

312, ¶2. Rockefeller, jr., to his father, Aug. 2, 1911, enclosing Gates's memo., Gates papers, copy W.P.

312, ¶4. Flexner, A., *I Remember*, p. 183.

313, ¶1. Barker, "Some Tendencies in Medical Education in the United States," *J. Am. Med. Assn.*, 1911, *57*, 613.

313–314, f.n. Welch to Osler, Aug. 30, 1904, Cushing papers, copy W.P.

314, ¶1. Osler to Welch, May 23, 1911. Osler to H. M. Thomas, April 18, 1911, in Cushing, *The Life of Sir William Osler*, Oxford, 1925, *2*, 270.

314, ¶2. Welch to MacCallum, Jan. 1, 1911, coll. MacCallum, copy W.P.

315, ¶1–316, ¶3. Welch, "The Relation of the Hospital to Medical Education and Research," at opening of new Jefferson Med. Coll. Hospital, Phila., June 7, 1907, *J. Am. Med. Assn.*, 1907, *49*, 531, *P. & A.*, *3*, 132. Welch, "Advantages to a Charitable Hospital of Affiliation with a University Medical School," at Presbyterian Hospital, Dec. 2, 1911, *Survey*, 1912, *27*, 1764, *P. & A.*, *3*, 146.

316, ¶4. Welch, "The Hospital in Relation to Medical Science," *J. Am. Med. Assn.,* 1912, *59,* 1667, *P. & A., 3,* 142.

317, ¶1. Welch, "Present Position of Medical Education, Its Development and Great Needs for the Future," at Univ. of Cincinnati Med. Coll., Jan. 16, 1914, *Lancet-Clinic,* 1914, *111,* 104, *P. & A., 3,* 111.

317, ¶2. Welch, Address at formal opening of the Peter Bent Brigham Hospital, Nov. 12, 1914, *Peter Bent Brigham Hosp. Pamphlet,* Boston, 1914, 8, *P. & A., 3,* 153.

317, ¶3. Welch to Gates, March 30, 1912, coll. Rockefeller, jr., copy W.P.

318, ¶1. Welch to Osler, Sept. 23, 1912, Cushing papers, copy W.P.

318, ¶2. Welch to Buttrick, Jan. 27, 1913, Gen. Educ. Bd. files, copy W.P.

318, ¶3. *Evening Sun,* Balto., June 6, 1913.

318, ¶4. Welch to E. W. Kellogg, March 13, 1913.

319, ¶1. McCrae, Thomas, *William H. Welch,* ms. Welch to E. W. Kellogg, Aug. 6, 11, 1910, Dec. 29, 1911, June 10, 1914. Welch to F. C. Walcott, Jan. 29, 1930, coll. Walcott, copy W.P.

319, ¶2. Welch to E. W. Kellogg, July 11, Aug. 8, 1913.

319, ¶3. Welch to E. W. Kellogg, Aug. 27, 1913. Welch to F. C. Walcott, Sept. 7, 1913.

320, ¶1. *The Sun,* Balto., June 6, 7, 1913. Welch to MacCallum, Feb. 21, 1913, coll. MacCallum, abstract W.P.

320, ¶2. Welch to E. W. Kellogg, June 10, 1914.

320, ¶3. Welch to the Gen. Educ. Bd., Oct. 21, 1913, Gen. Educ. Bd. files, copy W.P.

321, ¶2. Buttrick to Welch, Oct. 29, 1913, Hopkins Univ. files, copy W.P.

321, ¶4. Sabin, Florence R., ms. account of interview with Welch, Dec. 9, 1933.

321, ¶5. *The News,* Balto., Oct. 25, 1913. *The Sun,* Balto., Oct. 26, 1913.

322, ¶1. "Two Munificent Gifts to Medical Education," *Boston Med. & Surg. J.,* 1913, *169,* 689. "Full-Time Professors," *Med. Record,* 1914, *85,* 850. "Full-Time, Salaried Clinical Professors," *J. Am. Med. Assn.,* 1913, *61,* 1906. "A New Departure in Clinical Teaching," *ibid.,* 1914, *62,* 853.

322, f.n. Welch to E. W. Kellogg, July 23, 1907.

323, ¶1–3. Vaughan, Victor C., "Reorganization of Clinical Teaching," *J. Am. Med. Assn.,* 1915, *64,* 785.

324, ¶1. Welch to S. Flexner, March 1, 1915, coll. S. Flexner, abstract W.P.

324, ¶3. Welch to Barker, Jan. 13, 1914; Welch to Howland, Jan. 13, 1914; Welch to Halsted, Jan. 13, 1914, handwritten drafts.

325, ¶1–2. Welch to Janeway, April 28, 29, 1914, Janeway papers, copies W.P.

325, ¶3. Statement by Gen. Educ. Bd., for release July 6, 1914.

326, ¶1. Halsted to A. Flexner, April 19, 1915; Howland to A. Flexner, April 16, 1915; Janeway to A. Flexner, April 20, 1915, Gen. Educ. Bd. files, copies W.P.

326, ¶2. Janeway, "Outside Professional Engagements by Members of Professional Faculties," *Educational Rev.,* March, 1918, p. 207, also *J. Am. Med. Assn.,* 1928, *90,* 1315. Janeway to Welch, Nov. 4, 1917, Janeway papers, copy W.P.

326, ¶4. Osler to Welch, Aug. 28, 1919. Osler to Gen. H. S. Birkett, Dean of the Medical Faculty, McGill Univ., Aug. 29, 1919, *Bull. No. 9 of Internat. Assn. of*

Med. Museums, Sir William Osler Memorial Number . . . , ed. by Maude E. Abbott, Montreal, 1926, pp. 591–92.

327, ¶2. "Full Time Teaching in Clinical Medicine," *J. Am. Med. Assn.*, 1940, *115*, 1888. Welch, *Report on Endowment of Univ. Med. Educ., op. cit.*

327, ¶3. Flexner, A., *The History of Full-Time Clinical Teaching, op. cit.*

CHAPTER XV   TEXT NOTES

1. Fifty of his scientific friends and admirers in Greater New York gave Welch a testimonial dinner on Dec. 31, 1906, after the annual meeting of the American Association for the Advancement of Science, of which Welch was president-elect.
2. One large example of the medallion was presented to the Johns Hopkins University and another to the Medical and Chirurgical Faculty of Maryland; a smaller reproduction in gold was given to Welch, and his associates subscribed for bronze facsimiles of the same size as Welch's gold one.
3. In the spring of 1927 Welch, after failing to answer several letters on the subject, promised Mrs. Biggs that he would prepare an introduction to C.-E. A. Winslow's life of Biggs. This meant taking a second suitcase full of papers across the ocean with him, which he did faithfully, but after that the story is one of continual letters, telegrams, and personal calls from Winslow and members of the Biggs family. He answered as few messages as he could, and when cornered promised that the introduction would be finished any day. That this procrastination was painful to the widow, who wrote that his failure "has just plunged me into the depths" (Winslow to Welch, Oct. 4, 1928), seems never to have occurred to Welch. He waited until the last moment, when the book was all set up by the publishers, and then finally wrote his piece. (Winslow, *The Life of Hermann M. Biggs*, Phila., 1929, ix.)

CHAPTER XV   SOURCE REFERENCES

329, ¶1. Welch to S. Flexner, Feb. 22, 1910, coll. S. Flexner, abstract W.P.

329, ¶2. Welch to sister, June 8, 1896. Welch to F. C. Walcott, Dec. 30, 1906. Welch to sister, May 26, 1905.

330, ¶1–2. Welch to S. Flexner, June 18, 1909, Rock. Inst. files, abstract W.P. Welch to E. W. Kellogg, March 28, 1910.

330, ¶3. *In Honour of William H. Welch*, Balto., 1910. Welch's address, somewhat edited, also in *P. & A.*, *3*, 360.

332, ¶3. Welch to E. W. Kellogg, April 4, 1910.

332, ¶4–5. Welch to F. C. Walcott, June 12, 1910.

333, ¶1–3. Welch to E. W. Kellogg, June 28, July 7, 1910. *The Sun*, Balto., July 11 and 12, 1910.

334, ¶2. W. C. Burket to Welch, Oct. 1, Nov. 26, 1922, April 10, 1926. Welch to Miss Stokes, April 20, 1923, coll. MacCallum, copy W.P. Diary No. 20, June 26, 28, 1924. Diary No. 21, Sept. 30, 1924. Freeman, A. W., *Memorandum on My Personal Memories of Doctor Welch*, April 22, 1936, p. 9, ms. Pres. Frank J. Goodnow to Welch, Oct. 29, 1927.

334, ¶3. Diary No. 24, May 17, 1927. Welch to A. C. Klebs, April 20, 1928, coll. Klebs, copy W.P. Rev. Samuel C. Bushnell to Welch, May 15, 1928. Diary No. 28, May 29, 1928. Halsted, W. S., *Surgical Papers*, Balto., 1924.

334, ¶4. Diary No. 32, Aug. 3, 9, 16, 26, 27, 28, 1930. MacCallum, W. G., *William Stewart Halsted, Surgeon*, Balto., 1930, v.

335, ¶1. *The Sun*, Balto., Sept. 4, 1939.

335, ¶2. Welch to E. W. Kellogg, Dec. 20, 1911, Dec. 24, 1908, Dec. 23, 1906, Dec. 19, 1912.

336, ¶1–2. Conversation between J. T. Flexner and Lois Kellogg Jessup and Emeline Kellogg Adams. Welch to T. S. Cullen, Nov. 28, 1922, coll. Cullen, copy W.P.

336, ¶3. S. M. Gunn to S. Flexner, April 20, 1940. Certificate of flight.

337, ¶1. Welch to W. W. Flexner, Dec. 26, 1909, coll. S. Flexner, abstract W.P. Welch to E. W. Kellogg, Dec. 23, 1906.

337, ¶2–3; 338, ¶1–2. Conversation between J. T. Flexner and Mrs. Jessup and Mrs. Adams.

338, ¶3. Welch to W. W. Flexner, Sept. 22, 1920, coll. S. Flexner, abstract W.P.

339, ¶1. Conversation between S. Flexner and Frederica Heimendahl Gittings, Jan. 1936.

339, ¶2–3. Welch to F. Gittings, June 25, 1924, coll. Gittings, copy W.P.

340, ¶1. Mary Simmons to Emma Welch Walcott, Nov. 1, 1902.

CHAPTER XVI   TEXT NOTES

1. Regular instruction in hygiene was evidently attempted in the University as early as 1883, when the Trustees offered a professorship in that subject to John S. Billings. However, the War Department would not permit Billings to accept a full professorship; he was only allowed to give lectures. "Within three or four years," he wrote Gilman (June 18, 1883, coll. Hopkins Library, copy W.P.) "I feel certain that you can get a man better qualified than I am to fill this professorship—while I can act as a temporary stop-gap, and probably supplement in some ways for a time the teaching of the gentleman whom you select. There is no man in this country who is fitted to fill the position and probably he is to be found in Great Britain rather than elsewhere. I think you would do well to talk over the matter with Mr. John Simon and with Dr. Buchanan of the Local Government Board who will undoubtedly know the most promising man in this line of work."

   For ten years or more Billings continued to hold the title of lecturer on hygiene, or municipal hygiene, in the Hopkins University. He gave lectures on the history of medicine as well, and in 1896 his title became lecturer on the history of medicine.

2. While working in Flügge's laboratory in 1888, Nuttall had discovered the remarkable ability of fresh blood to kill anthrax bacilli, an observation regarded as influencing the later discovery of humoral antitoxic immunity. Rubner, in whose hygienic laboratory Nuttall worked in 1893, was trained as a physiologist under Voit, an associate of von Pettenkofer. He investigated the specific dynamic action of foods on metabolism, using the animal body as a calorimeter.

   Nuttall became university lecturer on bacteriology at Cambridge in 1900; later he specialized in parasitology, making many important contributions to that subject. He was made Quick professor of biology in 1906, and in 1919 became head of the Molteno Institute devoted to the study of parasitology. In 1901 Nuttall founded the (English) *Journal of Hygiene,* and in 1908 the journal *Parasitology,* serving as editor of both these journals. He died in 1937. (Graham-Smith, G. S., and Keilin, D., "George Henry Falkiner Nuttall, 1862–1937," *Obituary Notices of Fellows of the Royal Society,* 1939, 2, 493.)

3. During the cholera epidemic, the quarantine methods of Dr. Jenkins, health officer of the port of New York, were publicly attacked; he seems to have stated that he was acting upon advice given by Welch. In an interview published on the front page of the *New York Evening Post,* Sept. 24, 1892, Welch denied that he had been consulted and expressed disapproval of Jenkins's methods. More significant, perhaps, is the fact that in an editorial published the same day, the *Post* said: "Prof. Welch is conceded on all sides to be the highest authority in

this country on quarantinable diseases and methods for their treatment, so that what he says may be taken literally as the final word on the subject."

4. The time was not distant when a far greater extension of public health laboratories was to take place; they were to become places of the manufacture of vaccines, of curative sera, even of curative specific drugs, and they were destined to serve the entire medical profession of the state through centralized and branch laboratories.

5. In this agitation Welch, Remsen, Gilman, and Billings took leading parts. Although the *Maryland Medical Journal* (1892–1893, *28,* 341) said that the movement owed its inception to Welch, Welch wrote Gilman that the original suggestion was made by Dr. Rohe when Commissioner of Health in 1890 (Welch to Gilman, Dec. 14, 1892, coll. Hopkins Library, copy W.P.). However, Welch wrote his sister on Dec. 22, 1892: "I am responsible for the agitation of the subject by an address which I gave at the Charity Organization Society and it really looks as if something were to be accomplished. Mr. Bonaparte is Chairman of the Committee, Mr. Gilman is also a member."

Welch served on a commission to select the site of the hospital, and in March, 1893, arrangements had so progressed that an ordinance appropriating $35,000 for the erection of the building was presented to the City Council. It was rejected by a vote of 11 to 10. (*Maryland Med. J.,* 1892–1893, *28,* 418.) The whole movement must have broken down at this time, for we know nothing further of it until in 1906, when Welch was attending meetings of a Joint Standing Committee on Ways and Means of the City Council to consider an appropriation for the hospital. The opening of the Sydenham Hospital on April 3, 1909, at last gave Baltimore its hospital for infectious diseases.

6. The truth of Welch's statement is shown by the fact that between 1906–1910 and 1938 the death rate from typhoid fever in Baltimore dropped from 35.1 per hundred thousand population to 1.5. One-third or more of the deaths represented by the lower figure were stated to be of non-residents. (*J. Am. Med. Assn.,* 1939, *112,* 1941.)

7. In a rare burst of discouragement, Welch wrote me on May 30, 1930 (coll. S. Flexner, abstract W.P.): "That big mental hygiene Congress which I attended recently in Washington was rather terrible as an example of arousing the public before the foundation of sound knowledge and doctrine has been laid. With good psychiatric and neurological institutes something might be done in mental hygiene, but it would have to be at first so elementary as to lack altogether the spectacular appeal now made for this subject." Usually, however, Welch was enthusiastic about the movement.

8. The hospital for mental diseases, which was planned by Phipps's own architect, Grosvenor Atterbury, cost $800,000. In 1923 the clinic was put on the full-time basis by an endowment of $2,000,000, half of it given by Mr. and Mrs. Phipps and the other half made up of gifts of $750,000 from the Rockefeller Foundation, $125,000 from E. S. Harkness, and $125,000 from citizens of Baltimore. (Meyer, Adolf, "Retrospect and Prospect," *Contributions Dedicated to Dr. Adolf Meyer,* Balto., 1938, p. 95.)

9. Concerning the commission headed by Walter Reed which demonstrated the insect transmission of yellow fever, Welch wrote the editor of the *Journal of the American Medical Association:* "In the all too generous appreciation of my work in the editorial in *The Journal,* April 9, it is intimated that my advice may have led to the creation of the Yellow Fever Commission. As all that relates to the history and work of this commission is highly important, permit me to say that the credit for the creation of this commission belongs solely to General Sternberg, who had previously so completely exhausted the purely bacteriological study of yellow fever that it was possible for the commission to follow the new direction which proved so fruitful in results." (*J. Am. Med. Assn.,* 1910, *54,* 1326.)

10. Also in 1908, Welch, at Stiles's request, interceded with President Theodore Roosevelt to have Stiles placed on the Country Life Commission, so that hookworm work might be carried on by that body. Although Roosevelt was unable to follow Welch's suggestion at that time, since the Commission was full, when

a vacancy occurred Stiles was appointed. (Stiles to Welch, Aug. 14, 1908; Welch to Stiles, Aug. 22, 1908; Rudolph Forster to Welch, Aug. 24, 1908, Stiles papers, copies W.P.) He was also attached to the Rockefeller Sanitary Commission in an advisory capacity.

11. The Rockefeller Sanitary Commission was made up of the group which met in Rockefeller's office, with the addition of P. P. Claxton, J. Y. Joyner, and, of course, Wickliffe Rose. (*Rockefeller Sanitary Commission for the Eradication of Hookworm Disease, 5th Ann. Rep., for 1914,* Wash., 1915.)

12. Welch was to quote a leading southern sanitarian as saying: "The South was fortunate in some respects in having hookworm infection, for hookworm disease has been the means of stimulating rural health work as nothing else could have done." (Welch, "The Services of Wickliffe Rose to Public Health," address at memorial meeting, Feb. 25, 1932, in *Wickliffe Rose, 1862–1931,* N.Y., 1932, p. 5.)

The original members of the International Health Commission were: Charles W. Eliot, S. Flexner, Gates, William C. Gorgas, Jerome D. Greene, Charles O. Heydt, David F. Houston, Murphy, Walter H. Page, Rockefeller, Jr., Rose, and Welch. (*Internat. Health Comm., First Ann. Rep., June 27, 1913–Dec. 31, 1914,* N.Y., 1915.)

13. In 1911, Welch tried to promote a department of hygiene at Columbia University, as is shown by a letter to MacCallum (March 5, coll. MacCallum, copy W.P.), then professor of pathology there: "I have been very much interested in talking with Dr. Dunbar of Hamburg, and have especial pleasure in handing him these lines of introduction. I have suggested to him that he should talk with you about the possibility of establishing a department of public hygiene at Columbia as I believe that he is admirably qualified to initiate work in this line. Certainly it would be a great service to the country if Columbia could take the lead in training health officers and supplying good courses in hygiene."

14. The committee of the General Education Board, comprising Abraham Flexner, Jerome D. Greene, and Wickliffe Rose, visited Harvard, the Massachusetts Institute of Technology, the Hopkins, the Universities of Pennsylvania and Chicago, Washington University, and Tulane University. They reported that the combined department of hygiene maintained by the Massachusetts Institute of Technology and Harvard under William T. Sedgwick, Milton J. Rosenau, and George C. Whipple covered the ground best, but added that the instruction there, although a distinct step forward, necessarily lacked unity, and that the department neither attempted the teaching of advanced students nor presented opportunities for research in hygiene. (*Rock. Found. Document of Record No. 65,* Jan. 26, 1916. Rose—A. Flexner correspondence, 1915. Rock. Found. files, abstracts W.P.)

After being graduated from the Sheffield Scientific School, William T. Sedgwick studied under Newell Martin at the Hopkins from 1879 to 1881, and in 1883 he was called to the chair of biology, later enlarged to include public health, at the Massachusetts Institute of Technology. Of him Welch said: "Although a useful contributor to science and an admirable writer, Sedgwick belongs to the class of great teachers whose fame is spread and perpetuated by his students and disciples and by personal tradition." (Welch, *Public Health in Theory and Practice,* New Haven, 1925, p. 2.)

15. Those present at the conference were: Abbott, Biggs, Wallace Buttrick, F. Cleveland, A. Flexner, S. Flexner, Gates, Greene, Victor G. Heiser, D. D. Jackson, Edwin O. Jordan, Murphy, William H. Park, Rose, M. J. Rosenau, E. C. Sage, Theobald Smith, Welch, George C. Whipple, C.-E. A. Winslow. (Minutes of the conference of Oct. 16, 1914. Rock. Found. files, abstract W.P.)

16. In his introduction to the first number of the *American Journal of Hygiene,* Welch wrote: "Since the establishment a quarter of a century ago by the editor of the present journal of the *Journal of Experimental Medicine*—the first in this country intended solely for the publication of original research in the medical sciences—nearly every one of these sciences has been provided with a scientific periodical of its own, and has been greatly stimulated thereby." He added that "the growing number of investigators and workers" and "the abundance of valuable contributions to hygienic knowledge available for publication in this

country" proved hygiene ready for a journal of its own. (*Am. J. Hygiene,* 1921, *1,* 1.)

17. Welch's seventieth birthday was also the occasion of his portrait being painted by Thomas C. Corner for the University Club of Baltimore. Burket had previously compiled a bibliography of Welch's writings: *Bibliography of William Henry Welch, M.D., LL.D.,* Balto., 1917.

18. It was not until 1939, when a Rockefeller Foundation appropriation made possible the appointment of a professor of preventive medicine in the Medical School, that the Johns Hopkins Hospital was brought actively into relation with the School of Hygiene and Public Health. The new grant enables the Medical School to extend instruction in preventive medicine throughout the four years of the medical course.

19. Only one virtually complete set of lecture notes remains; it covers the academic year 1920–1921. In addition there are odd pages of notes for other years as well as work cards and sheets.

20. The term "miasmatic contagium" was coined in 1885 by von Liebermeister to account for the supposed manner of transmission of cholera, typhoid fever, dysentery, and fellow fever. The first three diseases are of bacillary origin, the last of virus origin. (Von Liebermeister, C., "Cholera Asiatica et Nostras," in *Spec. Path. u. Therap.,* Nothnagel, Vienna, 1896, Pt. 1, vol. 4.)

21. Russell was successively Rose's successor as director general of the International Health Board and professor of preventive medicine and hygiene at the Harvard Medical School.

22. Three of Welch's addresses given in 1920–1922 and preserved only in manuscript or stenographic report are of special interest: *The Training of Students in Schools of Hygiene and Public Health,* before the Conference of State and Provincial Health Authorities of North America in Washington, May 25, 1920; *The Training of Public Health Officials,* before the American Congress on Internal Medicine, Baltimore, Feb. 23, 1921; *Remarks as Chairman of the Conference on the Future of Public Health in the United States,* Washington, March 14, 1922. These addresses were devoted to explaining the new school, its organization, faculty, and courses, and in expounding the kind of training it offered.

CHAPTER XVI   SOURCE REFERENCES

341, ¶1. Welch to Gilman, Dec. 18, 1884, Hopkins Univ. files, copy W.P.

341, ¶3. Garrison, F. H., *John Shaw Billings, a Memoir,* N.Y., 1915, pp. 248, 342. Pepper, William, "Memoir of Dr. Alexander Crever Abbott," *Tr. College Physn. Phila.,* 1936, *3* (4th s.), xxx.

342, ¶1. Welch to Nuttall, June 23, Sept. 28, 1894, Nuttall papers, copies W.P.

342, ¶2. Welch to Abbott, Oct. 11, 13, 1896, Abbott papers, copies W.P. A. M. Chesney to S. Flexner, June 8, 1939.

343, ¶1. Welch, "On Some of the Humane Aspects of Medical Science," at 10th anniv. of Hopkins Univ., April 26, 1886, *Johns Hopkins Univ. Cir.,* 1886, *5,* 101; *P. & A., 3,* 3. "Modes of Infection," annual address before Med. and Chir. Fac., April 27, 1887, *Tr. Med. & Chir. Fac. Maryland,* 1887, 67, *P. & A., 1,* 549. "Some of the Advantages of the Union of Medical School and University," at Yale, June 26, 1888, *N. Eng. & Yale Rev.,* 1888, *13,* 145, *P. & A., 3,* 26. "Considerations Concerning Some External Sources of Infection in Their Bearing on Preventive Medicine," address on state medicine before A. M. A. at Newport, R. I., June 28, 1889, *Med. News,* 1889, *55,* 29, *P. & A., 1,* 567. "State Medicine," before A. M. A. at Indianapolis, 1903, *Indiana Med. J.,* 1903, *21,* 510 (abstr.), ms.

343, ¶2. Winslow, C.-E. A., *The Life of Hermann M. Biggs,* Phila., 1929, pp. 91–106.

343, ¶3. Welch, "Asiatic Cholera in Its Relations to Sanitary Reforms," *Pop. Health Mag.,* 1893–1894, *1,* 6, *P. & A., 1,* 599.

344, ¶1. Welch, "Relations of Laboratories to Public Health," address before Amer. Pub. Health Assn., Minneapolis, Oct. 31—Nov. 3, 1899, *Am. Pub. Health Assn. Rep., 1899*, Columbus, 1900, *25*, 460, *P. & A., 1,* 615.

344, ¶2. Welch, "Sanitation in Relation to the Poor," address before Charity Organization Soc., Balto., Nov. 14, 1892, *Charities Review*, Feb. 1893, *P. & A., 1,* 588.

344, ¶3. Welch to stepmother, March 7, 1893.

345, ¶1–3. Welch, "The Relation of Sewage Disposal to Public Health," at a joint meeting of the Med. and Chir. Fac. & the Maryland Pub. Health Assn., Nov. 19, 1897, *Maryland Med. J.*, 1897–1898, *38*, 199, *P. & A., 1,* 607.

345, ¶4. Sherwood, Harry S., "A First Citizen of the Scientific World," *Scribner's Mag.*, Nov., 1927, p. 686. (Courtesy of the editors.)

346, ¶1. Welch to Abbott, Oct. 1, 1901, Abbott papers, copy W.P.

346, ¶2. Ford, W. W., "The Public Health Work of Dr. William H. Welch in Maryland," *Johns Hopkins Alumni Mag.*, 1937, *25*, 97.

347, ¶1. Sherwood, *op. cit.*

347, ¶2. Welch to sister, Nov. 23, 1909.

348, ¶1–2. Welch, "What May Be Expected from More Effective Application of Preventive Measures against Tuberculosis," address in Albany, N.Y., Jan. 27, 1908, *Albany Med. Ann.*, 1908, *29*, 256, *P. & A., 1*, 632. (See also: Welch, Opening remarks as president of the Section on Path. and Bacter., 6th Internat. Cong. of Tuberc., Wash., Dec. 28, 1908, *Tr. VI Internat. Cong. Tuberc.*, Phila., 1908, *1*, Sect. I, 2, *P. & A., 1*, 629. "Considerations Relating to the Control of Tuberculosis," before Nat. Assoc. for the Study and Prevent. of Tuberc., Washington, May 14, 1909, *Tr. Nat. Assn. Study & Prev. Tuberc.*, 1909, *5*, 34, *P. & A., 1*, 637. "The Significance of the Great Frequency of Tuberculous Infection in Early Life for Prevention of the Disease," president's address, Nat. Assoc. for the Study and Prevent. of Tuberc., Denver, June 20, 1911. *Tr. Nat. Assn.*, 1911, *7*, 17, *P. & A., 1*, 640. "Control of Bovine Tuberculosis," same Assoc. meeting, June 21, 1911, *ibid.*, *7*, 367, 374, *P. & A., 1*, 651.) Knopf, S. Adolphus, *A History of the National Tuberculosis Association*, N.Y., 1922, pp. 22–32. Homer Folks to Welch, April 1, 1925. Barker, ms. notes on talk with Welch, July 17, 1933, copy W.P.

348, ¶3. Farrand, Livingston, in *William Henry Welch at Eighty*, ed. by Victor O. Freeburg, N.Y., 1930, 23. See also Appendix B.

348, ¶4. Beers, Clifford W., *A Mind That Found Itself*, N.Y., 1935. Paul O. Komora to S. Flexner, May 19, 1941.

349, ¶1. Beers to S. Flexner, April 3, 1936.

349, ¶2. Welch, Introd. to *Twenty-Five Years After*, ed. by Wilbur L. Cross, N.Y., 1934, xv. Henry Phipps to Welch, May 18, 22, 1908.

349, ¶3. Phipps to Welch, June 13, 1908. Phipps to Welch, June 12, 1908, copy W.P.

350, ¶1–2. Theodore Roosevelt to Welch, Feb. 24, 1904, with copy of letter of same date to Rear Admiral John C. Walker.

350, ¶3. Welch to Cushing, Aug. 26, 1922, Cushing papers, copy W.P. Kelly, H. A., *Walter Reed and Yellow Fever*, Balto., 1923, pp. 324–31.

351, ¶1. Smillie, W. G., and Rhoads, C. P., "Hookworm Disease," *Cyclopedia of Medicine, Surgery and Specialties*, Phila., 1939.

351, ¶2. Sullivan, Mark, *Our Times, United States, 1900–1925, 3, Pre-War America*, N.Y., 1930, pp. 290–324. Nevins, Allan, *John D. Rockefeller*, N.Y., 1940, *2*, pp. 649–54. Rockefeller, jr., to members of group meeting in his office, Oct. 26, 1909, copy W.P. See also: Björkman, F. M., "The Cure for Two Million Sick," *World's Work*, 1909, *18*, 11607. "A New Emancipation for the South" (editorial), *ibid.*, *19*, 12316.

352, ¶1. Flexner, S., "Wickliffe Rose, 1862–1931," *Science*, 1932, *75*, 504.

352, ¶2. Welch, "The Services of Wickliffe Rose to Public Health," address at memorial meeting, Feb. 25, 1932, *Wickliffe Rose, 1862–1931*, N.Y., 1932, 5.

352, ¶4. *Rock. Found. Ann. Rep.*, 1916, p. 53.

353, ¶2. Minutes of Rock. Found. meetings of Dec. 30, 1913, Jan. 21, 1914, Rock. Found. files, abstract W.P.

353, ¶3–355, ¶1. Minutes of confer., Oct. 16, 1914, Rock. Found. files, abstract W.P.

355, ¶2. Rose to A. Flexner, Oct. 27, 1914, Rock. Found. files, abstract W.P.

355, ¶3. Rose to Welch, Nov. 2, 1914; Rose to A. Flexner, March 13, 1915; Welch to Rose, March 17, 1915; Rose to Welch, April 12, 1915; Welch to Rose, April 25, 1915, originals or carbons, Rock. Found. files, copies or abstracts, W.P.

355, ¶4. Rose to Welch, May 12, 1915, carbon Rock. Found. files, copy W.P.

356, ¶1. Welch and Rose, "An Institute of Hygiene," *Rock. Found. Ann. Rep.*, 1916, 415, *P. & A., 1*, 660.

356, ¶2. Charles W. Eliot to A. Flexner, Feb. 1, 1916, Rock. Found. files, copy W.P.

356, ¶3. A. Flexner to Eliot, Feb. 11, 1916, carbon Rock. Found. files, copy W.P. Eliot to A. Flexner, Feb. 18, 1916, Rock. Found. files, copy W.P.

356, ¶4. Recommendations of the com. (S. Flexner, J. D. Greene, and W. Rose) appointed by the Exec. Com. of the Rock. Found. on April 11, 1916, to confer with the Hopkins Univ. about plans for a school of hygiene, *Rock. Found. Document of Record No. 74*, May 24, 1916, abstract W.P.

357, ¶1. J. D. Greene to Pres. Frank J. Goodnow, June 12, 1916, carbon Rock. Found. files, abstract W.P. Welch, "The School of Hygiene and Public Health at the Johns Hopkins University," *Johns Hopkins Univ. Cir.*, 1916, *35*, 9, *P. & A., 1*, 669.

357, ¶2. Welch to Abbott, June 18, 1916, Abbott papers, copy W.P.

357, ¶3. *Report of the Fiftieth Reunion of the Class of 1870, Yale University*, New Haven, 1920, p. 10.

358, ¶1. Ames, Joseph S., ms. account of Welch.

358, ¶2. "School of Hygiene and Public Health, Preliminary Announcement," *Johns Hopkins Univ. Cir.*, 1918, No. 301, p. 5. *Rock. Found. Ann. Rep.*, 1918, p. 41.

359, ¶2. Halsted to S. Flexner, Jan. 12, 1920, coll. S. Flexner, abstract W.P.

359, ¶3. *Evening Post*, N.Y., March 1, 1922. News release sent out by Welch, March 1, 1922.

361, ¶2. Garrison, F. H., *Bull. Inst. History of Med.*, 1935, *3*, 1.

362, ¶2. Welch, "Duties of a Hospital to the Public Health," address before Nat. Confer. of Charities and Correction, Balto., May 14, 1915, *Proc. Nat. Confer. Char.*, Balto., 1915, 209, *P. & A., 1*, 621.

363, ¶1–2. F. F. Russell to S. Flexner, Aug. 7, 1939.

364, ¶1. *Rock. Found. Ann. Rep.*, 1916–1931. Welch to E. W. Kellogg, Oct. 28, 1927.

CHAPTER XVII   TEXT NOTES

1. The charter of the National Academy of Sciences had been enacted by Congress and approved by President Lincoln in 1863, and Academy members and committees had dealt actively with military and naval problems of the Civil War. (*National Research Council: Organization and Members*, Wash., 1939, p. 3.)
2. Since the war the Council, reorganized, at President Wilson's request, for peace-

time service, has devoted its energies to the promotion of scientific research in general, continuing to maintain close relationships with Government scientific bureaus. It is supported by grants from the Carnegie Corporation and the Rockefeller Foundation, the latter providing funds for fellowships in a number of branches of science. The Council's present membership is composed of representatives of more than eighty scientific and technical societies, representatives of research organizations and Government scientific bureaus, and some 220 members at large. (*Nat. Res. Council op. cit.*)

3. Welch was always interested in improving the quality of the education of trained nurses and gave two addresses on the subject: "The State Registration of Trained Nurses," before the Johns Hopkins Nurses Alumnae Assoc., Balto., 1903, *Johns Hopkins Nurses Alum. Mag.*, 1903, *2*, 155, *P. & A.*, *3*, 157; and "A Plea for Endowment of Training Schools for Nurses and Opportunities for Specialized Training," before graduating class of the Hopkins Hospital Training School for Nurses, Balto., May 24, 1916, *Johns Hopkins Nurses Alum. Mag.*, 1916, *15*, 140, *P. & A.*, *3*, 163.

4. The following record of Welch's military service is furnished by the Adjutant General's Office, War Department: Appointed Major, Medical Officers' Reserve Corps, July 16, 1917; ordered into active service Nov. 16, 1917; appointed Lieutenant Colonel, Feb. 20, 1918; Colonel, July 24, 1918; honourably discharged as Colonel, Medical Department, Dec. 31, 1918. During the war, he was on duty in the Surgeon General's Office in an advisory capacity. Appointed Colonel, Medical Reserve Corps, Feb. 24, 1919; Brigadier General, Medical Reserve, Dec. 23, 1921; transferred to the Auxiliary Reserve, Feb. 26, 1925, and was a Brigadier General, Auxiliary Reserve, at the time of his death. (Maj. Gen. C. R. Reynolds to S. Flexner, Nov. 12, 1935.)

5. A story in the *New York Times* of March 5, 1917, quotes Welch as saying that Germany "has flung down the gauntlet to the United States, and there is no honorable course open for us than to fight; and since war is inevitable, let it begin at once." This, however, did not represent his true attitude, as a letter from Welch to Hale (March 8, 1917, Hale papers, copy W.P.) shows: "Did you see in the New York Times that I have declared war against Germany? I did not say that, for I was trying to tell a reporter something about the Research Council, but all he seized on were some rather hot remarks which I made about the filibusters."

6. Gram's stain serves to separate two important groups of bacteria, one called Gram positive, the other Gram negative. The test is applied by staining the bacteria with basic triphenylmethane dyes, such as gentian violet, and then treating with iodine followed by alcohol. Under these circumstances the Bacillus influenzæ (Pfeiffer) becomes decolourized (Gram negative). When the reaction failed to appear in the specimens examined because water had been substituted for alcohol, Welch became alarmed and suspected a new and destructive kind of infection. In the highly fatal camp pneumonias the influenza bacilli were associated with Gram positive micrococci, a particularly severe and often fatal combination. Today we know that the specific germ or agent of influenza is not Pfeiffer's bacillus, but a virus.

7. According to the *Statement of Henry P. Davison, Chairman, on Behalf of the American Red Cross War Council on Its Retirement*, March 1, 1919 (pamphlet), gifts made to the American Red Cross during twenty-one months of war work exceeded $400,000,000, including cash and supplies.

Welch had other objects as well as the Red Cross in mind when he sailed for Europe. On March 14 he wrote Buttrick (Gen. Educ. Bd. files, copy W.P.): "I am glad of the opportunity of going over, as there are several matters of interest to the School of Hygiene and the Medical School which I can attend to on the other side."

8. Welch was influential in securing recognition of the League of Red Cross Societies in the Covenant of the League of Nations, but the statement which is sometimes made that he drafted the health provisions of that document is an exaggeration. (Th. Madsen and Ludwik Rajchman to Welch, March 27, 1930, in *William Henry Welch at Eighty*, N.Y., 1930, p. 29. Diary No. 13, March 30, 1919.)

9. C.-E. A. Winslow, director of the League's Department of Health, reported in that year: "It was the feeling of the Board . . . that the League as at present organized is too costly to be supported by the Red Cross Societies after the present funds are exhausted, and that vigorous measures of economy should be introduced during the year, so as to make existing resources last as long as possible, and to bring the budget of the League within limits which the Red Cross Societies can reasonably be expected to meet when they take over its support." (Annual report to . . . Medical Advisory Board, Dept. of Health, League of Red Cross Societies, June 1, 1921.) In his letter to Welch of June 17, 1921, Winslow said: "This reduction has been effected without any serious injury to the proper work of the League,—the service of Red Cross Societies." A pamphlet published by the League in 1926 explained: "The expenses of the activities of the Secretariat are met by contributions from national Red Cross Societies belonging to the League. Up to the present time, the greater part of these expenses has been borne by the American Red Cross, which in 1919 voted a substantial sum to constitute a guarantee fund during the first years of the League's existence. The other national Societies were first asked to contribute to the League's budget in 1922." (*The League of Red Cross Societies*, Paris, 1926, p. 7.)

10. The *London Times* of June 13, 1923, said that "in presenting Dr. W. H. Welch . . . the Public Orator recalled the hero of Virgil:

> On whom the fond, indulgent god
> His augury had fain bestowed,
> His lyre, his sounding bow.
> But he, the further to prolong
> A sickly parent's span,
> The humbler art of medicine chose,
> The knowledge of each herb that grows,
> Plying a craft unknown to song,
> An unambitious man. . . .

"They did not call him inglorious, as Virgil had, who had dedicated his whole life to medicine, and had not been content with traditional knowledge, but had worked to explore the secrets of nature and meet the disease ere it came. Such was the man before them—a Yale man born in Connecticut, the state that gave the norm to the United States. He was chief priest in that temple dedicated by Rockefeller in New York to Hygeia Propugnatrix."

11. On Nov. 17, 1922, Welch wrote Dr. E. Libman: "I am indeed glad to hear at first hand something about conditions which you found in Germany, and to know that the little that I could say or do in behalf of my friends over there had been of some comfort to them. I was never more touched than to receive recently from those starving Viennese a gold medal and diploma for helping the University. German science and art must survive for the good of the rest of the world, and nothing is more important than to aid in the continuance of the scientific work of Germany and Austria." (coll. E. Libman, copy W.P.)

12. A typical example of the basic entries on which Welch built his more elaborate calculations reads as follows:

Tuesday, June 19, London

I sold the 24 penny postage stamps (good only for postal cards in England) which Nuttall sent me (see foot-note p. 23) to boy in hotel for 2 shillings—so that I have received in cash as rebate on Smith's bill for academic gown 12 shillings. The remaining ⅙ was in usable 1½d. stamps. I sold the penny stamps to boy in office at hotel. My actual cash payment for gown etc. should appear as £21-1-6.

1. Bkft—(Strand Corner House) 2/5
2. Visa of Passport at German Consulate £2-5
   (21A. Bedford Place—see my account in diary of this date)
3. 4 cigars 2/1
   (2 at 7d.—2 at 5½d.) $0.48
4. Luncheon at "Ye Olde Cock Tavern") 4/3
   22 Fleet St.—opposite Chancery Lane founded 1549.
5. Russian Bath—Br. La. 3/9
   Poor

6. Dinner—Bar sort of Restaurant on Whitehall 4/9
7. Sundries 1/1
    Papers—Bus—Underground, etc.
8. Coliseum in evening—admission 2/4
                    Total for Day = £3-5-8
(Expense account, loose sheet for June 19, 1923)
13. Thorvald Madsen, director of the State Serum Institute at Copenhagen.

CHAPTER XVII   SOURCE REFERENCES

365, ¶1. Welch to E. W. Kellogg, July 27, 1914.

365, ¶3. Welch to F. C. Walcott, Aug. 12, 1914.

366, ¶3. M. C. Winternitz to S. Flexner, March 15, 1937.

366, ¶4. George E. Hale to Welch, July 13, 1915. Welch to Hale, July 14, 1915, Hale papers, copies W.P.

366, ¶5. Welch to Woodrow Wilson, April 23, 1916, handwritten draft.

367, ¶1. Hale, *Some Recollections of Dr. Welch,* Nov. 28, 1934, ms. Hale to Welch, July 3, 1916, Hale papers, copy W.P.

367, ¶2. Woodrow Wilson to Welch, July 24, 1916, copy in Hale, *Some Recollections of Dr. Welch,* p. 5.

367, ¶3. Hale, *op. cit.*

368, ¶1–3. Diary No. 7, Aug. 27, 21, Sept. 4, 1916. Welch to Hale, Sept. 12, 1916, Hale papers, copy W.P.

368, f.n. Welch to Hale, Oct. 16, 1917, Hale papers, copy W.P.

369, ¶1. Welch to Hale (telegram), March 8, 1917, Hale papers, copy W.P.

369, ¶2. Welch to Hale, June 16, 1917, Hale papers, copy W.P.

370, ¶1. *Report of the Fiftieth Reunion, Class of 1870, Yale University,* New Haven, 1920, p. 11.

370, ¶2. Welch to S. Flexner, July 18, 1917, coll. S. Flexner, abstract W.P. Welch to E. W. Kellogg, July 23, 1918.

370, ¶3–372, ¶1. Welch to S. Flexner, Oct. 25, 30, June 11, 1917, May 15, 1918, coll. S. Flexner, abstract W.P.

372, ¶2. Martin, Franklin H., *Digest of the Proceedings of the Council of National Defense,* Wash., 1934, p. 304.

372, ¶4. *Report of the Fiftieth Reunion,* p. 12. Welch to S. Flexner, Jan. 12, 1918, coll. S. Flexner, abstract W.P.

373, ¶1. Welch to S. Flexner, Dec. 16, 1917, coll. S. Flexner, abstract W.P.

373, ¶2. Welch to S. Flexner, Dec. 29, 1917, Jan. 2, 1918, coll. S. Flexner, abstracts W.P.

374, ¶2. Welch to S. Flexner, Nov. 27, 1917, coll. S. Flexner, abstract W.P.

374, ¶3. F. F. Russell to S. Flexner, Sept. 25, 1935.

375, ¶1. Welch to S. Flexner, Nov. 23, 1917, coll. S. Flexner, abstract W.P.

375, ¶3. F. F. Russell to S. Flexner, Sept. 25, 1935. Welch to E. W. Kellogg, July 23, 1918.

375, ¶4. Welch to S. Flexner, Sept. 7, 1918. Welch to Helen Thomas Flexner, Oct. 4, 1918, coll. S. Flexner, abstracts W.P.

376, ¶1. Welch to H. A. Kelly, June 7, 1917, coll. Kelly, copy W.P.

376, ¶2–377, ¶1. Rufus Cole to S. Flexner, May 26, 1936.

377, ¶2. Welch to Helen Thomas Flexner, Oct. 4, 1918. Welch to S. Flexner, Jan. 2, 1919, coll. S. Flexner, abstracts W.P.

378, ¶2. Welch, "Remarks at Opening of Medical Conference of Red Cross Societies," *Proceedings of the Medical Conference, Cannes* . . . , Geneva, 1919, p. 24, *P. & A., 1,* 672.

378, ¶3. Diary No. 13, March 31, April 1, 1919.

378, ¶4–379, ¶1. League of Red Cross Societies, *The Cannes Medical Conference* (pamphlet), Geneva, 1920. *Proceedings* . . . Diary No. 13, April 10–13, 1919.

380, ¶1. Welch, "Scope of the Proposed Health Activities of the League of Red Cross Societies," *Proceedings* . . . , p. 50, *P. & A., 1,* 674. Stockton Axson to Welch, June 3, 1919.

380, ¶2. Welch to G. E. Vincent, April 4, 1919, Rock. Found. files, copy W.P. Welch to S. Flexner, Aug. 15, 1920, coll. S. Flexner, abstract W.P.

380, ¶3. *The League of Red Cross Societies,* Paris, 1926.

381, ¶1. Welch to Nuttall, May 18, 1919, Nuttall papers, copy W.P.

382, ¶2. Diary No. 13, April 23, 1919.

383, ¶1. *Ibid.,* April 25, 1919.

383, ¶2. *Ibid.,* April 29, 30, May 2, 1919.

384, ¶2. Diary No. 17, June 10–13, 1923. Welch to Nuttall, May 19, June 14, 1923, Nuttall papers, copy W.P. *Nature,* 1923, *111,* 900.

384, ¶3. Diary No. 17, May 19–26, 1923. Welch, Remarks at American Pasteur celebration at the Sorbonne, May 22, 1923, ms.

384, ¶4. Diary No. 17, June 5–8, 1923. *St. Bartholomew's Hosp. J.,* 1923, *30,* 157. See also: *Brit. Med. J.,* 1923, *1,* 1032.

385, ¶1. Diary No. 18, June 19, 21, 1923.

385, ¶2. *Ibid.,* June 28, 30, 1923.

386, ¶1–387, ¶1. *Ibid.,* June 29–30, 1923.

387, ¶2. *Ibid.,* July 2, 13, 1923.

388, ¶1. *Ibid.,* July 25–26, 1923.

388, ¶2. *Ibid.,* July 27–31, 1923.

389, ¶1. *Ibid.,* Aug. 3–10, 1923.

389, ¶2. Diary No. 19, Aug. 16–29, 1923. Welch to sister, Aug. 12, 1909.

389, ¶3–390, ¶1. Diary No. 19, Aug. 28, Sept. 13, 1923.

390, ¶2. Diary No. 26, Oct. 23, 31, 1927.

390, ¶3. Diary No. 19, 1923, p. 101.

391, ¶3. Diary No. 20, pp. 3–4, Welch to E. W. Kellogg, July 7, 1924. Freeman, A. W., *Memorandum* . . . *on My Personal Memories of Doctor Welch,* April 22, 1936.

392, ¶1–2. Diary No. 20, Aug. 7, 8, 9, 1924.

392, ¶3. Freeman, *op. cit.,* p. 15.

393, ¶1. Diary No. 20, July 27, 1924.

393, ¶2. Freeman, *op. cit.,* pp. 18–19.

393, ¶3. Garrison, F. H., "In Memoriam: William Henry Welch," *Scientific Monthly*, 1934, *38*, 579. Freeman, *op. cit.*, p. 17.

393, ¶4. Diary No. 20, Aug. 7, 1924.

394, ¶1–2. *Ibid.*, Aug. 12, 1924. Freeman, *op. cit.*, p. 20.

394, ¶3. Diary No. 21, Aug. 16, 1924.

394, ¶4. *Ibid.*, Aug. 30, 31, Sept. 1, 1924.

395, ¶1–2. *Ibid.*, Sept. 4, 5, 22–23, 1924.

CHAPTER XVIII TEXT NOTES

1. In 1921, the younger Rockefeller said that his father, "feeling that perhaps by seeking to assist in the establishment of higher educational standards the greatest service could be rendered to the Chinese people, . . . made possible the sending of a commission from the University of Chicago to study the educational conditions of China. The commission, composed of Dr. Ernest D. Burton, Professor of Theology, and Dr. Thomas C. Chamberlin, Professor of Geology, after thorough study, recommended the establishment at Peking of an educational institution for the teaching of the natural sciences." Because of the size of the undertaking, a second commission was sent in 1914, consisting of Dr. Harry Pratt Judson, president of the University of Chicago, Dr. Francis W. Peabody, and Roger S. Greene. "The commission returned convinced of the wisdom of the conclusion already reached and recommending the establishment of a medical school and hospital at Peking and a similar medical center in Shanghai." (Rockefeller, "Response for the Rockefeller Foundation," in *Addresses and Papers, Dedication Ceremonies and Medical Conferences, Peking Union Medical College*, Peking, 1922, p. 57.)
2. The delegation included Hata, who was with Ehrlich when Salvarsan was discovered and perfected; Shiga, who discovered the Japanese type of dysentery bacillus which bears his name; Miyajima, and others. Kitasato himself was perhaps the most international medical figure in Japan. An early pupil of Koch's, he carried bacteriology to Japan. The government at once gave him an Institute of Infectious Diseases modelled on Koch's in Berlin. That was in 1892; in 1914 he withdrew from that institution to set up the Kitasato Institute, his chief associates going with him to the new laboratory and hospital.
3. Western medicine was introduced to Japan by a group of remarkable physicians in the Dutch settlement at Nagasaki. During the nineteenth century they distributed a few Dutch books, chiefly of a medical and technical character, which conveyed such new ideas as anatomy and the Linnæan botanical system to a group of Japanese, among whom there were several physicians. (Terry, T. Philip, *Japanese Empire*, Boston, 1914, p. 664. Fujikawa, Y., *Geschichte der medizin in Japan*. . . . Tokyo, 1911.)
4. Dr. Franklin C. McLean, who was active in the selection of the faculty, writes: "Most of the first faculty were Americans. A number had had previous experience in China, some at the old P.U.M.C., and they were given fellowships for study in the United States or Europe before taking up their new duties." (McLean to S. Flexner, Jan. 7, 1941.)

CHAPTER XVIII SOURCE REFERENCES

397, ¶1. *Rock. Found. Ann. Rep.*, 1915, pp. 17–23, 245–64.

397, ¶2. Diary No. 1, Aug. 13, 1915. Welch to E. W. Kellogg, July 29, 1915.

398, ¶1–2. Welch to F. C. Walcott, Aug. 22, 1915.

398, ¶4. Diary No. 1, Aug. 23, 25, 26, 1915.

399, ¶1–3. *Ibid.*, Sept. 1, 1915.

400, ¶1–3. Welch to E. W. Kellogg, Sept. 11, 1915.

401, ¶1–402, ¶1. Diary No. 1, Sept. 11, to Diary No. 2, Sept. 18, 1915.

404, ¶2. Welch, "Spirit of Experimental Science in Education and Opportunities for Scientific Medicine and Service in China," address at Yale-in-China, Changsha, Oct. 17, 1915, *P. & A., 3,* 174.

405, ¶2–3. Diary No. 2, Sept. 20, Oct. 6, 1915.

406, ¶1–3. *Ibid.,* Sept. 21, 25–26, Oct. 3.

407, ¶1–2. *Ibid.,* Sept. 24, Oct. 4, 6.

408, ¶1–2. *Ibid.,* Oct. 7, 9.

410, ¶1–2. Diary No. 4, Nov. 26, 1915.

411, ¶1. Diary entry for Dec. 8, 1915, on loose sheets.

411, ¶2. Rockefeller, jr., to Welch, Feb. 24, 1921. Diary No. 15, Aug. 11, 1921.

411, ¶3. *Addresses and Papers, Dedication Ceremonies and Medical Conferences, Peking Union Medical College,* Peking, 1922, p. 14. Welch to E. W. Kellogg, Oct. 30, 1921.

412, ¶1. Welch to Kellogg, Oct. 30, 1921. Rockefeller, jr., to S. Flexner, March 20, 1936.

412, ¶2. Quotation from Dean, Sam, "Singing Craftsmen of Peking," *Asia,* Aug. 1921, in Rockefeller, "Response for the Rockefeller Foundation," *Addresses and Papers,* p. 57.

413, ¶1. Welch, "The Advancement of Medicine and Its Contribution to Human Welfare," and "Pathological Problems in the Orient," *Addresses and Papers, op. cit.,* pp. 148, 377.

413, ¶2. Diary No. 15, Sept. 24–27, 1921.

414, ¶1. Rockefeller to S. Flexner, March 20, 1936.

414, ¶7. Freeman, A. W., *Memorandum . . . on My Personal Memories of Doctor Welch,* April 22, 1936, p. 13.

414, ¶8. Balme, Harold, *China and Modern Medicine,* London, 1921, pp. 107–133.

414, ¶9. *Peiping Union Medical College, Annual Announcement,* 1940–1941, pp. 52–65. *Peiping Union Medical College Hospital, Annual Report of Supt.,* 1938–1939, p. 6.

CHAPTER XIX   TEXT NOTES

1. To mark Welch's seventy-fifth birthday, his friends and pupils presented to the Johns Hopkins University a portrait bust of Welch executed by the Russian sculptor, Sergei T. Konenkov. (Committee to Welch, April 7, 1925. Welch to Rufus Cole (chmn. of the com.), April 8, 1925, copy W.P.)
2. An undated memorandum of Weed's, which internal evidence tells us must have been written between 1922 and 1924, contains a plea for a million and a half dollars for the construction of a central medical library at the Hopkins, to be presided over by Garrison as librarian and professor of the history of medicine. This memorandum does not mention Welch, and states that if Garrison were to refuse "it seems hardly possible to find another such man."
3. On his desk calendar for May 26, 1925, Welch noted: "Conference with A. Flexner, 2:30 p.m., re my acceptance of chair of History of Medicine." The next day Flexner wrote Weed: "He will, I think, enter with enthusiasm on the professorship of the history of medicine." (A. Flexner to Weed, May 27, 1925, carbon Gen. Educ. Bd. files, abstract W.P.)
4. In February, 1927, the General Education Board appropriated $750,000 for land,

construction, and equipment for the library, agreeing further to give for not more than five years after the completion of the building the income on $250,000 for maintenance; this capital would become the property of the University if it could raise $500,000 before the end of that time. (*Johns Hopkins Univ. Cir.*, 1927, No. 384, p. 610.)

5. Billings was scheduled to give a series of lectures on medical history at the University in 1876, but did not do so until the fall of 1877, when he was officially the lecturer on history of medicine. In 1896, and for several years thereafter, he was listed in the faculty of the Medical School as lecturer on history and literature of medicine. (Billings to Gilman, Feb. 24, March 31, April 14, 1876, Nov. 6, 1877, coll. Hopkins Library, copies W.P. Chesney, A. M., "Two Papers by John Shaw Billings on Medical Education," *Bull. Inst. Hist. of Med.*, 1938, *6*, 285 *Johns Hopkins Univ. Cir.*, May, 1896, p. 72.)

6. In his Commemoration Day address, Feb. 22, 1929, Welch said: "Our Medical Historical Club was founded within a year after the opening of the Hospital. We owe that, as we owe the stimulus and, to a very large extent, the direction of our interest in medical history, to one of the most eminent, not only of physicians, but of medical historians, Dr. Osler." (*Johns Hopkins Alumni Mag.*, 1929, *17*, 374.)

7. A new interest in the club grew out of the Institute of the History of Medicine; Welch again became president in December, 1929. Although the organization, whose name has been changed to Johns Hopkins Medical History Club, is still largely under the influence of the hospital, it is now also associated with the institute. (MacCallum to S. Flexner, May 12, 1941. Program of 50th anniv., Johns Hopkins Med. Hist. Club, Nov. 18, 1940.)

8. A year before, as presiding officer of the same association at its meeting in New York, Welch had said: "Medicine has been called the mother of sciences. There was a time when the leading cultivators of natural science were physicians and when the medical faculties of universities were the homes of about all the science that then existed. In subsequent history physicians have played no small part in the development of the natural and physical sciences." (Welch, "Position of Natural Science in Education," *Proc. Am. Assn. Adv. Sc.*, 1906–1907, *56–57*, 617, *P. & A.*, *3*, 83.)

9. At the time of his appointment to his new professorship, Welch did not belong to any important medico-historical societies. On Jan. 15, 1927, Garrison wrote him that at Oliver's suggestion he had put him up for the London, Paris, and international societies. He suggested that Klebs or Streeter propose him for the Italian society, and asked if Welch wished to join the Charaka Club in New York.

10. In Philadelphia on May 14, 1929, Welch said: "The Leipzig Institute, inadequately housed in the lower floors of the Mineralogical Institute, . . . centers about an excellent reference library which has been built up on the principle of affording opportunities for research rather than the accumulation of medical rarities. The library covers related historical topics (e. g. mathematics and other sciences), as it is impossible to separate the history of medicine from the other histories of the same period. . . . Each student is assigned a place and attends lectures and seminars as well as pursuing individual research. More emphasis is placed on the seminars than the lectures. These are given at stated periods but without any idea of covering the whole subject in a given semester. A different subject may be taken up each semester; Dr. Sigerist, the present Director, being especially fond of Medieval history . . . Sudhoff still has quarters in the building and is again working at his monumental work on Paracelsus. . . . Sudhoff takes the point of view that no single medical historian can properly include in the field of his own studies the history of science after Galileo, as it then becomes too extensive and specialized. The Institute is now supported by the Saxon government, as the original foundation became entirely inadequate after the fall of the financial value of the mark. Both Sudhoff and Sigerist show a remarkable knowledge of the whereabouts of the important manuscripts and early medical books throughout Europe. . . . There are several journals devoted to the subject [history of medicine] published from the Institute. For instance, the *Archiv für Geschichte der Medizin*, the *Studien, Beiträge* and the *Jahrbuch*. The *Mit-*

teilungen belongs to the Society of the History of Medicine of Germany." (*Annals of Med. Hist.*, 1929, n.s. *1*, 731.)

11. The first purchase recorded in his diary was made on July 27, in Amsterdam. (Diary No. 25, p. 105.)

12. En route to Budapest, Welch attended the opening of Richard Koch's Institute of the History of Medicine and Anatomy in Frankfurt, and stopped off in Munich "to see my old friend, Friedrich Müller." During a few days in Vienna, when he was supposed to be attending a League of Nations Health Committee conference on infant mortality at von Pirquet's clinic, he spent most of his time in bookshops. (Welch to Sir Arthur Newsholme, Oct. 6, 1927, copy W.P. Welch to E. W. Kellogg, Oct. 28, 1927.)

13. Sir George Newman had written Welch about the tercentenary celebration of the publication of Harvey's *De Motu Cordis*, saying, "It is most important that the head of the medical profession in America should be present on this occasion." (Newman to Welch, Feb. 13, 1928.) At the Guildhall banquet on May 16, which he called "a really magnificent occasion," Welch responded to the toast to the delegates. (*Lancet,* 1928, *1,* 1090. *Brit. Med. J.*, 1928, *1,* 910. Diary No. 28, May 16, 1928.)

14. MacCallum wrote Welch, probably in March, asking him to recommend someone for librarian. On May 9, Weed cabled: "Imperative to answer MacCallum's letter," and in a letter mailed two days later wrote: "MacCallum is tremendously disturbed because he has not had from you an expression of opinion regarding the type of librarian." Although Welch had previously written Klebs that "Garrison would come," and although Singer had strongly recommended Garrison, Welch made no move until he landed in New York, and then he wrote MacCallum: "I really had no suggestion to make about a librarian. If you have not selected one, we will talk the matter over when I get back to Baltimore towards the end of next week." After the faculty committee on the library had recommended Garrison, Welch made the formal offer. (Weed to Welch, May 9 (cable), 11, 1928. Welch to Klebs, April 20, 1928, coll. Klebs, copy W.P. Diary No. 28, May 13, 1928. Welch to MacCallum, Sept. 27, 1928, coll. MacCallum, copy W.P. Welch to Garrison, Jan. 6, 1930, Garrison papers, copy W.P.)

15. On June 18, 1932, Welch wrote his niece: "I have to write by way of introduction to a three volume 'Festschrift' an article on 'Emanuel Libman and Mt. Sinai Hospital,' which involves considerable research. Dr. Libman is a kind of hero-worshipper—thinks I helped him in his professional career—gave $10,000 to Johns Hopkins for a lectureship when I was made professor of the history of medicine—has endowed the William H. Welch Lectureship at Mt. Sinai Hospital—etc. etc." In his introduction, Welch praised Libman's interest in the history of medicine and stated: "No one has recognized more clearly than he the importance of the cultivation of clinical medicine as science and art by its own methods of observation and experiment." (Welch, "Emanuel Libman," introduction to *Contributions to the Medical Sciences in Honor of Dr. Emanuel Libman by His Pupils, Friends and Colleagues,* N.Y., 1932, *1,* xiii.)

16. Welch's reference here, of course, is to Prohibition, a law which he had disapproved of from the first. In 1916, he had written Kelly: "While I do not believe in prohibition for Baltimore—it would not work where there are so many opposed to it—I am strongly for temperance and education on the evils of alcohol. I feel this is the direction in which we should work. . . . It is a mistake to identify the political movement for prohibition with the cause of temperance. The political movement, I think, has been a demoralizing one in our legislature." (Nov. 8, 1916, coll. H. A. Kelly, copy W.P.)

Welch was willing to break laws upon occasion. We have a letter to MacCallum written in Welch's hand although signed by Ernest Gittings: "I shall be delighted if you will join us in a small criminal dinner which I am giving at the Maryland Club at 7:30 tomorrow—Wednesday—night. Lest the gang should be raided I am asking the participants in the crime not to dress for dinner. The particular crime is indulging in canvass-back ducks in violation of the State law. Hoping you will become *particeps criminis* . . ." (coll. MacCallum.)

17. In his talk as chairman of the dedication exercises of the department of history

of medicine (Oct. 18, 1929), Welch expanded on this theme: "I think also that there should be workers specifically interested in the ideas, in the conceptions of medicine. As far as I know, there is really no history of medicine written from such a point of view. It would be a very different kind of medical history, for some of the figures now given great emphasis would be reduced to a sentence or two while others having a paragraph would occupy a good deal of space." (Welch, Remarks at inauguration of Dept. of History of Med., stenographic report, p. 5.)

18. Welch made his Commemoration Day address from hardly more than a page of notes; the text from which we have quoted is probably an unedited stenographic transcript.

19. The international celebration, to which the New York Academy of Medicine and the University Club of Baltimore had added dinners, naturally brought a flood of congratulatory messages from institutions and from Welch's friends and colleagues all over the world. These were bound together into three huge volumes which were presented to Welch nine months later at a testimonial dinner over which Rockefeller, jr., presided. (Kingsbury to S. Flexner, Sept. 5, 1935.)

20. Welch received the Harben gold medal at the meeting of the Royal Institute of Public Health in Frankfurt; he attended the hundredth anniversary of the Harveian Society and the International Congress of the History of Science and Technology in London; the four-hundredth anniversary of the Collège de France in Paris; and the International Neurological Congress at Berne, where he and Pavlov were the guests of honour. (Diary No. 37, May 19, 1931. Diary entry for June 11 (loose sheets). Diary No. 38, June 28—July 4, June 18–21. Diary No. 39, Aug. 29—Sept. 4.)

CHAPTER XIX   SOURCE REFERENCES

416, ¶1. Welch to S. Flexner, Jan. 1, 1925, coll. S. Flexner, abstract W.P.

416, ¶2. Frank J. Goodnow to Welch, April 23, 1925.

416, ¶3. Welch to S. Flexner, May 26, 1924, coll. S. Flexner, abstract W.P. W. H. Wilmer to S. Flexner, Sept 20, 1935. Welch to Wilmer, Feb. 10, 1925, Wilmer papers, copy W.P. Donations received after the close of the campaign reduced the deficit to be met by the University by nearly half. Welch to Rockefeller, jr., Feb. 10, 1925, coll. Rockefeller, jr., copy W.P.

417, ¶1. Garrison to Welch, April 21, 1925. Flexner, A., *Reminiscences of Dr. Welch*, May 16, 1934, ms.

418, ¶1. Welch to Garrison, April 22, 1925, Garrison papers, copy W.P.

418, ¶2. Welch to E. W. Kellogg, May 15, 1927.

419, ¶1. A. Flexner to Welch, April 28, 1925, W.P. Welch to Cushing, April 12, 1926, Cushing papers, copy W.P.

419, ¶2. *Gen. Educ. Bd. Ann. Rep.*, 1926–1927, pp. 11–12. *Johns Hopkins Univ. Cir.*, 1927, No. 384, p. 609. L. H. Weed to Welch (cable), May 9, 1928.

419, ¶3. Welch to E. W. Kellogg, Jan. 3, 1907. Welch to Raymond Pearl, March 22, 1927, coll. Pearl, copy W.P.

420, ¶1. Welch to sister, Aug. 8, 1906. Frederick R. Huber to H. A. Kelly, Feb. 16, 1933, coll. Kelly, copy W.P. Shriver, A. J., Address at memorial meeting for Welch, May 22, 1934, ms.

420, ¶2. Kellogg, E. W., ms. account of Welch. Cortissoz, Royal, summary of Welch's remarks, *Experience as a Sitter for the Sargent Portrait*, at presentation of portrait to University, Jan. 19, 1907, *Johns Hopkins Univ. Cir.*, 1907, *26*, 19, *P. & A.*, *3*, 355.

420, ¶3. Welch to E. W. Kellogg, Dec. 29, 1911.

421, ¶1. Welch, Address before the William Welch Soc., Univ. and Bellevue Hosp. Med. Coll., Feb. 25, 1930, *Bellevue Violet*, 1930, *6*, 192.

421, ¶2. Chesney, A. M., "Two Papers by John Shaw Billings on Medical Education," *Bull. Inst. Hist. of Med.*, 1938, *6*, 285. Welch, "Some of the Advantages of the Union of Medical School and University," *New Eng. & Yale Rev.*, 1888, *13*, 145, *P. & A.*, *3*, 26.

421, ¶3. Cole, Rufus, Remarks at New York Academy of Medicine dinner in honour of Welch's eightieth birthday, April 4, 1930, *William Henry Welch at Eighty*, ed. by Victor O. Freeburg, N.Y., 1930, p. 59.

422, ¶2. Welch, "Landmarks in the History of Pathology," N.Y. Acad. of Med. anniv. address, Nov. 17, 1898, *Med. Record*, 1898, *54*, 778, ms., W.P. Welch, Address at presentation of Ernst Ziegler library to Medical School, Univ. of Pittsburgh, Dec. 5, 1913, *Bull. Inst. Hist. Med.*, 1935, *3*, 1.

422, ¶3. McCrae, Thomas, *William H. Welch*, 1935, ms. Oliver, J. R., "William Henry Welch: Humanist," *Johns Hopkins Alumni Mag.*, 1935, *23*, 107. Riesman, David, "William Henry Welch, Scientist and Humanist," *Scientific Monthly*, 1935, *41*, 251.

423, ¶1. S. Flexner's notes of conversation with J. McKeen Cattell, Dec. 12, 1936. Welch, "The Interdependence of Medicine and Other Sciences of Nature," *Science*, 1908, *27*, 49, *P. & A.*, *3*, 315. Garrison, Dedication of the Welch Bibliophilic Society edition of *The Interdependence of Medicine with Other Sciences of Nature*, Balto., 1934, p. 5.

423, ¶2–424, ¶1. Vesalius, Andreas, *De Fabrica Humani Corporis*, 1543. Welch, "The Times of Vesalius," address before Johns Hopkins Hosp. Hist. Club, Feb. 8, 1915, *Bull. Johns Hopkins Hosp.*, 1915, *26*, 118, *P. & A.*, *3*, 428.

424, ¶2. Welch to E. W. Kellogg, May 27, 1927.

424, ¶3. *Ibid.* Klebs to Welch, June 8, 1927.

425, ¶1. Welch to E. W. Kellogg, May 27, 1927.

425, ¶2. *Ibid.* Diary No. 29, Aug. 19, 1928. Welch to Klebs, Sept. 30, 1924, coll. Klebs, copy W.P.

425, ¶3. Welch to Klebs, June 29, 1927, coll. Klebs, copy W.P.

426, ¶1. Welch to S. Flexner, Dec. 2, 1927, coll. S. Flexner, abstract W.P. Welch to A. Flexner, Aug. 10, 1927. Diary No. 24, July 22, 1927. Van Rijnberk, G., in *Nederlandsch Tijdschrift voor Geneeskunde*, 1927, July 30, p. 506.

426, ¶2. Diary No. 24, July 18, 20, 1927. Welch, "The Relation of the Hospital to Medical Education and Research," *J. Am. Med. Assn.*, 1907, *49*, 531, *P. & A.*, *3*, 132.

427, ¶1. Diary No. 24, July 20, June 19, June 12, July 13, 1927.

427, ¶2. Welch to F. C. Walcott, Sept. 17, 1927, coll. Walcott, copy W.P. Diary No. 25, Aug. 15, 18, 1927. Welch to A. Flexner, Aug. 10, 1927.

428, ¶1. Welch to Klebs, June 6, Oct. 26, 1927, coll. Klebs, copies W.P. Diary No. 26, Sept. 15, 1927. Diary No. 28, May 17, 1928. Welch to Weed, Nov. 21, 1927, coll. Weed, copy W.P.

428, ¶2. Weed to A. Flexner, Sept. 16, 1927, Gen. Educ. Bd. files, abstract W.P. A. Flexner to Weed, Sept. 19, 1927, copy Gen. Educ. Bd. files, abstract W.P. A. Flexner to Welch, Sept. 17, 1927 (cable). Welch to Weed, Nov. 21, 1927, coll. Weed, copy W.P. Diary No. 28, June 12, 1928. Welch to A. Flexner, June 12, 1928.

428, ¶3. Diary No. 26, Sept. 16–22, 1927. Welch to Weed, Nov. 21, 1927, coll. Weed, copy W.P.

429, ¶1. Welch to Sir Arthur Newsholme, Oct. 26, 1927, copy W.P. Diary No. 26, Oct. 1, 1927.

429, ¶2. Diary No. 26, Oct. 10, 7, 1927.

429, ¶3. *Ibid.*, Sept. 30, Oct. 1, 1927.

430, ¶1. Welch to Weed, Nov. 21, 1927, coll. Weed, copy W.P. Frank J. Goodnow to Welch, Jan. 12, 1928.

430, ¶2. Welch to E. W. Kellogg, Oct. 28, 1927.

430, ¶3. Welch to S. Flexner, Dec. 2, 1927, coll. S. Flexner, abstract W.P. Welch to F. F. Russell, Nov. 17, 1927, coll. Russell, copy W.P. Diary No. 26, Nov. 28, 1927.

431, ¶1. Welch to F. C. Walcott, Dec. 11, 1927, coll. Walcott, copy W.P.

431, ¶2. Welch to J. J. Walsh, Dec. 19, 1927, coll. N. Y. Acad. Med., copy W.P. Walsh, *Laughter and Health*, N.Y., 1928.

432, ¶2. Welch to A. Flexner, undated (May 30?), 1928. Diary No. 28, June 12, 1928.

432, ¶3. Diary No. 28, June 28, 1928, W.P. Welch to Klebs, July 19, 1928, coll. Klebs, copy W.P.

433, ¶1. Diary No. 28, July 1, 1928. Diary No. 24, July 7, 1927.

433, ¶2. Diary No. 27, Feb. 16, 1928. Diary No. 29, Sept. 12, 1928. Welch to Weed, Nov. 21, 1927, coll. Weed, copy W.P.

433, ¶3. Welch to Weed, Nov. 21, 1927, Feb. 19, 1928, coll. Weed, copies W.P. Diary No. 27, April 3, 1928.

434, ¶1. Welch to F. C. Walcott, Sept. 7, 1928, coll. Walcott, abstract W.P.

434, ¶2. Welch to G. E. Vincent, March 16, 1928, Rock. Found. files, copy W.P. Diary No. 29, Sept. 14, 1928.

434, ¶3. Welch to Weed, Nov. 21, 1927, coll. Weed, copy W.P. Cole, Rufus, in *Welch at Eighty*, N.Y., 1930. Conversation between Klebs and S. Flexner, Feb. 3, 1937, ms.

435, ¶1. Diary No. 29, Aug. 19, 1928.

435, ¶2. Welch, Remarks at inauguration of the Department of the History of Medicine, Oct. 18, 1929, *The William H. Welch Medical Library*, Balto., 1930, p. 91. Welch to Klebs, Aug. 26, 1928, coll. Klebs, copy W.P.

436, ¶2. Welch to Klebs, Aug. 26, 1928. Pearce, R. M., memo. of conversation between Welch, Trevor Arnett, and Pearce, Oct. 1, 1928; Memo.: A proposal for establishment of an institute of the history of medicine at the Johns Hopkins University, enclosed with Joseph S. Ames to Trevor Arnett, Nov. 15, 1929; Pearce to Welch, Dec. 2, 1929, Gen. Ed. Bd. files, copies & abstracts W.P. Welch to E. Libman, Dec. 19, 1929, coll. Libman, copy W.P. Weed, in *The William H. Welch Medical Library*, p. 3.

436, ¶3. Welch, Address on Commemoration Day, Feb. 22, 1929, *Johns Hopkins Alumni Mag.*, 1929, *17*, 374.

438, ¶1. Welch to Cushing, July 8, 1929, Cushing papers, copy W.P. *The William H. Welch Medical Library*, p. 98.

438, ¶2. Kingsbury to S. Flexner, Sept. 5, 1935. Kingsbury to Welch, Oct. 24, 1929.

438, ¶3. Welch to Kingsbury, Oct. 23, 1929, coll. Kingsbury, copy W.P.

438, ¶4. Welch to S. Flexner, April 16, 1930, coll. S. Flexner, abstract W.P. For committee members, see: *William Henry Welch at Eighty*.

439, ¶1. W. W. Brierley to Joseph S. Ames, date unknown, copy in Diary No. 31, June 23, 1930. Welch to Sir D'Arcy Power, June 11, 1930, as summarized Diary No. 31, June 11, 1930. Welch to John R. Oliver, June 1, 1930. *Johns Hopkins Univ. Cir.*, 1930, No. 418, p. 124.

439, ¶2. Diary No. 31, 1930, p. 5, W.P. Welch to S. Flexner, Sept. 11, 1930, coll. S. Flexner, abstract W.P.

439, ¶3. Max Farrand to S. Flexner, March 6, 1936. Welch to F. C. Walcott, July 23, 1930, coll. Walcott, copy W.P.

440, ¶1. Welch to Max Farrand, Sept. 15, 1930, coll. Farrand, copy W.P.

440, ¶2–441, ¶1. Diary No. 31, June 25, 23, 1930.

441, ¶2. Welch to F. C. Walcott, July 23, 1930, coll. Walcott, copy W.P.

441, ¶3. *Johns Hopkins Univ. Cir., op. cit.,* pp. 124–5. Welch to Cushing, Feb. 1, 1931, Cushing papers, copy W.P.

441, ¶4. Joseph S. Ames to Cushing, Dec. 1, 1930, Cushing papers, copy W.P. Cushing to Ames, Dec. 3, 1930, copy W.P. Welch to Cushing, Feb. 1, 1931, Cushing papers, copy W.P. Cushing to Welch, Feb. 4, 1931. Charles Singer to Welch, March 27, 1931. Cushing to Welch, Nov. 23, 1931.

442, ¶1. Welch to Klebs, Aug. 19, 1931, coll. Klebs, copy W.P.

442, ¶2. Cushing, *Welch Memorabilia, 4,* p. 70, Cushing papers, copy W.P.

442, ¶3. Cushing to Welch, Nov. 23, 1931. Diary No. 37, May 31, 1931. Welch to Henry E. Sigerist, Dec. 31, 1931, May 6, 1932, coll. Sigerist, copy W.P. Conver. between Welch and S. Flexner, Sept. 15, 1933, S. Flexner diary notes, copy W.P.

443, ¶1. Welch to Mrs. George H. Williams, Jan. 5, 1933, coll. Mrs. Williams, copy W.P.

443, ¶2. Sidney Licht to Welch, April 2, 1929. Licht to S. Flexner, Dec. 17, 1936. M. Pijoan to S. Flexner, Oct. 4, 1937, S. Flexner files, abstract W.P. Welch, *The Interdependence of Medicine with Other Sciences of Nature,* Balto., 1934. A. Flexner to Welch, March 25, 1933.

CHAPTER XX   TEXT NOTE

1. Welch retired from organizations in which he had been active in the following years:
International Health Board—1927 (because of reorganization)
China Medical Board—1928
Maryland State Board of Health—1929
Peking Union Medical College—1931
Johns Hopkins University faculty—June, 1931
Milbank Memorial Fund (as chairman of Advisory Board)—1932
Rockefeller Institute (Boards of Trustees and of Scientific Directors)—1933

CHAPTER XX   SOURCE REFERENCES

444, ¶1. Welch, Address before the William Welch Soc., Univ. & Bellevue Hosp. Med. Coll., Feb. 25, 1930, *Bellevue Violet,* 1930, *6,* 192.

444, ¶2. Welch to A. J. Shriver, March 26, 1934, Shriver papers, copy W.P.

445, ¶1. Shriver, Address at memorial meeting for Welch, Univ. Club, Balto., May 22, 1934, ms.

445, ¶2. Pratt, Joseph H., "A Tribute to Dr. William Henry Welch," *New Eng. J. Med.,* 1934, *210,* 1038.

445, ¶3. Welch to E. W. Kellogg, Dec. 25, 1931. Welch to H. A. Kelly, Jan. 6, 1932, coll. Kelly, copy W.P.

446, ¶1. Welch to Kingsbury, Nov. 21, 1932, coll. Kingsbury, copy W.P.

446, ¶2. Welch to F. C. Walcott, Dec. 3, 1932, coll. Walcott, abstract W.P. Welch to Kingsbury, Dec. 12, 1932, coll. Kingsbury, copy W.P.

446, ¶3. Minutes of Milbank Memorial Fund meeting, March 17, 1932, excerpt W.P. Welch, "Duties of a Hospital to the Public Health," *Proc. Nat. Confer. Char.,* 1915, 209, *P. & A., 1,* 621.

446, ¶4. S. Flexner's diary notes, June 26, 1932, copy W.P. Welch to Helen Thomas Flexner, Oct. 20, 1932, coll. S. Flexner, abstract W.P.

447, ¶1. Cushing, ms. account of showing of film at the Rock. Inst., Jan. 18, 1933, *Welch Memorabilia, 4,* p. 81, Cushing papers, copy W.P.

448, ¶1. Welch to MacCallum, June 21, 1932, coll. MacCallum, copy W.P.

448, ¶2. S. Flexner's diary notes, June 30, 1932, coll. S. Flexner, abstract W.P.

448, ¶3–449, ¶3. Welch's desk calendar, June 6—Oct. 1, 1932. Welch to Shriver, Oct. 7, 1932, coll. F. C. Walcott, copy W.P. Welch to E. Libman, Oct. 3, 1932, coll. Libman, copy W.P. Welch, "Emanuel Libman," intro. to *Contributions to the Medical Sciences in Honor of Dr. Emanuel Libman by His Pupils, Friends and Colleagues,* N.Y., 1932, *1,* xiii. Welch to Mrs. L. F. Barker, June 22, 1932, coll. Barker, copy W.P. Cushing, *Welch Memorabilia, 4,* p. 77, copy W.P.

449, ¶4. Welch, *Nathan Smith,* Beaumont Lecture, to have been delivered at Yale, Dec. 16, 1932, ms. notes. Welch, *Relation between Doctrines Held at Various Periods Concerning the Origin and Nature of Disease* . . . , before the Twentieth Century Club of Hartford, Conn., Dec. 14, 1932, ms. notes. Welch to M. C. Winternitz, Oct. 31, 1932, coll. Winternitz, copy W.P. Welch to Cushing, Oct. 25, 1932, Cushing papers, copy W.P. Welch to Kingsbury, Dec. 12, 1932, coll. Kingsbury, copy W.P.

450, ¶1. M. S. Sherman to F. C. Walcott, Dec. 15, 1932, coll. F. C. Walcott, copy W.P.

450, ¶2. Welch to Winternitz, Dec. 15, 1932, coll. Winternitz, copy W.P. Flexner, S., ms. account of visit to Norfolk, Aug. 9–11, 1937, p. 7.

450, ¶3–451, ¶1. Welch to Kingsbury, Dec. 19, 1932, coll. Kingsbury, copy W.P. Shriver, Address at memorial meeting, *op. cit.*

451, ¶2. Longcope, Warfield T., ms. account of Welch's last illness, Sept. 11, 1935, p. 3.

452, ¶1. Welch to F. C. Walcott, June 30, 1933, coll. Walcott, abstract W.P. Welch to Cushing, June 22, 1933, Cushing papers, copy W.P. Longcope, *op. cit.,* pp. 6–7.

452, ¶2–4. Longcope, *op. cit.,* pp. 7–8. Barker, ms. notes on Welch's last illness, copy W.P. S. Flexner's diary notes on visits to hospital, abstracts W.P.

453, ¶1. Barker to S. Flexner, July 3, 1933. Longcope to S. Flexner, Sept. 14, 1933. Longcope, ms. account of Welch's illness, p. 9.

453, ¶2. S. Flexner's diary notes, May 30, 1934, abstract W.P. Barker, ms. account of Welch, July 11, 1934.

453, ¶3. Barker, ms. notes on Welch's last illness, July 17, 1933, copy W.P.

454, ¶1. Longcope to S. Flexner, Nov. 25, 1933.

454, ¶2. F. C. Walcott to S. Flexner, Dec. 17, 1933. Longcope to S. Flexner, Dec. 26, 1933.

454, ¶3. S. Flexner's diary notes, Feb. 26, 1934, abstract W.P.

455, ¶1. Longcope, ms. account of Welch's last illness, pp. 14, 15, 16.

455, ¶2. MacCallum, "Dr. Welch, April 8, 1850—April 30, 1934," *Bull. Johns Hopkins Hosp.,* 1934, *54,* 383. Longcope, *op. cit.,* pp. 14, 13.

Index